Current Common Dilemmas in Colorectal Surgery

Christopher M. Schlachta • Patricia Sylla
Editors

Current Common Dilemmas in Colorectal Surgery

Springer

Editors
Christopher M. Schlachta
University Hospital
London Health Sciences Centre
London, ON, Canada

Patricia Sylla
Mount Sinai School of Medicine
New York, NY, USA

ISBN 978-3-030-09934-3   ISBN 978-3-319-70117-2 (eBook)
https://doi.org/10.1007/978-3-319-70117-2

Softcover re-print of the Hardcover 1st edition 2018

Printed on acid-free paper

This Springer imprint is published by Springer Nature
The registered company is Springer International Publishing AG
The registered company address is: Gewerbestrasse 11, 6330 Cham, Switzerland

For Paul, Jonah, Ariel, Mark, William, and Mary Lynn.

Preface

In April 2015, the Society of American Gastrointestinal and Endoscopic Surgeons (SAGES) sponsored a symposium at the annual meeting, held in Nashville, Tennessee, entitled "Current Common Dilemmas in Colorectal Surgery." The symposium was divided into three sessions that tackled common controversies related to selecting the most appropriate surgical treatment for various colorectal pathologies, the role of novel technologies and techniques to assist in their surgical management, and intraoperative strategies to overcome complications during routine and complex colorectal surgery. The success of the symposium inspired this textbook, which has the objective of providing a comprehensive and up-to-date overview by experts of current recommendations and strategies in the management of common colorectal pathologies.

Following the introduction of laparoscopic colon surgery, it has often been heard that the surgical community is waiting for the "next big thing." The reality is that, like all scientific advancements, major change occurs through a series of small steps. The evolution of care for patients with colorectal disease continues to evolve dramatically on several fronts prompting us to deliver this text in nine sections.

From optimizing preoperative bowel preparation to adoption of enhanced recovery pathways, the various strategies to minimize the perioperative morbidity of colorectal surgical procedures are extensively reviewed, with emphasis on the current standards and controversies in the endoscopic management of colorectal neoplasia. With respect to colorectal emergencies such as perforated diverticulitis and *Clostridium difficile* colitis, the role of minimally invasive and organ-preserving strategies is reviewed including various intraoperative strategies to optimize outcomes.

With respect to common pelvic floor disorders encountered in colorectal practice such as obstructed defecation, rectal prolapse, and fecal incontinence, the diagnostic workup and therapeutic options are reviewed, as are dilemmas regarding the role of surgery and optimal surgical approach when appropriate. With respect to other common colorectal pathologies such as symptomatic parastomal hernia, the role of hernia prevention and optimal strategies for repair is covered, as are recent trends in minimally invasive techniques applied to colorectal surgery, including the techniques and impact of intracorporeal anastomosis and natural orifice specimen extraction.

Finally, current controversies regarding the management of rectal cancer, including dilemmas related to selection and impact of neoadjuvant therapies, are extensively reviewed. The various strategies for sphincter preservation and abdominoperineal resection (APR), as well as various techniques to perform total mesorectal excision (TME), are reviewed at length, including the evolving role of transanal TME (taTME).

London, ON, Canada — Christopher M. Schlachta
New York, NY, USA — Patricia Sylla

Acknowledgments

We would like to share our mutual admiration and respect that developed while co-chairing the SAGES 2015 Current Common Dilemmas in Colorectal Surgery Symposium and which has grown into an incredible partnership in this project. We would also like to thank Michael Griffin from Springer who has guided us in harnessing the success of the symposium and helping infuse it back into this textbook. We would also like to thank SAGES for supporting high-quality educational symposia and initiatives and for its unwavering commitment to support general and colorectal surgeons in bridging the gap in adopting minimally invasive surgery. Finally, we would like to acknowledge our families who generously allow us to take time away from them to be applied to these passionate academic pursuits.

Contents

Contributors

Nawar A. Alkhamesi Department of Surgery, University Hospital, London Health Sciences Centre, London, ON, Canada

Nicholas Gerard Berger Department of Surgery, Division of Colorectal Surgery, Medical College of Wisconsin, Froedtert Memorial Lutheran Hospital, Milwaukee, WI, USA

Joshua I.S. Bleier Department of Surgery, PENN Presbyterian Medical Center, Philadelphia, PA, USA

Luigi Boni Department of General and Emergency IRCCS-Ca' Granda-Policlinico Hospital, University of Milan, Milan, Italy

Marylise Boutros Division of Colon & Rectal Surgery, Jewish General Hospital, McGill University, Montreal, QC, Canada

Liliana Bordeianou Department of General Surgery, Massachusetts General Hospital, Boston, MA, USA

Carl J. Brown Department of Surgery, St. Paul's Hospital, University of British Columbia, Vancouver, BC, Canada

Maria Emilia Carvalho e Carvalho Division of Colorectal Surgery, Mater Dei Hospital, Belo Horizonte, MG, Brazil

Daniel T. Chang Department of Radiation Oncology, Stanford Cancer Institute, Stanford, CA, USA

Quentin Denost Department of Colorectal Surgery, Magellan Centre, Bordeaux University Hospital, Pessac, France

Tony Dixon Department of Colorectal Surgery, North Bristol NHS Trust, Southmead Hospital Bristol, Bristol, UK

Liane S. Feldman Department of Surgery, McGill University Health Centre, Montréal, QC, Canada

Abe Fingerhut Department of Surgery, University Hospital of Graz, Graz, Austria

James Fleshman Department of Surgery, Baylor University Medical Center, Dallas, TX, USA

Morris E. Franklin Jr. Minimally Invasive Surgery, Texas Endosurgery Institute, San Antonio, TX, USA

Krishna C. Gurram Department of Gastroenterology, Winthrop University Hospital, Mineola, NY, USA

Brooke H. Gurland Department of General Surgery, Division of Colorectal Surgery Stanford University, Palo Alto, CA, USA

Kristina L. Guyton Department of Surgery, The University of Chicago Hospitals, Chicago, IL, USA

Viktor Justin Department of Surgery, Section for Surgical Research, Medical University of Graz, Graz, Austria

Angelita Habr-Gama Department of Surgery, Angelita and Joaquim Gama Institute, São Paulo, Brazil

Birgitta M.E. Hansson Department of Surgery, Canisius-Wilhelmina Hospital Nijmegen, Nijmegen, The Netherlands

Miguel A. Hernández Minimally Invasive Surgery, Texas Endosurgery Institute, San Antonio, TX, USA

Torbjörn Holm Section of Coloproctology, Department of Surgical Gastroenterology, Karolinska University Hospital, Stockholm, Sweden

Roel Hompes Department of GI and Oncologic Surgery, Academic Medical Center Amsterdam, Amsterdam, The Netherlands

Neil H. Hyman Department of Surgery, The University of Chicago Hospitals, Chicago, IL, USA

Steven H. Itzkowitz Division of Gastroenterology, Icahn School of Medicine at Mount Sinai Hospital, New York, NY, USA

John T. Jenkins Department of Surgery, St. Marks Hospital, London, UK

Maria Abou Khalil Division of General Surgery, McGill University, Montréal, QC, Canada

Albert C. Koong Department of Radiation Oncology, MD Anderson Cancer Center, Houston, TX, USA

Lawrence Lee Department of Surgery, McGill University Health Centre, Montréal, QC, Canada

François Letarte Department of Surgery, St. Paul's Hospital, University of British Columbia, Vancouver, BC, Canada

Paula Loughlin Department of Surgery, Altnagelvin Hospital, Derry, UK

Kirk A. Ludwig Department of Surgery, Division of Colorectal Surgery, Medical College of Wisconsin, Froedtert Memorial Lutheran Hospital, Milwaukee, WI, USA

James F. Marion Division of Gastroenterology, Icahn School of Medicine at Mount Sinai, New York, NY, USA

John H. Marks Marks Colorectal Surgical Associates, Lankenau Institute for Medical Research, Wynnewood, PA, USA

Division of Colorectal Surgery, Lankenau Medical Center, Wynnewood, PA, USA

Elisabeth C. McLemore General Surgery, Kaiser Permanente, Los Angeles Medical Center, Los Angeles, CA, USA

John Migaly Department of Surgery, Duke University Medical Center, Durham, NC, USA

Peter Alexander Newman Department of Colorectal Surgery, North Bristol NHS Trust, Southmead Hospital Bristol, Bristol, UK

O.N.M. Panton Division of General Surgery, Vancouver General Hospital, Vancouver, BC, Canada

Ian M. Paquette Division of Colon and Rectal Surgery, University of Cincinnati Medical Center, Cincinnati, OH, USA

Srikanth Parsi Marks Colorectal Surgical Associates, Lankenau Institute for Medical Research, Wynnewood, PA, USA

Division of Colorectal Surgery, Lankenau Medical Center, Wynnewood, PA, USA

Marta Penna Department of Colorectal Surgery, Oxford University Hospital, Oxford, UK

Rodrigo Oliva Perez Department of Surgery, Angelita and Joaquim Gama Institute, São Paulo, Brazil

Andrea M. Petrucci Department of Colorectal Surgery, Cleveland Clinic Florida, Weston, FL, USA

Nicolas D. Prionas Department of Radiation Oncology, Stanford Cancer Institute, Stanford, CA, USA

Teresa C. Rice Department of Surgery, University of Cincinnati Medical Center, Cincinnati, OH, USA

Timothy J. Ridolfi Department of Surgery, Division of Colorectal Surgery, Medical College of Wisconsin, Froedtert Memorial Lutheran Hospital, Milwaukee, WI, USA

Cecilia Beatriz Rossi Department of Surgery, Angelita and Joaquim Gama Institute, São Paulo, Brazil

Eric Rullier Department of Colorectal Surgery, Magellan Centre, Bordeaux University Hospital, Pessac, France

Patrick Vincent Saitta Department of Internal Medicine, Division of Gastroenterology, Winthrop University Hospital, Mineola, NY, USA

Jean Salem Marks Colorectal Surgical Associates, Lankenau Institute for Medical Research, Wynnewood, PA, USA

Division of Colorectal Surgery, Lankenau Medical Center, Wynnewood, PA, USA

Barry Salky Department of Surgery, Mount Sinai Health System, New York, NY, USA

Julia Saraidaridis Division of Colon and Rectal Surgery, Lahey Clinic, Burlington, MA, USA

Guilherme Pagin São Julião Department of Surgery, Angelita and Joaquim Gama Institute, São Paulo, Brazil

Shailja C. Shah Division of Gastroenterology, Icahn School of Medicine at Mount Sinai Hospital, New York, NY, USA

Nishit Shah Rhode Island Hospital, Providence, RI, USA

Skandan Shanmugan Department of Surgery, PENN Presbyterian Medical Center, Philadelphia, PA, USA

Stavros N. Stavropoulos Division of Digestive and Liver Diseases, Columbia University Medical Center, New York, NY, USA

Division of Gastroenterology, Hepatology, & Nutrition, NYU Winthrop Hospital, Mineola, NY, USA

Adam T. Stearns Department of Surgery, Norfolk and Norwich University Hospitals NHS Foundation Trust, Norwich, Norfolk, UK

Zhifei Sun Department of Surgery, Duke University Medical Center, Durham, NC, USA

Joana Torres Division of Gastroenterology, Icahn School of Medicine at Mount Sinai Hospital, New York, NY, USA

Megan Turner Department of Surgery, Duke University Medical Center, Durham, NC, USA

Ryan C. Ungaro Department of Gastroenterology, Icahn School of Medicine at Mount Sinai, New York, NY, USA

Selman Uranues Department of Surgery, University Hospital of Graz, Graz, Austria

Bruna Borba Vailati Department of Surgery, Angelita and Joaquim Gama Institute, São Paulo, Brazil

Katerina Wells Department of Surgery, Baylor University Medical Center, Dallas, TX, USA

Steven D. Wexner Department of Colorectal Surgery, Cleveland Clinic Florida, Weston, FL, USA

Albert M. Wolthuis Abdominal Surgery, University Hospital Leuven, Leuven, Belgium

Susana Wu General Surgery, Kaiser Permanente, Los Angeles Medical Center, Los Angeles, CA, USA

Part I

Perioperative Preparation and Care

To Prep or Not to Prep

1

Nishit Shah

Introduction

Oral mechanical bowel preparation (OMBP) has been employed for elective colorectal surgery for many years. The rationale for its use, based on early observational data as well as long-standing expert and intuitive opinion, was that by removing the fecal load from the colon lumen prior to surgery, infectious complications and overall morbidity would be lowered. This led to the widespread adoption of OMBP, a clinical practice which is still in place for the majority of colorectal surgeries in the United States today [1].

Since approximately 2000, however, the role of OMBP has come under increasing scrutiny. Aside from patient complaints of OMBP often not being well tolerated and potential issues with dehydration and electrolyte imbalances, investigators have perhaps more importantly questioned whether OMBP is as effective as traditionally thought in terms of reducing surgical site infection (SSI) rates.

Multiple randomized clinical trials over the last two decades failed to show any benefit from OMBP in terms of overall infectious complications and more specifically anastomotic leak rates [2–5]. The largest study evaluating 1343 patients randomized to OMBP or no OMBP found no significant differences in overall complications (24.5% OMBP vs. 23.7% no OMBP) nor in general infectious complications (7.9% OMBP vs. 6.8% no OMBP) [5]. Several meta-analyses have corroborated these findings (see Table 1.1) [6–8]. Indeed, the most recent Cochrane review in 2011, evaluating 18 trials, found no significant difference in wound infection, anastomotic leak rates, noninfectious complications, or mortality [9]. This has led to both European and Canadian surgical societies to recommend against routine

N. Shah (✉)
Rhode Island Hospital, Providence, RI, USA
e-mail: nshah@usasurg.org

C.M. Schlachta, P. Sylla (eds.), *Current Common Dilemmas in Colorectal Surgery*,
https://doi.org/10.1007/978-3-319-70117-2_1

Table 1.1 Pairwise meta-analysis results for the comparison of OMBP versus enema or no preparation

Outcome	Comparison	*N* studies (*N* events/*N* patients, per group)	OR (95% Cl)	Between-study variance (95% Crl)
All-cause mortality	OMBP ± enema vs enema/no prep	14 (45/2550 vs 44/2544)	1.17 (0.67–2.67)	0.12 (0.00–1.99)
	OMBP ± enema vs no prep	10 (38/2024 vs 40/2014)	1.09 (0.57–2.99)	0.17 (0.00–2.61)
	OMBP ± enema vs enema	4 (7/526 vs 4/530)	1.99 (0.27–18.45)	0.82 (0.00–3.76)
Anastomotic leakage	OMBP ± enema vs enema/no prep	16 (126/2702 vs 124/2680)	1.08 (0.79–1.63)	0.08 (0.00–0.72)
	OMBP ± enema vs no prep	12 (102/2176 vs 103/2150)	1.06 (0.73–1.73)	0.09 (0.00–0.95)
	OMBP ± enema vs enema	4 (24/526 vs 21/530)	1.24 (0.38–4.72)	0.61 (0.00–3.59)
Wound infection	OMBP ± enema vs enema/no prep	16 (266/2612 vs 239/2603)	1.19(0.93–1.63)	0.04 (0.00–0.41)
	OMBP ± enema vs no prep	12 (218/2086 vs 190/2073)	1.27 (0.95–1.88)	0.05 (0.00–0.50)
	OMBP ± enema vs enema	4 (48/526 vs 49/530)	1.04 (0.37–3.34)	0.52 (0.00–3.46)
Peritonitis/ intra-abdominal abscess	OMBP ± enema vs enema/no prep	14 (51/2381 vs 70/2362)	0.84 (0.50–1.66)	0.25 (0.00–1.77)
	OMBP ± enema vs no prep	10 (45/1855 vs 64/1832)	0.84 (0.45–2.00)	0.38 (0.00–2.74)
	OMBP ± enema vs enema	4 (6/526 vs 6/530)	0.99 (0.21–4.68)	0.42 (0.00–3.51)
Reoperation	OMBP ± enema vs enema/no prep	8 (124/1967 vs 119/1945)	1.14 (0.57–2.65)	0.38 (0.00–3.23)
	OMBP ± enema vs no prep	6 (117/1742 vs 111/1723)	1.15 (0.73–2.50)	0.09 (0.00–1.82)
	OMBP ± enema vs enema	2 (7/225 vs 8/222)	0.50 (0.03–6.12)	2.49 (0.27–3.93)
SSI	OMBP ± enema vs enema/no prep	7 (206/1279 vs 197/1230)	1.19 (0.56–2.63)	0.64 (0.11–2.91)
	OMBP ± enema vs no prep	5 (173/1087 vs 171/1040)	1.10 (0.41–3.05)	0.76 (0.10–3.39)
	OMBP ± enema vs enema	2 (33/192 vs 26/190)	1.50 (0.24–10.42)	1.20 (0.02–3.79)

OR values <1 indicate that events are less common among OMBP-treated groups (ie, that OMBP is beneficial). *Crl* credibility interval, *no prep* no OMBP and no enema, *OMBP* oral mechanical bowel preparation, *SSI* surgical site infection

Reprinted with permission from [8]

use of OMBP undergoing elective colon surgery [10, 11]. The Canadian Society did however deem the evidence insufficient to support or refute use of OMBP in elective rectal cancer surgery.

We recently undertook a systematic review of these studies (Fig. 1.1) [8]. We found that these studies used a variety of OMBP regimens, and this lack of standardization might have affected the validity of the findings. Furthermore, although almost all of the trials reported adjunct use of parenteral antibiotics perioperatively, the vast majority omitted oral nonabsorbable antibiotics. The role of gut decontamination with oral antibiotics will be expanded on below. In addition, we found there was some indication for between-study heterogeneity, particularly in the comparison of OMBP with or without enema versus enema alone for rectal surgery (Table 1.2). Details on the surgical indications (cancer vs. diverticular disease vs. inflammatory bowel disease), surgical approach (laparoscopic vs. open surgery), as well as operation types were generally poorly reported. This is relevant as numerous studies have recently found that surgical site infection (SSI) in colorectal surgery is influenced by primary disease diagnosis as well as the use of laparoscopy. The Mayo Clinic group noted that operations for diverticular disease were associated with more superficial SSI, whereas ulcerative colitis patients had more deep/organ space SSIs.

The benefits of laparoscopic surgery in reducing SSI have been clearly demonstrated. In a prospective study from Hong Kong of over 1000 patients, the rate of SSI was significantly higher following open surgery (5.7% open vs. 2.7% laparoscopic, $p < 0.05$) [12]. This benefit is further amplified in our growing obese patient population. It is uncertain whether the results of OMBP trials involving predominantly open surgical procedures can be extended to laparoscopic operations, particularly as from a technical standpoint prepped bowel may be easier to manipulate during a laparoscopic resection.

A note should be made regarding elective rectal surgery. It has been well documented that the risk of anastomotic leaks is greater in this setting compared to colon surgery, particularly when associated with low extraperitoneal anastomoses [13]. Indeed, a recent observational analysis involving patients undergoing resection surgery for colorectal surgery found that rectal resections were independently associated with an increased likelihood of both superficial and deep/organ space SSI [14]. With respect to stratification by surgical site in the trials we analyzed, only one randomized trial has been published exclusively enrolling patients undergoing rectal surgery, and only two studies looked specifically at left-sided colorectal operations. The GRECCAR III randomized trial from France showed a significant increase in infectious complications in the absence of OMBP (34% no OMBP vs. 16% OMBP, $p = 0.005$) but no difference in anastomotic leak rates, major morbidity, nor mortality rate [15]. A subgroup analysis of a large multicenter randomized OMBP trial examining outcomes of 449 patients who had undergone a low anterior resection with a primary anastomosis also revealed no difference in anastomotic leak rates, irrespective of whether a diverting ileostomy was created [16]. Furthermore, a recent meta-analysis also confirmed that OMBP had no impact on SSI, anastomotic leak rates, nor overall morbidity and mortality in patients

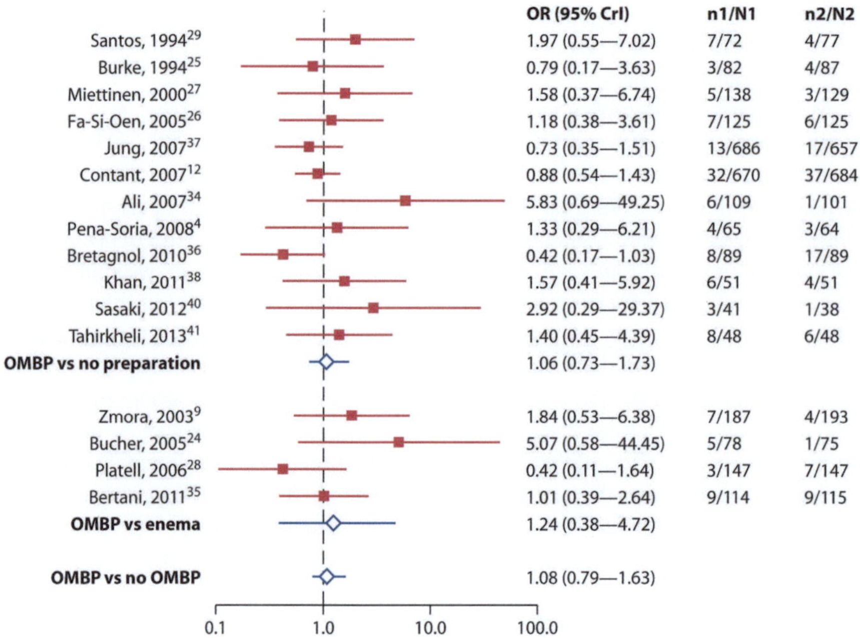

Fig. 1.1 Anastomotic leakage meta-analysis results for studies comparing OMBP (with or without enema) versus enema or no preparation. Reprinted with permission from [8]

Table 1.2 Meta-regression results for studies comparing OMBP (with or without enema) versus enema or no preparation

Outcome	Potential modifier	rOR (95% Crl)
All-cause mortality	ROB for randomized sequence generation (low vs moderate/high/unclear)	0.33 (0.07–1.40)
	ROB for allocation concealment (low vs moderate/high/unclear)	0.88 (0.23–4.39)
	Year of publication	0.98 (0.90–1.04)
Anastomotic leakage	ROB for randomized sequence generation (low vs moderate/high/unclear)	0.72 (0.35–1.56)
	ROB for allocation concealment (low vs moderate/high/unclear)	0.45 (0.23–0.86)[a]
	Year of publication	0.98 (0.91–1.05)
Wound infection	ROB for randomized sequence generation (low vs moderate/high/unclear)	0.90 (0.51–1.72)
	ROB for allocation concealment (low vs moderate/high/unclear)	0.64 (0.38–1.08)
	Year of publication	1.00 (0.97–1.03)

[a]Results are suggestive of an association

Crl credibility interval, *ROB* risk of bias, *rOR* relative OR, *SSI* surgical site infection

Reprinted with permission from [8]

undergoing a proctectomy [17]. In our recent review regarding OMBP and rectal surgery, we found that although there was no evidence of any beneficial effect of OMBP, this summary estimate was imprecise. The small number of studies in this setting was often underpowered with heterogeneous subgroup definitions, with the level of the anastomosis and use of protective diverting stomas often unclear [8].

Despite this ostensibly compelling data on the lack of its efficacy, the vast majority of US surgeons performing colorectal surgery still currently employ OMBP. Indeed, this ongoing debate has been revisited over the last couple of years, with the results of several large US studies seemingly swinging the pendulum back in favor of OMBP. Several recent National Surgical Quality Improvement Program (NSQIP) retrospective studies concluded that OMBP combined with oral antibiotics resulted in reduced SSI as well anastomotic leak rates after elective colorectal surgery [18, 19]. In thc largest study by Kiran et al., over 8000 patients were divided into three groups: no OMBP (27%), OMBP but no oral antibiotics (45%), and OMBP with oral antibiotics (28%). On multivariate analysis, OMBP with oral antibiotics, but not without, was independently associated with lower SSI, reduced anastomotic leak rates, as well as shorter postoperative ileus. The authors acknowledged that the no OMBP group did have more patients with sepsis, ascites, steroid use, disseminated cancer, and ASA class greater than 3, as well as fewer laparoscopic resections. Although their multivariate analysis tried to account for these differences, it is unclear to what extent these comorbidities may have contributed to the poorer results in the no OMBP group [18].

If there is some validity to these NSQIP reports, however, how do we reconcile these seemingly discrepant findings with those of the many randomized trials previously discussed? A closer examination of the OMBP literature suggests the role oral antibiotics may play in determining outcomes. The use of oral antibiotics to lower the bacterial load in the colon was popularized following the seminal study by Nichols in 1972 which demonstrated a reduction in SSIs in patients treated with a combination of OMBP and an oral neomycin-erythromycin regimen. Although their use gradually declined over the next couple of decades, there has been renewed interest in the value of oral antibiotics recently. A double-blind, randomized controlled trial by Lewis revealed that patients receiving both oral and intravenous antibiotics had a marked decrease in SSI (RR = 0.29, $p < 0.01$) and a much lower incidence of colonic bacteria in the surgical wound at the end of the case, compared to those receiving intravenous antibiotics alone, both groups having undergone OMBP [20]. In two more recent retrospective reviews from the Veterans Affairs (VA) NSQIP database and from the Michigan Surgical Collaborative, patients receiving both oral and parenteral antibiotics had dramatically lower SSI rates compared to patients receiving parenteral antibiotics alone [21, 22]. A closer breakdown of the VA study of over 9900 patients undergoing colorectal surgery showed that patients receiving preoperative oral antibiotics alone had similar SSI rates to those receiving oral antibiotics plus OMBP (8.3 vs. 9.2%). In addition, those patients receiving no OMBP had similar SSI rates compared to those receiving OMBP alone without oral antibiotics (18% vs. 20%) [21]. Moreover, in another NSQIP analysis of over 8400 colorectal operations, Morris reported that oral antibiotics reduced SSI rates compared to the no OMBP and OMBP alone groups (6.5% vs. 14.9%, vs.12.0%, respectively, $p < 0.001$) and resulted in lower anastomotic leak rates [19]. Similar to the VA study, there was no significant difference in SSI rates in the oral antibiotic plus OMBP group to those patients given oral antibiotics alone, though the latter group constituted only 8% of the patients. Putting these results together, it is evident that gut decontamination with oral nonabsorbable antibiotics may play a significant role in reducing infectious complications in colorectal surgery. Yet in our review of the many trials comparing the efficacy of OMBP to no bowel preparation, although we found no evidence of any benefit with OMBP use, we only noted three studies in which oral antibiotics were administered. Furthermore, although the traditional, intuitive opinion has been that oral antibiotics can only be administered after completion of a mechanical bowel preparation, the VA NSQIP and Morris studies suggest that even without an OMBP the benefits of oral antibiotics in reduction of SSI may persist.

Conclusion

Although we found no definitive evidence that OMBP is beneficial in elective colorectal surgery, the evidence on which this assumption is based was weak and of low quality. Moreover, many of these published studies do not reflect changes in the current practice of colorectal surgery, such as the increased popularity of laparoscopic surgery and enhanced recovery pathways. We propose there is an important need for a large randomized controlled trial examining all combinations of using or withholding OMBP, with and without oral antibiotics. Such a study should not be difficult due to the large volume of elective colorectal operations performed annually. A noninferiority design could be used to examine whether omission of OMBP does not worsen clinical outcomes, while a factorial design could readily determine the interaction between OMBP and oral antibiotics with a careful breakdown of anatomic location (colon vs. rectum) and the approach used (open vs. laparoscopic).

References

1. Zmora O, Wexner SD, Hajjar L, et al. Trends in preparation for colorectal surgery: survey of the members of the American Society of Colon and Rectal Surgeons. Am Surg. 2003;69:150–4.
2. Bucher P, Gervaz P, Soravia C, et al. Randomized clinical trial of mechanical bowel preparation versus no preparation before elective left-sided colorectal surgery. Br J Surg. 2005;92:409–14.
3. Contant CM, Hop WC, van't Sant HP, et al. Mechanical bowel preparation for elective colorectal surgery: a multicenter randomized trial. Lancet. 2007;370:2112–7.
4. Fa-Si Oen PR, Roumen R, Buitenweg J, et al. Mechanical bowel preparation or not? Outcome of a multicenter, randomized trial in elective open colon surgery. Dis Colon Rectum. 2005;48:1509–16.

5. Jung B, Pahlman L, Nystrom PO, Nilsson E, Mechanical Bowel Preparation Study Group. Multicentre randomized clinical trial of mechanical bowel preparation in elective colon resection. Br J Surg. 2007;94:689–95.
6. Cao F, Li J, Li F. Mechanical bowel preparation for elective colorectal surgery: updated systematic review and meta-analysis. Int J Color Dis. 2012;27:803–10.
7. Slim K, Vicaut F, Launay-Savary MV, Contant C, Chipponi J. Updated systematic review and meta-analysis of randomized clinical trials on the role of mechanical bowel preparation before colorectal surgery. Ann Surg. 2009;249:203–9.
8. Dahabreh I, Steele DW, Shah N, Trikalinos TA. Oral mechanical bowel preparation for colorectal surgery: systematic review and meta-analysis. Dis Colon Rectum. 2015;58:698–707.
9. Guenaga KE, Matos D, Wille-Jorgensen P. Mechanical bowel preparation for elective colorectal surgery. Cochrane Database Syst Rev. 2011;9:CD001544.
10. Prevention, diagnosis and management of colorectal anastomotic leakage. The Association of Coloproctology of Great Britain and Ireland. 2016.
11. Eskicioglu C, Forbes SS, Fenech DS, McLeod RS. Preoperative bowel preparation for patients undergoing elective colorectal surgery: a clinical practice guideline endorsed by the Canadian Society of Colon and Rectal Surgeons. Can J Surg. 2010;53:385–95.
12. Poon JT, Law WL, Wong IW, et al. Impact of laparoscopic colorectal resection on surgical site infection. Ann Surg. 2009;249:77–81.
13. Vignali A, Fazio VW, Lavery IC, et al. Factors associated with the occurrence of leaks in stapled rectal anastomoses. J Am Coll Surg. 1997;185:105–13.
14. Adelaide Murray AC, Pasam R, Estrada D, Kiran RP. Risk of surgical site infection varies based on location of disease and segment of colorectal resection for cancer. Dis Colon Rectum. 2016;59:493–500.
15. Bretagnol F, Panis Y, Rullier E, et al. Rectal cancer surgery with or without bowel preparation: the French GRECCAR III multicenter single-blinded randomized trial. Ann Surg. 2010;252:863–8.
16. Van't Sant HP, Weidema WF, Hop WC, et al. The influence of mechanical bowel preparation in elective lower colorectal surgery. Ann Surg. 2010;251:59–63.
17. Courtney DE, Kelly ME, Burke JP, Winter DC. Postoperative outcomes following mechanical bowel preparation before proctectomy: a meta-analysis. Color Dis. 2015;17:862–9.
18. Kiran RP, Murray AC, Chiuzan C, et al. Combined preoperative mechanical bowel preparation with oral antibiotics significantly reduces surgical site infection rates, anastomotic leak and ileus after colorectal surgery. Ann Surg. 2015;262:416–25.
19. Morris MS, Graham DI, Chu JA, et al. Oral antibiotic bowel preparation significantly reduces surgical site infection rates and readmission rates in elective colorectal surgery. Ann Surg. 2015;261:1034–40.
20. Lewis RT. Oral versus systemic antibiotic prophylaxis in elective colon surgery. Can J Surg. 2002;45:173–80.
21. Cannon JA, Altom LK, Deierhoi RJ, et al. Preoperative oral antibiotics reduce surgical site infection following elective colorectal resections. Dis Colon Rectum. 2012;55:1160–6.
22. Englesbe MJ, Brooks L, Kubus J, et al. A statewide assessment of surgical site infection following colectomy: the role of oral antibiotics. Ann Surg. 2010;252:514–9.

Practice Guidelines and Future Directions of Bowel Preparation: Science and History

2

Megan Turner, Zhifei Sun, and John Migaly

Introduction

Intestinal antisepsis has been a principle of health intervention since antiquity [1–3]. Bowel preparation and antisepsis have become a surgical interest with Jacques Lisfranc successfully performing the first perineal resection in 1826 and John Miles performing the first abdominoperineal resection in 1908 [4]. As sophistication of operative techniques, pharmacology, and perioperative care increased in the 1900s, the use of evidence-based practices for bowel preparation became an effective preoperative intervention for decreasing postoperative complications. This review will present basic scientific principles and key historical developments in the use of preoperative bowel preparation. Descriptions of combined mechanical, oral, and parenteral preparation are to follow, concluding with the current best practice guidelines and queries for future areas of study.

Basic Scientific Principles

At baseline, the colon has a high bacterial load, with up to 10^7 aerobic colony-forming units (CFU) per milliliter of irrigation and 10^8 anaerobic CFU per milliliter of irrigation [5]. Wound studies following colonic operations show a predominance of mixed aerobic-anaerobic growth, largely composed of *Bacteroides fragilis* and *Escherichia coli* [5]. In the early 1900s, nearly 80% of postoperative patients suffered from infectious complications with a 20% mortality [4]. Postoperative infections were attributed to colonic bacteria introduced into the surgical site following resection with gross or microscopic spillage, not introduced from the skin flora or

M. Turner (✉) • Z. Sun • J. Migaly
Department of Surgery, Duke University Medical Center, Durham, NC, USA
e-mail: megan.turner@dm.duke.edu; zhifei.sun@dm.duke.edu; John.Migaly@dm.duke.edu

C.M. Schlachta, P. Sylla (eds.), *Current Common Dilemmas in Colorectal Surgery*,
https://doi.org/10.1007/978-3-319-70117-2_2

surgical team. In an attempt to decrease infectious morbidity, methods to decrease bacterial load were developed including mechanical bowel preparation and the use of antibiotics.

Mechanical preparations of bulking agents were popularized to facilitate evacuating the entirety of the intestinal tract, frequently followed by enemas to ensure complete cleanliness. The dogma of early intestinal surgery was that no anastomosis should be made with residual fecal contents present.

In the 1940s, nonabsorbable sulfonamides were tested for impact on colonic bacterial counts. Little effect on postoperative infectious outcomes was found with sulfonamide use given the narrow spectrum of activity, bacteriostatic nature, and the associated multiday mechanical bowel preparation [6–8]. Sensitivity studies that followed examined single-agent antibiotic preparations compared to multiple-agent antibiotic preparations. Single-agent therapies were found to be inferior to combination therapies in the reduction of colonic bacteria and subsequent postoperative sepsis [9, 10]. A decrease in colonic bacterial counts of up to 10^5 was observed in all major colonic bacterial groups following oral combination antimicrobial therapy [5].

Early studies examined the emergence of single organism overgrowth and bacterial resistance in fecal flora following antimicrobial therapy. Single-agent preparations were associated with increased growth of isolated organisms, leading to diarrhea and pseudomembranous colitis [6, 11]. The use of combination therapy prevented the emergence of overgrowth, and resistant strains were avoided [5, 12].

History of Bowel Preparation

1860s–Early1900s

In the late 1860s, the quest for medical antisepsis began with the established relationship between bacteria and disease. Halsted is known for his work in antiseptic surgical technique in the 1890s, which was not widely adopted until well into the twentieth century. In parallel with development of techniques for aerobic and anaerobic cell culture came clinical studies evaluating the efficacy of mechanical bowel preparation on reducing bacterial burden. Historically, preoperative bowel preparation was guided by the principle of complete colonic emptying by starvation and purgation. Surgeons of the 1900s used bulking agents and stimulants to empty the bowel of its contents [13]. Mechanical bulking agents, such as vegetable matter, increased the volume of stool and allowed easier passage. Castor oil (a stimulant of peristalsis through its conversion to ricinoleic acid in the duodenum) was a choice purgative. It was believed clearing the bowel of fecal material would decrease the total bacterial burden, decreasing the risk of infection.

Surgical experiments at this time were performed primarily in animals and focused on the integrity of intestinal anastomoses, specifically evaluating dehiscence and leak [14]. The leading theory was that an unprepared bowel would be unable to heal an intestinal anastomosis. However, as early as the 1920s, the doctrine of complete bowel emptying prior to anastomosis formation was challenged with the advent of antibiotics [15]. The discovery of nonabsorbable enteral antibiotics led to experimentation of intestinal antisepsis in both animals and humans.

1940s–1970s

With the introduction of antibiotics, surgeons began to use enteral antibiotic formulations in addition to mechanical preparation to reduce postoperative morbidity. Early studies examined the impact of preoperative enteral preparations on surgical site infection, correlating cultures from colonic specimens and subsequent wound infections [9, 10, 16]. Through these studies, it was apparent that appropriate prophylaxis required coverage of both aerobes and anaerobes to obtain clinical effectiveness [11, 17, 18]. Given the bacteriostatic nature of the available antibiotics, they were administered in combination with mechanical bowel preparations over several days preoperatively. Nichol's 1973 landmark prospective randomized control trial, and subsequent retrospective analysis, compared mechanical preparation to mechanical preparation plus nonabsorbable enteral antibiotics. A dramatic decrease in surgical site infection with combination therapy was observed. Thus, the combination was termed the "Nichols prep" and has continued use in modern practice [19].

Similarly, the 1977 prospective randomized control trial by Clarke et al. showed a decrease in postoperative septic complications in patients who received both enteral antibiotics and mechanical bowel preparation [20]. Subsequent trials provided additional evidence that enteral antibiotics improved outcomes with decreased anastomotic dehiscence and surgical site infections independent of mechanical bowel preparation [5, 21]. Even in these early studies, the authors have suggested that mechanical preparation alone will become obsolete. Studies in pathophysiology showed that intestinal anastomoses without preoperative antibiotic therapy were healed by secondary intention as seen with superficial contaminated wounds, whereas anastomoses protected by enteral antibiotics were healed by primary intention [6, 12].

As a result of the trials by Nichols and Clark, the combination of enteral antibiotics and mechanical preparation was widely implemented and based in substantial evidence. By the end of the 1970s, it was the standard of care for elective colorectal procedures. The availability of broad-spectrum parenteral antibiotics became the next frontier in battling postoperative complications for colorectal surgery.

1980s–1990s

Combination of mechanical and enteral antibiotic bowel preparation was well established in the 1980s [22]. However, the role of parenteral antibiotics was unclear. Surgeons sought to maintain low rates of postoperative complications while streamlining preoperative antisepsis interventions. Burke et al. describe the use of parenteral antibiotics in patients randomized to a mechanical preparation compared to no preparation. No difference in anastomotic dehiscence or wound infections was found [23]. Petrelli et al. utilized mechanical preparation and oral antibiotics and randomized their patients to receive parenteral antibiotics. Their findings concluded that parenteral antibiotics provided no additional benefit, with equal distribution of anastomotic and infectious complications [24]. Conversely, a large prospective randomized trial by Schoetz et al. showed dramatic improvement in infectious complications in patients who received parenteral antibiotics in addition to oral antibiotics and mechanical preparation [25]. Despite early conflicting evidence, by the late 1990s, the consensus of practicing colorectal surgeons was the use of mechanical preparation and parenteral and enteral antibiotics in preparation for elective colorectal surgery [26, 27].

2000–2010

Following over 100 years of strict adherence to elective intestinal anastomoses being performed in mechanically cleansed bowels, data from trauma surgery in the early 2000s challenged these practices [28–30]. Curran et al. performed a meta-analysis of 35 studies including 5400 penetrating colon injuries to better define the consequences of primary repair in the setting of trauma [29]. Their findings were a low rate of anastomotic leak, concluding colonic injury may be managed by primary repair in select circumstances. This analysis was further supported by a subsequent prospective multicenter trial by Demetriades et al. which compared outcomes between patients with penetrating colon injury who underwent primary repair with and without diversion [30]. They found no difference in intra-abdominal complications between the two groups accumulating evidence for the safety of performing anastomoses in an un-prepped colon. This data was extrapolated to elective colorectal surgery as evidence for the possibility of a safe anastomosis without mechanical preparation.

Randomized trials during this same time period examined the need for mechanical preparation with the use of parenteral antibiotics in elective colorectal surgery. Zmora et al. randomized 380 patients to either mechanical bowel preparation or no preparation for elective colon resection. All patients received enteral and parenteral antibiotics. They found no difference in infectious or anastomotic complications leading to the conclusion that anastomoses can be safely created in a nonmechanically prepped bowel with enteral and parenteral antibiotics [31]. This was complemented by a larger multicenter trial by Contant et al. randomizing 1400 patients to parenteral antibiotics with or without mechanical preparation, and they found no difference in anastomotic integrity [32]. In 2002, Lewis et al. performed a randomized, placebo-controlled prospective trial examining the impact of combination mechanical, enteral, and parenteral antibiotic preparation compared to mechanical and parenteral antibiotics alone. They concluded the combination of systemic and enteral antibiotic prophylaxis was superior to systemic antibiotics alone [33]. Additionally, their meta-analysis of studies through the 1990s corroborated their conclusions.

The Cochrane Review guidelines of 2009 recommended enteral and parenteral antibiotics prior to elective colorectal surgery with a reduction in infectious complications by 75% [34]. In their meta-analysis, improved surgical site infectious outcomes with combination of enteral and parenteral antibiotics over either therapy alone were observed. No outcome differences were seen between different regimens of antibiotics, providing the patients had adequate aerobic and anaerobic coverage. Length of antibiotic therapy did not lead to a difference in outcomes, but concerns arose regarding the development of resistant organisms and *Clostridium difficile* (*C. diff*) infection with prolonged use.

The association between antibiotic prophylaxis for colorectal surgery and *C. diff* has garnered limited enthusiasm for newer studies despite worse outcome implications for postoperative patients infected with *C. diff*. In 2005 Wren et al. retrospectively examined the impact of enteral antibiotics, in addition to parenteral antibiotics and mechanical preparation, finding higher incidences of *C. diff* infections in those receiving enteral prophylaxis [35]. Their cohort did not have differences in surgical site infection or anastomotic breakdown. A larger follow-up study was performed in 2011 by the Michigan Surgical Quality Colectomy Project, which did not find a difference in rates of *C. diff* among patients who underwent mechanical bowel preparations versus preparations with enteral antibiotics [36]. Based on the clear benefit of enteral antibiotic use on overall outcomes for elective colorectal resections, the use of enteral antibiotics continues to be the standard of care. Minimizing the incidence of *C. diff* infection rates remains a challenge in the postoperative period.

Best Practice Guidelines

Despite the large body of data surrounding the use of various preparations in combination, in 2011, Englesbe et al. published the first study to compare patients receiving parenteral antibiotic prophylaxis without mechanical preparation or enteral antibiotics to those receiving combined mechanical preparation and enteral and parenteral antibiotics. Using the Michigan Surgical Quality Collaborative-Colectomy Best Practices Project database, patients undergoing elective colon resections were evaluated in propensity-matched groups to evaluate outcomes between the un-prepped cohort and the combination prepped cohort [37]. Their primary outcomes evaluated surgical site infection, *C. diff* colitis, prolonged ileus, as well as National Surgical Quality Improvement Project (NSQIP) outcomes. In their unadjusted analysis, no differences were observed in rates of surgical site infection with or without mechanical preparation. However, among propensity-matched patients, significant outcome differences were seen; specifically, surgical site infections were lower with enteral antibiotic use. Correspondingly, superficial wound infections and organ space surgical site infections were lower with enteral antibiotic use. Additionally, the use of enteral antibiotics was associated with reduced rates of prolonged ileus, without an increase in the risk for *C. diff*.

In 2014, Nelson et al. provided recommendations in an updated Cochrane Review; the quality of the existing evidence was such that the recommendations are unlikely to change significantly with future studies. No benefit was found with mechanical bowel preparation alone, and there was significant benefit to combined preparation of mechanical, enteral, and parenteral antibiotic prophylaxis. While there was robust data that no benefit exists with mechanical preparation alone, given the support for nonabsorbable enteral antibiotic use, many surgeons continued to use mechanical preparation as no studies determined the efficacy of enteral antibiotics in an un-prepped colon [38].

Our group addressed the concerns outlined above with a retrospective study of the National Surgical Quality Improvement Project data to conclude that combined mechanical, enteral, and parental antibiotic preparations prior to elective colorectal surgery had improved outcomes [39]. Specifically, the use of enteral antibiotics in a mechanically prepped colon and an un-prepped colon is addressed. The primary outcomes measured were incisional surgical site infection, anastomotic leak, and mortality. We found that the combination of mechanical preparation and enteral and parenteral antibiotics had lower incidence of incisional surgical site infection, lower incidence of anastomotic leak, shorter postoperative length of stay, and lower readmission rates compared to patients with no preparation [39]. In general, there was no significant difference in outcomes between patients who received mechanical preparations and parenteral antibiotics or enteral and parenteral antibiotic preparations without mechanical preparation and patients who received parenteral antibiotics alone. The improved effect of enteral antibiotics in combination with mechanical preparation is attributed to decreases in fecal bulk increasing the delivery of the antibiotics to the colonic mucosa.

Future Directions

In the last decade, our understanding of commensal bacteria on human immunology and tissue healing has led to reevaluation of antibiotic prescriptive practices. This increase in knowledge spurred the National Institute of Health to sponsor the Human Microbiome Project Roadmap Initiative to catalogue the human microbiome to better characterize the impact of these organisms on human health and disease. With regard to colorectal surgery, the Nichols preparation of preoperative, nonabsorbable, enteral antibiotics is based on historic fecal culture data. These studies have not been repeated with newer techniques, namely, genomic sequencing; thus, there is an incomplete understanding of the bacterial community of the colon. There is strong evidence for the use of broad-spectrum, nonabsorbable, preoperative antibiotics in the prevention of anastomotic leak; however, given the incomplete catalog of bacteria at the site, the mechanism of this phenomenon is incompletely understood. The newest data regarding anastomotic healing examines the impact of bacteria on induction of human immune factors both systemically and at the site of the anastomosis [40, 41]. Additionally, under postoperative stress, pathogenic bacterial factors are produced with unknown consequences on tissue healing [40, 42, 43].

As the impact of the bacterial communities within the colon is further understood, preoperative enteral antibiotic regimens will need to be developed with increasing specificity to optimize outcomes following resection and anastomosis.

The findings from the large-scale retrospective studies of our group and Morris et al. elucidate the need for a prospective randomized trial to increase the robustness of data surrounding the benefit of combined mechanical preparation with enteral and parenteral antibiotics [44]. The impact of combined preparations on *Clostridium difficile* infections and outcomes has yet to be fully examined and will likely be impacted by the choice and timing of antibiotic preparations. Surgeon prescriptive practices for preoperative antibiotic prophylaxis will need to be responsive to discoveries that result from the Human Microbiome Project. Additionally, in retrospective studies, significant variability is observed in prescribed preparations in current practice [39]. Examination of variability and adherence to best practice guidelines are important in improving postoperative morbidity metrics on a national level.

Conclusions

The use of combined enteral antibiotics, mechanical preparation, and parenteral antibiotic prophylaxis, while arduous, leads to improved postoperative outcomes compared to streamlined preparations in elective colorectal surgery. Further directions of study include optimization of antibiotic timing and comprehensive characterization of colonic bacterial communities. Prescription variability and adherence to best practice guidelines remain as challenges in moving forward.

References

1. Tresilian F. Intestinal antisepsis. Br Med J. 1900;1(2036):45–6.
2. Ernst HC. Intestinal antisepsis. Boston Med Surg J. 1892;126(7):157–9.
3. Kinsman DN. Intestinal antisepsis. J Am Med Assoc. 1886;VII(1):5–11.
4. Glenn F, McSherry CK. Carcinoma of the distal large bowel: 32-year review of 1,026 cases. Ann Surg. 1966;163(6):838–49.
5. Bartlett JG, Condon RE, Gorbach SL, Clarke JS, Nichols RL, Ochi S. Veterans administration cooperative study on bowel preparation for elective colorectal operations: impact of oral antibiotic regimen on colonic flora, wound irrigation cultures and bacteriology of septic complications. Ann Surg. 1978;188(2):249–54.
6. Poth EJ. Intestinal antisepsis in surgery. J Am Med Assoc. 1953;153(17):1516–21.
7. Poth EJ. Modern concepts of intestinal antisepsis. Am Surg. 1952;18(6):572–8.
8. Firor WM, Poth EJ. Intestinal antisepsis, with special reference to sulfanilylguanidine. Ann Surg. 1941;114(4):663.
9. Cohn I Jr, Longacre AB. Novobiocin and novobiocin-neomycin for intestinal antisepsis. Ann Surg. 1957;146(2):184–9.
10. Cohn I Jr, Longacre AB. Erythromycin and erythromycin-neomycin for intestinal antisepsis. Am J Surg. 1957;94(3):402–8.
11. Poth EJ. The practical application of intestinal antisepsis to surgery of the colon and rectum. Dis Colon Rectum. 1960;3:491–6.
12. Poth EJ. The role of intestinal antisepsis in the preoperative preparation of the colon. Surgery. 1960;47:1018–28.

13. Ivy AC, Isaacs BL. Karaya gum as a mechanical laxative an experimental study on animals and man. Am J Dig Dis. 1938;5(5):315–21.
14. Flint JM. The healing of gastro-intestinal anastomoses. Ann Surg. 1917;65(2):202–21.
15. Mitchell WEM. The preparation of patients for operation. Lancet. 1927;210(5423):270–2.
16. Cohn I Jr. Intestinal antisepsis. Am Surg. 1959;25(7):498–502.
17. Poth EJ, Mc NJ, et al. The healing of bowel as influenced by sulfasuxidine and streptomycin. Surg Gynecol Obstet. 1948;86(6):641–6.
18. Finegold SM. Studies on antibiotics and the normal intestinal flora. Tex Rep Biol Med. 1951;9(3):432–44.
19. Nichols RL, Broido P, Condon RE, Gorbach SL, Nyhus LM. Effect of preoperative neomycin-erythromycin intestinal preparation on the incidence of infectious complications following colon surgery. Ann Surg. 1973;178(4):453–62.
20. Clarke JS, Condon RE, Bartlett JG, Gorbach SL, Nichols RL, Ochi S. Preoperative oral antibiotics reduce septic complications of colon operations: results of prospective, randomized, double-blind clinical study. Ann Surg. 1977;186(3):251–9.
21. Matheson DM, Arabi Y, Baxter-Smith D, Alexander-Williams J, Keighley MR. Randomized multicentre trial of oral bowel preparation and antimicrobials for elective colorectal operations. Br J Surg. 1978;65(9):597–600.
22. Guglielmo BJ, Hohn DC, Koo PJ, Hunt TK, Sweet RL, Conte JE Jr. Antibiotic prophylaxis in surgical procedures. A critical analysis of the literature. Arch Surg. 1983;118(8):943–55.
23. Burke P, Mealy K, Gillen P, Joyce W, Traynor O, Hyland J. Requirement for bowel preparation in colorectal surgery. Br J Surg. 1994;81(6):907–10.
24. Petrelli NJ, Conte CC, Herrera L, Stulc J, O'Neill P. A prospective, randomized trial of perioperative prophylactic cefamandole in elective colorectal surgery for malignancy. Dis Colon Rectum. 1988;31(6):427–9.
25. Schoetz DJ Jr, Roberts PL, Murray JJ, Coller JA, Veidenheimer MC. Addition of parenteral cefoxitin to regimen of oral antibiotics for elective colorectal operations. A randomized prospective study. Ann Surg. 1990;212(2):209–12.
26. Nichols RL, Smith JW, Garcia RY, Waterman RS, Holmes JW. Current practices of preoperative bowel preparation among North American colorectal surgeons. Clin Infect Dis. 1997;24(4):609–19.
27. Solla JA, Rothenberger DA. Preoperative bowel preparation. A survey of colon and rectal surgeons. Dis Colon Rectum. 1990;33(2):154–9.
28. Conrad JK, Ferry KM, Foreman ML, Gogel BM, Fisher TL, Livingston SA. Changing management trends in penetrating colon trauma. Dis Colon Rectum. 2000;43(4):466–71.
29. Curran TJ, Borzotta AP. Complications of primary repair of colon injury: literature review of 2,964 cases. Am J Surg. 1999;177(1):42–7.
30. Demetriades D, Murray JA, Chan L, Ordonez C, Bowley D, Nagy KK, et al. Penetrating colon injuries requiring resection: diversion or primary anastomosis? An AAST prospective multicenter study. J Trauma. 2001;50(5):765–75.
31. Zmora O, Mahajna A, Bar-Zakai B, Rosin D, Hershko D, Shabtai M, et al. Colon and rectal surgery without mechanical bowel preparation: a randomized prospective trial. Ann Surg. 2003;237(3):363–7.
32. Contant CM, Hop WC, van't Sant HP, Oostvogel HJ, Smeets HJ, Stassen LP, et al. Mechanical bowel preparation for elective colorectal surgery: a multicentre randomised trial. Lancet. 2007;370(9605):2112–7.
33. Lewis RT. Oral versus systemic antibiotic prophylaxis in elective colon surgery: a randomized study and meta-analysis send a message from the 1990s. Can J Surg. 2002;45(3):173–80.
34. Nelson RL, Glenny AM, Song F. Antimicrobial prophylaxis for colorectal surgery. Cochrane Database Syst Rev. 2009;1:CD001181.
35. Wren SM, Ahmed N, Jamal A, Safadi BY. Preoperative oral antibiotics in colorectal surgery increase the rate of Clostridium difficile colitis. Arch Surg. 2005;140(8):752–6.
36. Krapohl GL, Phillips LR, Campbell DA Jr, Hendren S, Banerjee M, Metzger B, et al. Bowel preparation for colectomy and risk of *Clostridium difficile* infection. Dis Colon Rectum. 2011;54(7):810–7.

37. Englesbe MJ, Brooks L, Kubus J, Luchtefeld M, Lynch J, Senagore A, et al. A statewide assessment of surgical site infection following colectomy: the role of oral antibiotics. Ann Surg. 2010;252(3):514–9. discussion 9–20.
38. Nelson RL, Gladman E, Barbateskovic M. Antimicrobial prophylaxis for colorectal surgery. Cochrane Database Syst Rev. 2014;5:CD001181.
39. Scarborough JE, Mantyh CR, Sun Z, Migaly J. Combined mechanical and oral antibiotic bowel preparation reduces incisional surgical site infection and anastomotic leak rates after elective colorectal resection: an analysis of colectomy-targeted ACS NSQIP. Ann Surg. 2015;262(2):331–7.
40. Shogan BD, Smith DP, Christley S, Gilbert JA, Zaborina O, Alverdy JC. Intestinal anastomotic injury alters spatially defined microbiome composition and function. Microbiome. 2014;2:35.
41. Krezalek MA, Alverdy JC. The role of the microbiota in surgical recovery. Curr Opin Clin Nutr Metab Care. 2016;19:347.
42. Shogan BD, Belogortseva N, Luong PM, Zaborin A, Lax S, Bethel C, et al. Collagen degradation and MMP9 activation by enterococcus faecalis contribute to intestinal anastomotic leak. Sci Transl Med. 2015;7(286):286ra68.
43. Zaborin A, Smith D, Garfield K, Quensen J, Shakhsheer B, Kade M, et al. Membership and behavior of ultra-low-diversity pathogen communities present in the gut of humans during prolonged critical illness. MBio. 2014;5(5):e01361-14.
44. Dellinger EP. Should a scheduled colorectal operation have a mechanical bowel prep, preoperative oral antibiotics, both, or neither? Ann Surg. 2015;261(6):1041–3.

Enhanced Recovery Pathways: Is It Laparoscopy or Is It Everything Else?

3

Lawrence Lee and Liane S. Feldman

Introduction

The management of patients undergoing colorectal surgery has undergone two important paradigm shifts: first, laparoscopy and other minimally invasive techniques changed the way the surgery itself was performed, and second, enhanced recovery pathways (ERP) altered the way these patients were managed in the perioperative period. By minimizing surgical trauma, laparoscopy has been demonstrated to diminish the surgical stress response, decrease postoperative pain, hasten gastrointestinal function and accelerate return to independence, which have translated into improved clinical outcomes [1]. In view of these benefits, as well as equivalence of long-term oncologic outcomes, laparoscopic colorectal surgery has largely become the standard of care, with the majority of elective colonic operations in the USA now performed laparoscopically [2]. Despite this, an important number of patients still experience significant postoperative morbidity and delayed recovery [3]. The reasons for this are multifactorial and complex. Many patient risk factors are non-modifiable or are not affected by surgical technique alone. Postoperative recovery is poorly understood, and recovery to functional independence may be significantly delayed even in the absence of postoperative morbidity [4, 5].

There are limitations in what surgical technique alone can achieve. Many other aspects of perioperative care play an important role in the surgical stress response and subsequent postoperative trajectory of patients undergoing surgery (Fig. 3.1). Perioperative management has been traditionally dictated according to dogma and each individual specialist's preferences, with little communication between care providers. This has led to variability in outcomes and suboptimal care as practices such as prolonged fasting and routine use of drains have remained in clinical care [6]. Resistance

L. Lee • L.S. Feldman (✉)
Department of Surgery, McGill University Health Centre, Montréal, QC, Canada
e-mail: larry.lee@mail.mcgill.ca; liane.feldman@mcgill.ca

C.M. Schlachta, P. Sylla (eds.), *Current Common Dilemmas in Colorectal Surgery*,
https://doi.org/10.1007/978-3-319-70117-2_3

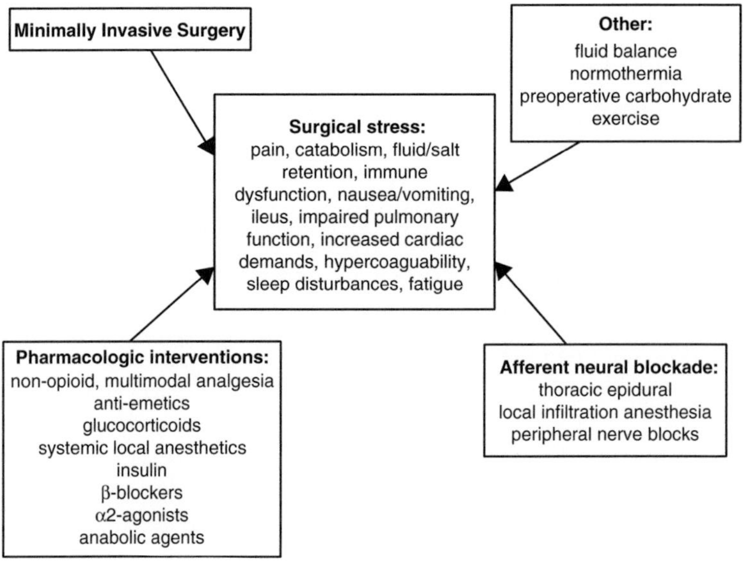

Fig. 3.1 Perioperative interventions that affect the surgical stress response. Modified from Kehlet and Wilmore [7]

to change has prevented the introduction of best available evidence. In the past decade, 'conventional' perioperative management has slowly given way to enhanced recovery principles, which aim to integrate all aspects of perioperative care into a multidisciplinary care pathway to diminish surgical stress and improve outcomes (Table 3.1). The concept of 'enhanced recovery' was first introduced in the mid-1990s and has since developed into well-established care bundles incorporating 20 different evidence-based interventions in all perioperative phases [7, 8]. Randomized trials comparing ERPs to conventional perioperative management have proven the benefits of ERP: acceleration of recovery of gastrointestinal function and decreased complications and length of stay without increased readmissions and mortality [9]. (Fig. 3.1)

The goals of laparoscopy and ERPs are the same: minimizing the surgical stress response to improve clinical outcomes and accelerate postoperative recovery. Indeed, many ERP elements were already part of 'conventional' perioperative care, such as antibiotic prophylaxis and thromboprophylaxis. A multinational study from the ERAS Compliance Group reported that laparoscopy was the most important independent predictor of length of stay and the second most important independent predictor of complications in patients managed by ERP (excluding non-modifiable patient risk factors) [10]. Given the similar benefits between these two modalities, there is controversy as to the relative benefit of an ERP for laparoscopic surgery. Initial randomized trials comparing ERP to conventional perioperative management only included patients undergoing open operations [9]. Pooled data from these early trials of open surgery show that the magnitude of change for length of stay and complications are much stronger in favour of ERP over conventional perioperative care for open colorectal surgery than for laparoscopic surgery. Indeed, for open surgery, the magnitude of difference with ERP is even higher than in trials

Table 3.1 Components of an enhanced recovery programme

Perioperative phase	Component
Preoperative	• Patient education • Smoking cessation • Prehabilitation • Reduced fasting • Carbohydrate loading
Intraoperative	• Minimally invasive surgery • Postop nausea and vomiting prophylaxis • Nerve blocks • Fluid balance • Normothermia • Euglycaemia • Short-acting opioids
Postoperative	• Ileus prophylaxis • Multimodal opioid-sparing analgesia • Early nutrition • Early mobilization • Avoidance/early removal of drains and catheters • Standardized daily care maps • Discharge criteria and post-discharge planning

Table 3.2 Pooled data from meta-analyses of randomized trials

	Pooled data from RCTs only (95% CIs)		
	ERP vs. CC (open surgery) [9]	ERP vs. CC (laparoscopic surgery) [11]	Laparoscopic vs. open colorectal cancer surgery [12]
Primary length of stay	WMD −2.94 days (−3.69, −2.19)	WMD −1.22 (−1.57, −0.87)	WMD −1.73 days (−2.26, −1.20)
Overall complications	RR 0.52 (0.38, 0.71)	RR 0.68 (0.44, 1.04)	RR 0.74 (0.55, 1.00)
Mortality	RR 0.53 (0.12, 2.38)	RR 1.51 (0.29, 7.77)	RR 0.33 (0.16, 0.72)

RCT randomized controlled trial, *CI* confidence interval, *ERP* enhanced recovery pathway, *CC* conventional perioperative care, *WMD* weighted mean difference, *RR* relative risk

comparing laparoscopic and open colorectal surgery (Table 3.2). Since the benefits of ERP over conventional care in patients undergoing laparoscopic surgery are much less clear, this early data led some to question whether ERP alone can confer the short-term advantages of laparoscopy without the need for additional specialized training and equipment. On the other hand, laparoscopic surgery already provides several of the advantages of ERPs, including reduced ileus and pain, which facilitates earlier feeding, mobilization and discharge.

Improving Postoperative Recovery

Given that the goal of both modalities is to improve recovery, it is useful to define 'postoperative recovery' and identify important relevant outcomes in order to adequately assess the effectiveness of ERPs and laparoscopy. Recovery after surgery is a complex multidimensional construct that includes the physical, psychological, social and economic domains. It follows a natural trajectory characterized by an immediate postoperative deterioration, continuing into a period of gradual rehabilitation to baseline function [5], which can last much longer than expected. A significant proportion of elderly patients still experienced protracted disability compared to preoperative status at 6 months after major abdominal surgery [4]. Even patients undergoing relatively 'minor' procedures have important disruptions in their physical activity 1 month postoperatively [13]. Postoperative recovery can also be categorized into three main periods, early, intermediate and late recovery, each with their own relevant outcomes (Table 3.3). Clinicians are mainly interested in the early and intermediate stages of recovery, i.e. until the patient is discharged from the hospital. Recuperation of basic bodily functions, such as freedom from nausea and vomiting, return of GI function and mobility are important in this phase [19], but the traditional clinical outcomes of length of stay, morbidity and mortality are the most commonly reported. However, these outcomes may not be as relevant to patients, who define recovery as the return to their preoperative baseline function [20], and therefore are also interested in the late phase of recovery. During their late recovery, patients are especially concerned with their ability to carry out their daily routine, fatigue, energy level and general physical endurance [21, 22]. Late recovery is most often measured through health-related quality of life using generic- or

Table 3.3 Stages of recovery

Phase of recovery	Definition	Time frame	Threshold	Outcomes	Examples of existing instruments
Early	From OR to discharge from PACU	Hours	Safety (sufficiently recovered from anaesthesia and safe to go to floor)	Physiologic and biologic	Aldrete Postanaesthetic Recovery Score [14]
Intermediate	From PACU to discharge from hospital	Days	Self-care (able to care for self at home)	Symptoms and impairment in ADL	Quality of Recovery Score [15]
					Abdominal Surgery Impact Scale [16]
Late	From hospital discharge to return to usual function and activities	Weeks to months	Return to normal (baseline or population norms)	Functional status and health-related quality of life	Six-minute walk test [17]
					Community Health Activities Model Program for Seniors (CHAMPS) [13]
					SF-6D [18]

ADL activities of daily living, *OR* operating room, *PACU* postanaesthetic care unit
Reproduced from [5]

disease-specific instruments. However these questionnaires have their own limitations as very few of them have been specifically validated for the construct of postoperative recovery [23]. It is helpful to use this framework and understand the limitations of the outcomes to adequately assess the effectiveness of interventions advocated to improve postoperative recovery.

Early and Intermediate Recovery

There is unequivocal level I evidence supporting the clinical benefits of ERPs, especially in the context of open surgery. Therefore, the important question to ask is whether laparoscopy confers additional advantage within an ERP in patients undergoing colorectal surgery. Several important randomized trials have compared laparoscopy and open colorectal surgery within an ERP (Table 3.4). Four of the five studies originated from Europe [24–26, 28] and a single study from China [27].

Table 3.4 Characteristics of RCTs comparing laparoscopic and open colorectal surgery within an enhanced recovery programme (ERP)

Study	Lap *N*/ open *N*	Extent of surgery	No. of ERP elements	Details	Main outcomes (lap vs. open)
Basse et al. [24]	30/30	Colonic	14	Single centre, Denmark	*LOS* (mean): 3.8 vs. 3.9 days, p = NS
					Cx: 27 vs. 20%, p = NS
King et al. [25]	41/19	Colorectal	12	Single centre, UK	*LOS* (median): 5 vs. 8 days, $p = 0.006$
					Cx (major): 14 vs. 26%, $p = 0.208$
Vlug et al. [26] (LAFA)	100/93; 109/98[a]	Colonic	18	Multicentre, Netherlands	*LOS* (median): 5 vs. 7 days, $p = 0.008$; 6 vs. 7 days, $p = 0.010$[a]
					Cx: 34% vs. 46%, $p = 0.20$; 34% vs. 41%, $p = 0.20$[a]
Wang et al. [27]	40/41; 40/42[a]	Colonic	16	Single centre, China	*LOS* (mean): 5.2 vs. 6.5 days, $p < 0.05$; 6.3 vs. 7.4 days, $p < 0.05$[a]
					Cx: 8 vs. 17%, $p < 0.05$; 15 vs. 24%, p = NS[a]
Kennedy et al. [28] (EnROL)	103/101	Colorectal	18	Multicentre, UK	*LOS* (median): 5 days vs. 7 days, $p = 0.033$
					Cx: 32 vs. 36%, $p = 0.55$

Cx complications, *LOS* length of stay
[a]Conventional perioperative care groups

Two studies compared laparoscopic and open surgery within ERP and conventional perioperative care [26, 27].

Most of the data relates to intermediate recovery. Pooled analysis from these five randomized trials reported that total hospital stay (which includes primary hospitalizations and any readmissions within 30 days of surgery) was 1.92 days (95% CI −2.61, −1.23) lower in favour of laparoscopy, although there was no difference in primary hospital stay when readmissions were excluded (weighted mean difference −1.01 days; 95% CI −2.14, 0.12), but this was largely due to data from Basse et al. [24], which was the only study that demonstrated higher primary length of stay in the laparoscopy group [29]. There were no differences in the incidence of complications (pooled RR 0.81; 95% CI 0.64, 1.04), readmissions (pooled RR 0.73; 95% CI 0.39, 1.36) or mortality (pooled RR 0.53; 95% CI 0.19, 1.44) [29].

The LAFA trial deserves particular mention, as Vlug et al. randomized patients to four groups: laparoscopy versus open and ERP versus conventional perioperative care, allowing for direct comparisons [26]. In this study, laparoscopy combined with ERP had the lowest length of stay, at least 1 day (median) shorter than the other three groups. There were no differences between any of the four groups in the incidence of overall, minor or major morbidity, readmission rate and mortality. Patients in the lap/ERP group also met the five discharge criteria (pain control with oral medication, tolerating solid food, absence of nausea, passage of flatus/stool and mobilization as preoperative) faster than patients in the lap/conventional group and recovered gastrointestinal function quicker than the open/ERP group. Importantly, patients in the open/ERP group were able to tolerate solid food and mobilize quicker than patients in the lap/conventional group. During the first 72 h after surgery, immune function was best preserved in the lap/ERP group, but no difference in surgical stress hormone levels was found [30]. Wang et al. also measured immunologic response in postoperative day 1, 3 and 5 and found that immunologic function was better preserved in patients managed by ERP, regardless of surgical approach, while inflammatory markers were lowest in the lap/ERP group [27]. Observational data are generally in keeping with these results [31].

Basse et al. measured pain, fatigue, pulmonary function, quality of sleep, physical activity and mental function on each postoperative day in the first week (and up to 1 month with varying frequency in the case of pain and fatigue) [24]. Small statistically significant differences in pain, pulmonary function and quality of sleep were found between patients in the laparoscopic and open groups, but the clinical relevance of these findings is unknown, and any differences disappeared after the first 24 h after surgery. King et al. measured sleep and continuous pulse oximetry in the first 3 days after surgery and found no differences in sleep quality between laparoscopic and open surgery, but improved pulse oximetry assessments in the laparoscopic group [25]. In this study, performance tests to assess balance, gait and lower extremity strength and endurance were also undertaken at 2 and 12 days and again at 6 and 12 weeks after surgery. On postoperative day 2, patients in the laparoscopic group had a significantly higher performance score than the open group, but neither group returned to preoperative baseline by 12 weeks. Although not strictly a recovery measure, medical costs were also addressed by two studies, demonstrating no difference between laparoscopic and open surgery within an ERP [25, 26].

Late Recovery

Late recovery is generally poorly reported in the ERP literature, as a systematic review of outcome reporting in studies comparing ERP to conventional perioperative care in abdominal surgery identified only seven studies reporting postdischarge outcomes, none of which reported outcomes after 30 days [32]. Four of the five randomized trials comparing laparoscopic and open surgery within an ERP reported outcomes relevant to late recovery. Basse et al. found no difference in the proportion of patients that returned to normal daily activities at 30 days [24]. A long-term follow-up study of the initial King et al. trial assessed health-related quality of life, physical performance tests and functional outcomes up to 12 months after surgery [33]. There were no differences in quality of life, as measured using the European Organisation for Research and Treatment of Cancer (EORTC) QLQ-C30 generic and colorectal-specific QLQ-CR38 questionnaires, or in physical performance, but surprisingly both groups had not yet reached their preoperative performance by 12 months. Patients undergoing laparoscopic surgery felt fully recovered much quicker than patients in the open group, and at 1 year 90% of laparoscopic patients felt fully recovered compared to only 58% of open patients ($p = 0.016$). The LAFA trial did not find any differences in quality of life, as measured using the generic Short-Form 36 (SF-36) and disease-specific Gastrointestinal Quality of Life Index (GIQLI) instruments, at 2 and 4 weeks after surgery in any of their four comparison groups [26]. Lastly, the EnROL trial reported a patient-reported measure of fatigue assessed at 30 days, measured using the physical fatigue domain of the Multidimensional Fatigue Inventory 20 (MFI-20), as the primary outcome of the study [28]. Other relevant late recovery measures in this study included the remaining measures in the MFI-20, SF-36 and physical performance indicators (balance, walking and lower limb strength). At 30 days, none of these outcomes demonstrated a difference between patients undergoing laparoscopic or open surgery.

However, late recovery outcomes may pose complexities for interpretation. Generic measures of health-related quality of life, such as the SF-36 and the EORTC QLQ-C30, are especially difficult to interpret as outside factors such as social and environmental stressors may affect patients' responses, as well as changes in patients' evaluation of their quality of life due to adaptation to their disease process ('response shift'). Content validity may also be lacking for many of these instruments, as they may not contain all of the relevant concepts of postoperative recovery [5]. Single domain measures such as physical performance also ignore the other important aspects of recovery. It is therefore not surprising that there is few data demonstrating any differences in late recovery measures favouring laparoscopic surgery [34] or ERPs [35].

Summary

Laparoscopy and ERPs are important modalities to improve recovery in patients undergoing colorectal surgery. Individually, they both demonstrate significant incremental gains over open surgery and conventional perioperative management. Level I evidence clearly demonstrates a reduction in hospitalization as a result of integration of laparoscopy within an ERP. Data comparing other intermediate and late recovery outcomes were also favourable. The use of an ERP provides additional benefits to the laparoscopic approach and is associated with reduced hospital stay. Laparoscopy should be considered a key component of an ERP, perhaps the most important. However, embedding laparoscopy within an ERP ensures that the remainder of perioperative care meets the same high standards as the operative approach and maximizes the benefits of minimally invasive surgery. Patients undergoing colorectal surgery should benefit from both of these interventions together.

References

1. Schwenk W, Haase O, Neudecker J, Muller JM. Short term benefits for laparoscopic colorectal resection. Cochrane Database Syst Rev. 2005;3:CD003145.
2. Moghadamyeghaneh Z, Carmichael JC, Mills S, Pigazzi A, Nguyen NT, Stamos MJ. Variations in laparoscopic colectomy utilization in the United States. Dis Colon Rectum. 2015;58(10):950–6.
3. Keller DS, Delaney CP, Hashemi L, Haas EM. A national evaluation of clinical and economic outcomes in open versus laparoscopic colorectal surgery. Surg Endosc. 2016;30:4220.
4. Lawrence VA, Hazuda HP, Cornell JE, et al. Functional independence after major abdominal surgery in the elderly. J Am Coll Surg. 2004;199(5):762–72.
5. Lee L, Tran T, Mayo NE, Carli F, Feldman LS. What does it really mean to "recover" from an operation? Surgery. 2014;155(2):211–6.
6. Delaney CP, Senagore AJ, Gerkin TM, et al. Association of surgical care practices with length of stay and use of clinical protocols after elective bowel resection: results of a national survey. Am J Surg. 2010;199(3):299–304. discussion 304
7. Kehlet H, Wilmore DW. Evidence-based surgical care and the evolution of fast-track surgery. Ann Surg. 2008;248(2):189–98.
8. Gustafsson UO, Scott MJ, Schwenk W, et al. Guidelines for perioperative care in elective colonic surgery: enhanced recovery after surgery (ERAS®) society recommendations. World J Surg. 2013;37(2):259–84.
9. Spanjersberg WR, Reurings J, Keus F, van Laarhoven CJ. Fast track surgery versus conventional recovery strategies for colorectal surgery. Cochrane Database Syst Rev. 2011;2:CD007635.
10. ERAS Compliance Group. The impact of enhanced recovery protocol compliance on elective colorectal cancer resection: results from an international registry. Ann Surg. 2015;261(6):1153–9.
11. Tan SJ, Zhou F, Yui WK, et al. Fast track programmes vs. traditional care in laparoscopic colorectal surgery: a meta-analysis of randomized controlled trials. Hepato-Gastroenterology. 2014;61(129):79–84.
12. Tjandra JJ, Chan MK. Systematic review on the short-term outcome of laparoscopic resection for colon and rectosigmoid cancer. Color Dis. 2006;8(5):375–88.
13. Feldman LS, Kaneva P, Demyttenaere S, Carli F, Fried GM, Mayo NE. Validation of a physical activity questionnaire (CHAMPS) as an indicator of postoperative recovery after laparoscopic cholecystectomy. Surgery. 2009;146(1):31–9.
14. Aldrete JA, Kroulik D. A postanesthetic recovery score. Anesth Analg. 1970;49(6):924–34.
15. Myles PS, Hunt JO, Nightingale CE, et al. Development and psychometric testing of a quality of recovery score after general anesthesia and surgery in adults. Anesth Analg. 1999;88(1):83–90.
16. Urbach DR, Harnish JL, McIlroy JH, Streiner DL. A measure of quality of life after abdominal surgery. Qual Life Res. 2006;15(6):1053–61.
17. Moriello C, Mayo NE, Feldman L, Carli F. Validating the six-minute walk test as a measure of recovery after elective colon resection surgery. Arch Phys Med Rehabil. 2008;89(6):1083–9.

18. Lee L, Elfassy N, Li C, et al. Valuing postoperative recovery: validation of the SF-6D health-state utility. J Surg Res. 2013;184:108.
19. Aahlin EK, von Meyenfeldt M, Dejong CH, et al. Functional recovery is considered the most important target: a survey of dedicated professionals. Perioper Med. 2014;3:5.
20. Kleinbeck SV, Hoffart N. Outpatient recovery after laparoscopic cholecystectomy. AORN J. 1994;60(3):394. 397–398, 401–392
21. Jakobsson J, Idvall E, Wann-Hansson C. Patient-reported recovery after enhanced colorectal cancer surgery: a longitudinal six-month follow-up study. Int J Color Dis. 2014;29(8):989–98.
22. Lee L, Dumitra T, Fiore JF Jr, Mayo NE, Feldman LS. How well are we measuring postoperative "recovery" after abdominal surgery? Qual Life Res. 2015;24(11):2583–90.
23. Kluivers KB, Riphagen I, Vierhout ME, Brolmann HA, de Vet HC. Systematic review on recovery specific quality-of-life instruments. Surgery. 2008;143(2):206–15.
24. Basse L, Jakobsen DH, Bardram L, et al. Functional recovery after open versus laparoscopic colonic resection: a randomized, blinded study. Ann Surg. 2005;241(3):416–23.
25. King PM, Blazeby JM, Ewings P, et al. Randomized clinical trial comparing laparoscopic and open surgery for colorectal cancer within an enhanced recovery programme. Br J Surg. 2006;93(3):300–8.
26. Vlug MS, Wind J, Hollmann MW, et al. Laparoscopy in combination with fast track multimodal management is the best perioperative strategy in patients undergoing colonic surgery: a randomized clinical trial (LAFA-study). Ann Surg. 2011;254(6):868–75.
27. Wang G, Jiang Z, Zhao K, et al. Immunologic response after laparoscopic colon cancer operation within an enhanced recovery program. J Gastrointest Surg. 2012;16(7):1379–88.
28. Kennedy RH, Francis EA, Wharton R, et al. Multicenter randomized controlled trial of conventional versus laparoscopic surgery for colorectal cancer within an enhanced recovery programme: EnROL. J Clin Oncol. 2014;32(17):1804–11.
29. Zhuang CL, Huang DD, Chen FF, et al. Laparoscopic versus open colorectal surgery within enhanced recovery after surgery programs: a systematic review and meta-analysis of randomized controlled trials. Surg Endosc. 2015;29(8):2091–100.
30. Veenhof AA, Vlug MS, van der Pas MH, et al. Surgical stress response and postoperative immune function after laparoscopy or open surgery with fast track or standard perioperative care: a randomized trial. Ann Surg. 2012;255(2):216–21.
31. Watt DG, McSorley ST, Horgan PG, McMillan DC. Enhanced recovery after surgery: which components, if any, impact on the systemic inflammatory response following colorectal surgery?: a systematic review. Medicine (Baltimore). 2015;94(36):e1286.
32. Neville A, Lee L, Antonescu I, et al. Systematic review of outcomes used to evaluate enhanced recovery after surgery. Br J Surg. 2014;101(3):159–70.
33. King PM, Blazeby JM, Ewings P, Kennedy RH. Detailed evaluation of functional recovery following laparoscopic or open surgery for colorectal cancer within an enhanced recovery programme. Int J Color Dis. 2008;23(8):795–800.
34. Dowson HM, Cowie AS, Ballard K, Gage H, Rockall TA. Systematic review of quality of life following laparoscopic and open colorectal surgery. Color Dis. 2008;10(8):757–68.
35. Khan S, Wilson T, Ahmed J, Owais A, MacFie J. Quality of life and patient satisfaction with enhanced recovery protocols. Color Dis. 2010;12(12):1175–82.

Part II

Endoscopic Approaches for Colorectal Neoplasia

Improving Endoscopic Detection of Dysplasia in Inflammatory Bowel Disease: Where Do We Stand?

4

Ryan C. Ungaro and James F. Marion

Patients with inflammatory bowel disease (IBD), either ulcerative colitis (UC) or Crohn's disease (CD) involving at least one-third of the colon, are at an increased risk of developing dysplasia and colorectal cancer. Earlier studies suggested that the risk of colorectal cancer in UC may be as high as 18–34% at 30 years [1, 2]. More recent studies suggest that the risk is not as marked and may have decreased over time possibly due to improved surveillance, increased endoscopic removal of dysplastic lesions, and advances in medical treatment that more effectively control inflammation [3]. However, UC patients are still 1.5–2.5 times more likely to develop colorectal cancer than the general population [3, 4]. Factors that are associated with a higher risk of colorectal cancer in patients with UC include older age, male sex, family history of colorectal cancer, young age at diagnosis, longer duration of disease, extensive colitis, personal history of dysplasia, strictures, pseudopolyps, primary sclerosing cholangitis (PSC), and increased severity of histologic inflammatory activity [4–6]. Due to the increased risk of colonic neoplasia in IBD patients, it is recommended that UC patients undergo regular surveillance colonoscopies to detect dysplasia and early colorectal cancer. Our understanding of how to best survey IBD patients and detect neoplasia on endoscopy has significantly improved over time.

The first consideration for dysplasia surveillance in IBD is determining the appropriate interval for performing endoscopy to detect dysplasia. The extent of colitis based on histology should be used to determine when to start surveillance since patients with proctitis have no increased risk of colorectal cancer and should follow standard average-risk screening guidelines [7]. Per the American Gastroenterology Association guidelines, patients with left-sided or extensive colitis should undergo a colonoscopy every 1–2 years starting 8 years after diagnosis [8]. This is because the relative risk for colorectal cancer appears to significantly increase 7–8 years after being diagnosed with IBD [4, 8]. If a patient has two negative consecutive examinations, the next surveillance examination can be performed

R.C. Ungaro (✉) • J.F. Marion
Division of Gastroenterology, Icahn School of Medicine at Mount Sinai, New York, NY, USA
e-mail: ryan.ungaro@mssm.edu; james.marion@mssm.edu

C.M. Schlachta, P. Sylla (eds.), *Current Common Dilemmas in Colorectal Surgery*,
https://doi.org/10.1007/978-3-319-70117-2_4

in 1–3 years until 20 years since diagnosis at which point subsequent examinations should return to every 1–2 years due to the increased risk associated with longer disease duration [8]. An important group of patients that warrant closer endoscopic surveillance are those with PSC. The risk of colorectal cancer in UC patients with PSC is up to five times greater than other UC patients, so it is recommended that surveillance begin at the time of diagnosis and continue annually [8]. It is important to note that there is no general international consensus on exactly how often surveillance endoscopies should be performed. European societies recommend stratifying surveillance intervals based on patients' risk factors. For example, lower-risk IBD patients (e.g., quiescent disease) should have a colonoscopy every 2–5 years depending on the guideline [7, 9]. A comparison of the most recent recommendations from major gastroenterology societies is presented in Table 4.1. Overall, more rigorous endoscopic surveillance appears to have decreased advanced and interval cancer incidence and increased detection of dysplasia and early cancer during the last 40 years [10]. For example, a retrospective study found that IBD patients who have had colonoscopy in the prior 3 years have a 35% decreased risk of colorectal cancer over 5–6 years of follow-up [11].

White-Light Endoscopy

While the importance of endoscopic surveillance in IBD patients is widely recognized, the techniques used to detect neoplasia are varied. Dysplasia and neoplastic lesions in UC can often be non-polypoid, flat, ill-defined, or multifocal. Given the concern that dysplastic lesions may be difficult to visualize in IBD, many have employed the random biopsy method during surveillance exams with white-light endoscopy (WLE). In addition to biopsying or removing any visible lesions (polypoid lesions, strictures, raised or irregular mucosa), random four-quadrant biopsies are taken every 10 cm starting in the cecum and continuing distally. This is a prevalent strategy that has been part of major society recommendations [7, 8]. Although the random biopsy method requires at least 32 biopsies to be taken, many endoscopists take fewer than the recommended number of biopsies [12]. In a study utilizing statistical modeling, 32 biopsies provide only 80% confidence that dysplasia involving ≥5% of the entire colon will be detected [13]. A retrospective study of 475 UC patients undergoing surveillance colonoscopy using conventional video colonoscopy found that in the 85 colonoscopies that found a neoplastic lesion, neoplasia was detected by random biopsies in only 5 colonoscopies (per-colonoscopy yield 6.9%) [14]. On a per biopsy analysis, random biopsies revealed neoplasia 0.2% of the time compared to targeted biopsies which found neoplastic changes 23% of the time. Of the 167 colonoscopies performed for surveillance purposes only (removing any symptomatic indication), only 1 colonoscopy (0.6%) led to a relevant clinical change in management due to invisible neoplasia found on random biopsy. The relatively low yield of random biopsies is concerning; however, most dysplastic lesions are visible using standard WLE and are able to be directly targeted. For example, a study of 2204 surveillance colonoscopies performed at St. Mark's Hospital in

Table 4.1 Overview of major colon cancer and dysplasia surveillance in IBD guidelines

Guideline	Major recommendations
American Gastroenterology Association (AGA) Institute Technical Review [8]	• All patients, regardless of the extent of disease at initial diagnosis, should undergo a screening colonoscopy a maximum of 8 years after onset of symptoms, with multiple biopsy specimens obtained throughout the entire colon, to assess the true microscopic extent of inflammation • Patients with extensive or left-sided colitis should begin surveillance within 1–2 years after the initial screening endoscopy • After two negative examinations (no dysplasia or cancer), further surveillance examinations should be performed every 1–3 years. Recent data suggest that increasing the frequency of surveillance colonoscopy to every 1–2 years after 20 years of disease is not needed for all patients but should be individualized according to the presence or absence of other risk factors • Patients with a history of colorectal cancer in first-degree relatives, ongoing active endoscopic or histologic inflammation, or anatomic abnormalities such as a foreshortened colon, stricture, or multiple inflammatory pseudopolyps may benefit from more frequent surveillance examinations • Representative biopsy specimens from each anatomic section of the colon is recommended

European Crohn's and Colitis Organisation (ECCO), European evidence-based consensus for endoscopy in inflammatory bowel disease [7]	• Screening colonoscopy should be offered at estimated 8 years after the onset of colitic symptoms to all patients to reassess disease extent
	• As there is no clear evidence for surveillance intervals, individualizing intervals based on risk stratification is recommended:
	  ○ Patients with high-risk features (stricture or dysplasia detected within the past 5 years, PSC, extensive colitis with severe active inflammation, or a family history of CRC in a first-degree relative at less than 50 years) should have next surveillance colonoscopy scheduled for 1 year
	  ○ Patients with intermediate-risk factors should have their next surveillance colonoscopy scheduled for 2–3 years. Intermediate-risk factors include extensive colitis with mild or moderate active inflammation, post-inflammatory polyps, or a family history of colorectal cancer in a first-degree relative at 50 years and above
	  ○ Patients with neither intermediate- nor high-risk features should have their next surveillance colonoscopy scheduled for 5 years
	  ○ All patients with dysplasia (within the past 5 years), irrespective of grade, should undergo annual colonoscopic surveillance
	• Pan-colonic methylene blue or indigo carmine chromoendoscopy should be performed during surveillance colonoscopy, with targeted biopsies of any visible lesion
	• If appropriate expertise for chromoendoscopy is not available, random biopsies (4 every 10 cm) should be performed

(continued)

Table 4.1 (continued)

Guideline	Major recommendations
National Institute for Health and Clinical Excellence (NICE), Colonoscopic Surveillance for Prevention of Colorectal Cancer in People with Ulcerative Colitis [9]	• Offer colonoscopic surveillance to people with inflammatory bowel disease (IBD) whose symptoms started 10 years ago and who have ulcerative colitis (but not proctitis alone) • Offer a baseline colonoscopy with chromoscopy and targeted biopsy of any abnormal areas to determine risk of developing colorectal cancer • Offer colonoscopic surveillance to people with IBD as defined based on their risk of developing colorectal cancer determined at the last complete colonoscopy o Low risk: 5-year interval o Intermediate risk: 3-year interval o High risk: 1-year interval • Risk groups: o Low risk: extensive but quiescent ulcerative colitis or left-sided ulcerative colitis (but not proctitis alone) o Intermediate risk: extensive ulcerative colitis with mild active inflammation that has been confirmed endoscopically or histologically or post-inflammatory polyps or family history of colorectal cancer in a first-degree relative aged 50 years or over o High risk: extensive ulcerative colitis with moderate or severe active inflammation that has been confirmed endoscopically or histologically or primary sclerosing cholangitis (including after liver transplant) or colonic stricture in the past 5 years or any grade of dysplasia in the past 5 years or family history of colorectal cancer in a first-degree relative aged under 50 years • Colonoscopy with chromoscopy is the method of surveillance

London between 1988 and 2002 found that 77.3% of neoplastic lesions were macroscopically visible [15]. Another retrospective study from Chicago found that 58.5% of dysplastic lesions and 80% of cancers were visible to the endoscopist on WLE [16]. It is important to note that these studies looked at exams prior to the wider adoption of high-definition (HD) colonoscopy technologies (1080p), which has significantly increased image resolution. HD equipment appears to further increase the number of visible lesions during colonoscopy compared to standard definition. A retrospective, matched cohort study of IBD patients with long-standing disease (greater than 7 years) who underwent surveillance exams compared the yield of standard definition to that of HD colonoscopy [17]. One hundred sixty standard WLE exams were compared to 209 HD colonoscopies. HD surveillance was more likely to detect any dysplastic lesion with an adjusted prevalence ratio of 2.21 (95% CI 1.09–4.45) compared to standard definition. Consistent with these data, around 20% of patients in standard-definition WLE studies had dysplasia detected by random biopsy, while in comparison, 1–1.5% of patients in HD colonoscopy studies would not have had dysplasia detected if random biopsies were not performed [18].

Chromoendoscopy

Although many neoplastic lesions are visible during WLE in IBD patients, a significant number may be difficult to detect, for example, non-polypoid or lesions with indistinct borders. Therefore, various methods to increase the identification of neoplastic lesions during colonoscopy in IBD patients have been studied. The most commonly used and well-studied enhanced visualization technique in IBD surveillance is chromoendoscopy (CE). CE involves spraying the colonic mucosa with a contrast dye, either methylene blue or indigo carmine, and then performing targeted biopsies. Methylene blue is preferentially absorbed by normal colonic epithelium but not inflamed or neoplastic mucosa, whereas indigo carmine collects within colonic crypts leading to greater delineation of abnormal mucosa [19]. The result is a more marked contrast between normal colon and neoplastic lesions (Figs. 4.1 and 4.2). One approach to perform CE involves mixing 5 cm^3 of methylene blue 1% (or

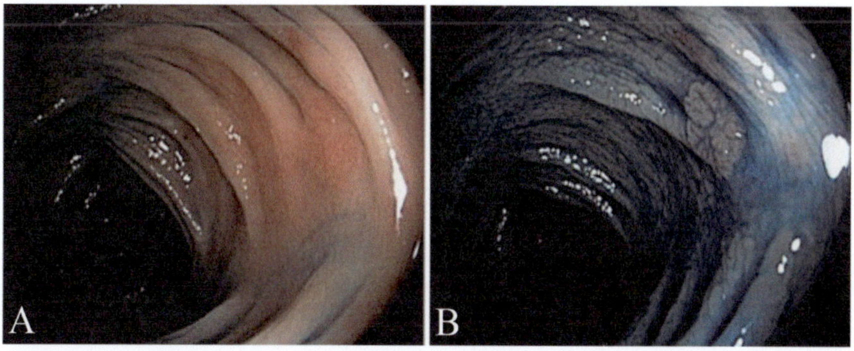

Fig. 4.1 Representative image of the same flat lesion with low-grade dysplasia, on white-light colonoscopy (**a**) and on chromoendoscopy (**b**). With permission from Deepak et al. [23]

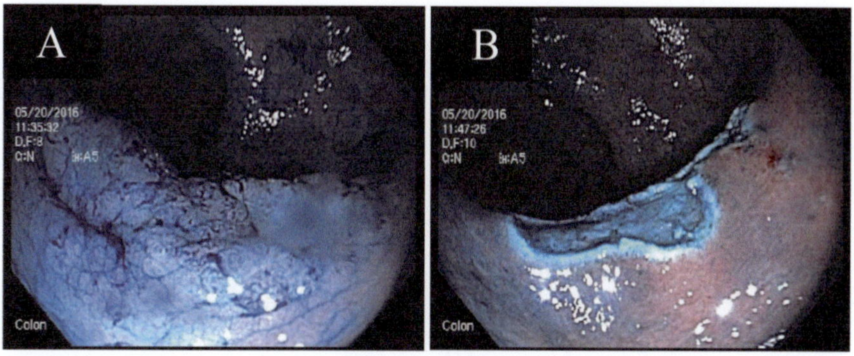

Fig. 4.2 Flat neoplastic lesion in ulcerative colitis patient found on chromoendoscopy (**a**) and after endoscopic mucosal resection (**b**). Images from personal image library of Dr. James F. Marion

10 cm^3 of indigo carmine 0.8%) in 500 cm^3 of water and placing into the colonoscope water spray bottle. The endoscopist then advances to the cecum and begins spraying the dye into the colon. The colonic mucosa should then be closely inspected either in a seesaw fashion (spray a segment while withdrawing and then advance back into that segment) or using a double withdrawal technique (the entire colon is sprayed, and then the colonoscope is advanced and withdrawn a second time). In order for the CE to be high quality, inflammation should be quiescent and the colon should have good or excellent preparation. Any identified endoscopically resectable lesions should then be removed. Any other lesions should be biopsied, tattooed, and referred to a surgeon or an endoscopist skilled at endoscopic mucosal resection (if feasible). Random biopsies do not need to be taken unless unable to perform a high-quality exam.

Multiple studies have compared surveillance using CE with WLE. A meta-analysis of eight studies comparing CE with standard-definition WLE found a significant increase in the detection of dysplastic lesions (RR 1.8, 95% CI 1.2–2.6) [18]. An overview of these studies is provided in Table 4.2. One of the first studies of CE by Rutter and colleagues performed "back to back" tandem colonoscopies (WLE with random and targeted biopsies immediately followed by CE with indigo

Table 4.2 Overview of major studies comparing chromoendoscopy (CE) and white-light endoscopy (WLE)

Study	Study design	Number of patients	RR (95% CI)	Absolute risk increase (95% CI)	Number of visible dysplastic lesions	Chromoendoscopy white-light
Kiesslich [32]	Randomized parallel group	165	2.1 (0.8–5.2)	8% (−2 to 18%)	32	10
Kiesslich [33]	Randomized parallel group	153	2.5 (0.8–7.5)	8% (−1 to 17%)	19	2
Marion [21]	Prospective tandem	102	1.8 (0.96–3.5)	10% (0–20%)	35	13
Rutter [20]	Prospective tandem	100	3.5 (0.8–16.4)	5% (−1 to 11%)	9	2
Matsumoto [34]	Prospective tandem	57	1.0 (0.5–2.0)	0% (−2 to 2%)	18	8
Hlvaty [35]	Prospective tandem and additional cohort	75	3.0 (0.6–15.4)	9% (−5 to 23%)	6	2
Gunther [36]	Retrospective two-group	100	5.0 (0.3–101.6)	4% (−3 to 11%)	2	0
Chiorean [37]	Prospective tandem	63	Not available	Not available	41	18

RR relative risk, *CI* confidence interval. Adapted from Laine et al. [18]

carmine) on 100 UC patients with long-standing disease [20]. Following application of indigo carmine spray, investigators found seven additional dysplastic lesions in five patients that were not seen on WLE. Another tandem colonoscopy study of 102 IBD patients found that methylene blue dye spray revealed significantly more dysplasia (16 patients with low grade and 1 patient with high grade) than random biopsies (3 patients with low grade, $p = 0.001$) [21]. A follow-up of 68 patients from this study (median follow-up 27.8 months) who had repeated examinations demonstrated that a negative result on an index CE exam was the best predictor of being colectomy-free [22]. CE at any time during the follow-up period was significantly more likely to detect dysplasia compared to random biopsy [22]. Performing CE after a WLE exam finds dysplasia may increase the yield of surveillance. A retrospective cohort study of 95 IBD patients looked at the yield of performing CE after an initial WLE found dysplasia on targeted biopsy (median 6 months later) [23]. Investigators found that CE found an additional 34 lesions in 50 patients that were not seen on the initial WLE. Most lesions were endoscopically resectable, but 14 patients underwent surgery based on the findings of the subsequent CE exam, which revealed two cases of colorectal cancer and three cases of high-grade dysplasia.

Despite the apparent improved performance of CE in multiple studies, there are still some areas of uncertainty that have limited its adoption thus far [24, 25]. For example, it has not been definitively shown that CE is superior to a high-quality HD colonoscopy exam, as the vast majority of studies have compared to standard-definition WLE. A retrospective study of 401 IBD patients undergoing surveillance with either CE or HD colonoscopy (with random and targeted biopsies) did not find any increase in dysplasia detection [26]. In contrast, one parallel group, randomized, controlled trial in which 103 patients with long-standing UC (>10 years) were randomized to either CE or HD colonoscopy found that CE detected significantly more dysplastic lesions per patient compared to HD colonoscopy (0.26 ± 0.6 versus 0.12 ± 0.4, $p = 0.04$) [27]. In addition, the lesions discovered by CE are often smaller or flatter, and the natural history of these lesions that were previously missed is an important question that remains to be determined [24]. What do these lesions become and how should we advise our patients? Lastly, CE is user dependent and requires experience at interpreting mucosal lesions which may vary based on training and local IBD surveillance exam volume. Further research and educational programs are needed to address these concerns.

Narrow Band Imaging

Other enhanced visualization techniques have been studied for IBD surveillance, but either has not shown benefit or still needs further research. Narrow band imaging (NBI) technology highlights vascular and pit patterns in the mucosa through light filters that provide bands of blue and green light wavelengths [19]. Studies comparing NBI to standard-definition and HD WLE have not demonstrated a significant difference in dysplasia detection [28, 29]. In addition, CE has outperformed NBI in studies (up to 22% greater proportion of patients found to have dysplasia with CE) and is therefore not recommended for surveillance by SCENIC [18]. Autofluorescence imaging (AFI), which creates CE-like images through processing of different emission spectra from normal and neoplastic tissue, decreased neoplasia miss rates compared to WLE in one tandem study but was not endorsed by SCENIC [30]. Two "virtual CE" technologies, Fuji Intelligent Chromoendoscopy (FICE, Fujinon) and i-Scan (Pentax), have been tested in average-risk colorectal cancer screening but have not been formally investigated in IBD patients [19]. Lastly, a new computer-aided diagnostic system that combines endocytoscopy, which provides high-magnification images of the mucosa, and NBI had high sensitivity (84.5%) and specificity (97.6%) for adenomatous lesions when tested using an image library and warrants further investigation [31].

Conclusions

Current gastroenterology society guidelines generally state that while CE is recommended for surveillance in IBD, WLE with random biopsies is an acceptable method since it is easy to perform and does not require the additional materials or expertise that are needed for other endoscopic surveillance techniques (Table 4.1). The SCENIC international consensus statement was created in order to provide more unified guidance on methods of dysplasia surveillance in IBD [18]. According to SCENIC, CE is now recommended as the preferred method for surveillance when performing WLE, while the use of CE is suggested when performing HD colonoscopy [18]. It is important to note that SCENIC left a number of areas unaddressed, including risk stratification of surveillance based on patient characteristics, suggested methods for follow-up surveillance exams, proper pit pattern interpretation, and recommendations about intervals between exams. Nevertheless, SCENIC was very helpful in that it moved to codify the current evidence on IBD dysplasia surveillance and proposed recommendations that can help standardize IBD patient care.

In conclusion, our ability to detect dysplasia and colorectal cancer in IBD has advanced greatly. Ensuring patients are following an appropriate surveillance program for dysplasia is a key element of IBD care. CE is becoming the preferred method for dysplasia surveillance with multiple studies demonstrating a higher yield of dysplastic lesions. Random biopsy technique has performed poorly in multiple prospective trials and should be abandoned. In settings where resources are low or there is unfamiliarity with CE, WLE using high-definition equipment with targeted biopsies is a reasonable alternative.

References

1. Eaden JA, Abrams KR, Mayberry JF. The risk of colorectal cancer in ulcerative colitis: a meta-analysis. Gut. 2001;48:526–35.
2. Greenstein AJ, Sachar DB, Smith H, Pucillo A, Papatestas AE, Kreel I, et al. Cancer in universal and left-sided ulcerative colitis: factors determining risk. Gastroenterology. 1979;77:290–4.

3. Jess T, Rungoe C, Peyrin-Biroulet L. Risk of colorectal cancer in patients with ulcerative colitis: a meta-analysis of population-based cohort studies. Clin Gastroenterol Hepatol. 2012;10:639–45.
4. Beaugerie L, Itzkowitz SH. Cancers complicating inflammatory bowel disease. N Engl J Med. 2015;373:195.
5. Rubin DT, Huo D, Kinnucan JA, Sedrak MS, McCullom NE, Bunnag AP, et al. Inflammation is an independent risk factor for colonic neoplasia in patients with ulcerative colitis: a case-control study. Clin Gastroenterol Hepatol. 2013;11:1601–8.e1.
6. Gupta RB, Harpaz N, Itzkowitz S, Hossain S, Matula S, Kornbluth A, et al. Histologic inflammation is a risk factor for progression to colorectal neoplasia in ulcerative colitis: a cohort study. Gastroenterology. 2007;133:1099–105. quiz 1340.
7. Annese V, Daperno M, Rutter MD, Amiot A, Bossuyt P, East J, et al. European evidence based consensus for endoscopy in inflammatory bowel disease. J Crohns Colitis. 2013;7:982–1018.
8. Farraye FA, Odze RD, Eaden J, Itzkowitz SH. AGA technical review on the diagnosis and management of colorectal neoplasia in inflammatory bowel disease. Gastroenterology. 2010;138:746–74. 774.e1.
9. Centre for Clinical Practice at NICE (UK). Colonoscopic surveillance for prevention of colorectal cancer in people with ulcerative colitis, crohn's disease or adenomas. National Institute for Health and Clinical Excellence: Guidance. London: National Institute for Health and Clinical Excellence (UK); 2011.
10. Choi C-HR, Rutter MD, Askari A, Lee GH, Warusavitarne J, Moorghen M, et al. Forty-year analysis of colonoscopic surveillance program for neoplasia in ulcerative colitis: an updated overview. Am J Gastroenterol. 2015;110:1022–34.
11. Ananthakrishnan AN, Cagan A, Cai T, Gainer VS, Shaw SY, Churchill S, et al. Colonoscopy is associated with a reduced risk for colon cancer and mortality in patients with inflammatory bowel diseases. Clin Gastroenterol Hepatol. 2015;13:322–329.e1.
12. Rodriguez SA, Eisen GM. Surveillance and management of dysplasia in ulcerative colitis by U.S. gastroenterologists: in truth, a good performance. Gastrointest Endosc. 2007;66:1070.
13. Awais D, Siegel CA, Higgins PDR. Modelling dysplasia detection in ulcerative colitis: clinical implications of surveillance intensity. Gut. 2009;58:1498–503.
14. Van den Broek FJC, Stokkers PCF, Reitsma JB, Boltjes RPB, Ponsioen CY, Fockens P, et al. Random biopsies taken during colonoscopic surveillance of patients with longstanding ulcerative colitis: low yield and absence of clinical consequences. Am J Gastroenterol. 2014;109:715–22.
15. Rutter MD, Saunders BP, Wilkinson KH, Kamm MA, Williams CB, Forbes A. Most dysplasia in ulcerative colitis is visible at colonoscopy. Gastrointest Endosc. 2004;60:334–9.
16. Rubin DT, Rothe JA, Hetzel JT, Cohen RD, Hanauer SB. Are dysplasia and colorectal cancer endoscopically visible in patients with ulcerative colitis? Gastrointest Endosc. 2007;65:998–1004.
17. Subramanian V, Ramappa V, Telakis E, Mannath J, Jawhari AU, Hawkey CJ, et al. Comparison of high definition with standard white light endoscopy for detection of dysplastic lesions during surveillance colonoscopy in patients with colonic inflammatory bowel disease. Inflamm Bowel Dis. 2013;19:350–5.
18. Laine L, Kaltenbach T, Barkun A, McQuaid KR, Subramanian V, Soetikno R, et al. SCENIC international consensus statement on surveillance and management of dysplasia in inflammatory bowel disease. Gastroenterology. 2015;148:639–651.e28.
19. Naymagon S, Marion JF. Surveillance in inflammatory bowel disease: chromoendoscopy and digital mucosal enhancement. Gastrointest Endosc Clin N Am. 2013;23:679–94.
20. Rutter MD, Saunders BP, Schofield G, Forbes A, Price AB, Talbot IC. Pancolonic indigo carmine dye spraying for the detection of dysplasia in ulcerative colitis. Gut. 2004;53:256–60.
21. Marion JF, Waye JD, Present DH, Israel Y, Bodian C, Harpaz N, et al. Chromoendoscopy-targeted biopsies are superior to standard colonoscopic surveillance for detecting dysplasia in inflammatory bowel disease patients: a prospective endoscopic trial. Am J Gastroenterol. 2008;103:2342–9.

22. Marion JF, Waye JD, Israel Y, Present DH, Suprun M, Bodian C, et al. Chromoendoscopy is more effective than standard colonoscopy in detecting dysplasia during long-term surveillance of patients with colitis. Clin Gastroenterol Hepatol. 2016;14:713–9.
23. Deepak P, Hanson GJ, Fletcher JG, Tremaine WJ, Pardi DS, Kisiel JB, et al. Incremental diagnostic yield of chromoendoscopy and outcomes in inflammatory bowel disease patients with a history of colorectal dysplasia on white-light endoscopy. Gastrointest Endosc. 2016;83:1005–12.
24. Marion JF, Sands BE. The SCENIC consensus statement on surveillance and management of dysplasia in inflammatory bowel disease: praise and words of caution. Gastroenterology. 2015;148:462–7.
25. Ananthakrishnan AN. Chromoendoscopy is better: so why am I not (yet) using it for routine inflammatory bowel disease surveillance? Clin Gastroenterol Hepatol. 2016;14:720–2.
26. Mooiweer E, van der Meulen-de Jong AE, Ponsioen CY, Fidder HH, Siersema PD, Dekker E, et al. Chromoendoscopy for surveillance in inflammatory bowel disease does not increase neoplasia detection compared with conventional colonoscopy with random biopsies: results from a large retrospective study. Am J Gastroenterol. 2015;110:1014–21.
27. Mohammed N, Kant P, Abid F, Rotimi O, Prasad P, Hamlin JP, et al. High definition white light endoscopy (Hdwle) versus high definition with chromoendoscopy (Hdce) in the detection of dysplasia in long standing ulcerative colitis: a randomized controlled trial. Gastrointest Endosc. 2015;81(5):AB148.
28. Dekker E, van den Broek FJ, Reitsma JB, Hardwick JC, Offerhaus GJ, van Deventer SJ, et al. Narrow-band imaging compared with conventional colonoscopy for the detection of dysplasia in patients with longstanding ulcerative colitis. Endoscopy. 2007;39:216–21.
29. Ignjatovic A, East JE, Subramanian V, Suzuki N, Guenther T, Palmer N, et al. Narrow band imaging for detection of dysplasia in colitis: a randomized controlled trial. Am J Gastroenterol. 2012;107:885–90.
30. Van den Broek FJC, Fockens P, van Eeden S, Reitsma JB, Hardwick JCH, Stokkers PCF, et al. Endoscopic tri-modal imaging for surveillance in ulcerative colitis: randomised comparison of high-resolution endoscopy and autofluorescence imaging for neoplasia detection; and evaluation of narrow-band imaging for classification of lesions. Gut. 2008;57:1083–9.
31. Misawa M, Kudo S-E, Mori Y, Nakamura H, Kataoka S, Maeda Y, et al. Characterization of colorectal lesions using a computer-aided diagnostic system for narrow-band imaging endocytoscopy. Gastroenterology. 2016;150:1531–1532.e3.
32. Kiesslich R, Fritsch J, Holtmann M, Koehler HH, Stolte M, Kanzler S, et al. Methylene blue-aided chromoendoscopy for the detection of intraepithelial neoplasia and colon cancer in ulcerative colitis. Gastroenterology. 2003;124:880–8.
33. Kiesslich R, Goetz M, Lammersdorf K, Schneider C, Burg J, Stolte M, et al. Chromoscopy-guided endomicroscopy increases the diagnostic yield of intraepithelial neoplasia in ulcerative colitis. Gastroenterology. 2007;132:874–82.
34. Matsumoto T, Nakamura S, Jo Y, Yao T, Iida M. Chromoscopy might improve diagnostic accuracy in cancer surveillance for ulcerative colitis. Am J Gastroenterol. 2003;98:1827–33.
35. Hlavaty T, Huorka M, Koller T, Zita P, Kresanova E, Rychly B, et al. Colorectal cancer screening in patients with ulcerative and Crohn's colitis with use of colonoscopy, chromoendoscopy and confocal endomicroscopy. Eur J Gastroenterol Hepatol. 2011;23:680–9.
36. Günther U, Kusch D, Heller F, Bürgel N, Leonhardt S, Daum S, et al. Surveillance colonoscopy in patients with inflammatory bowel disease: comparison of random biopsy vs. targeted biopsy protocols. Int J Color Dis. 2011;26:667–72.
37. Chiorean MV, Helper DJ, Saxena R, Cummings OW, Tabbey R, Johnson CS. Targeted biopsies using chromoendoscopy can replace random biopsies in patients with IBD at high risk for colorectal neoplasia. Gastroenterology. 2012;142(Suppl 1):S339.

Management of Dysplasia in IBD

5

Shailja C. Shah, Joana Torres, and Steven H. Itzkowitz

Introduction

Patients with long-standing inflammatory bowel disease (IBD) involving the colon, specifically ulcerative colitis (UC) or extensive Crohn's colitis, are at a higher risk of developing colorectal neoplasia (CRN)—i.e., colorectal dysplasia or colorectal cancer (CRC)—compared to the general population [1]. While a meta-analysis from 2001 suggested a cumulative risk for CRC in UC patients of 2% at 10 years, 8% at 20 years, and 18% at 30 years [2], more recent estimates suggest lower cumulative risks [3, 4]. A more recent meta-analysis of population-based studies found an absolute cumulative risk for CRC in UC of 1.15% after 15 years, 1.69% after 20 years, and 2.61% after 25 years of disease, which corresponds to a 2.4 (95% CI: 2.1–2.7)-fold increased risk for CRC in UC patients [5]. The cumulative risk for CRC in Crohn's colitis patients is thought to be at least similar to those with a history of extensive colitis [6, 7].

In IBD, CRC is thought to develop from a stepwise progression of inflammation to varying degrees of dysplasia before finally progressing to cancer. The primary goal of dysplasia surveillance with interval colonoscopic exams is to identify early neoplasia and implement an appropriate treatment or prevention strategy accordingly. Years ago, dysplasia in the setting of IBD colitis was managed surgically with either colectomy or sometimes segmental resection in the case of limited Crohn's colitis. Such a generalized approach is now less common in the current era, presumably due to improved medical therapies, enhanced endoscopic technology for dysplasia detection, and our ability to successfully manage dysplasia in IBD endoscopically. The decision to enter into a dysplasia surveillance program, rather

S.C. Shah (✉) • J. Torres • S.H. Itzkowitz
Division of Gastroenterology, Icahn School of Medicine at Mount Sinai Hospital, New York, NY, USA
e-mail: shailja.c.shah@vanderbilt.edu; joanatorres00@gmail.com; steven.itzkowitz@mountsinai.org

C.M. Schlachta, P. Sylla (eds.), *Current Common Dilemmas in Colorectal Surgery*, https://doi.org/10.1007/978-3-319-70117-2_5

than opting for colectomy when dysplasia is detected, must be a joint, well-informed decision between the patient and gastroenterologist. A successful surveillance program depends on open communication between both parties with routine office visits, colonoscopies, and, most importantly, patient adherence with medical therapy and surveillance exams.

Detection and Categorization of Dysplasia

Appropriate management of dysplasia in IBD colitis hinges on consistent definitions. The nomenclature and terminology used to classify dysplastic lesions seen on endoscopy, termed "visible dysplasia," or found on random biopsy during CRN surveillance, termed "invisible dysplasia," have evolved considerably in recent years, in parallel with the improvements in optic endoscopy and the use of chromoendoscopy [8]. Terms such as dysplasia-associated lesion or mass (DALM), adenoma-associated lesion or mass (ALM), and flat versus raised dysplasia, among others, are a source of confusion given their differing and inconsistent definitions between the IBD literature and general endoscopy literature, and even within the IBD literature alone. As an example, in the IBD literature, a "flat" lesion was historically used to describe any lesion not seen grossly, which is in comparison to the endoscopy literature where "flat" lesion referred to a slightly raised lesion (less than 2.5 mm in height) [9]. Given that most dysplasia is indeed visible using high-resolution methods (e.g., high-resolution white light endoscopy) or image-enhancing techniques like chromoendoscopy, new nomenclature for describing findings on colonoscopy was recently proposed by an international group of experts in the SCENIC statement [8]. This nomenclature incorporates descriptors that are used in the Paris classification [9] for CRN and bear prognostic value (Fig. 5.1). Polypoid lesions are defined as those protruding at least 2.5 mm into the lumen, while nonpolypoid lesions may range from superficially elevated (less than 2.5 mm) lesions to depressed lesions [9]. For nonpolypoid lesions, it is important to clearly define the borders, which may be facilitated by chromoendoscopy. The presence of depressed ulceration within lesions may imply underlying malignancy and should be reported as well.

Even with modern technology, detection of dysplasia in IBD can be difficult, as dysplastic lesions with less distinct borders are more common in the IBD colon compared to those without IBD. To optimize visualization, it is important to perform surveillance exams for dysplasia on an adequately cleansed bowel and ideally when inflammation is quiescent. Dysplasia detection can be confounded both macroscopically and microscopically by the presence of active inflammation. Active disease should not preclude performing the surveillance exam, but the extent and severity of disease activity should be clearly documented (especially if there are visible lesions), and the pathologist should be informed. Once medically optimized, consideration should be given to performing a repeat short-interval surveillance examination if in fact active inflammation made it difficult to discern neoplastic lesions. Even in quiescent disease, luminal abnormalities such as pseudopolyps and

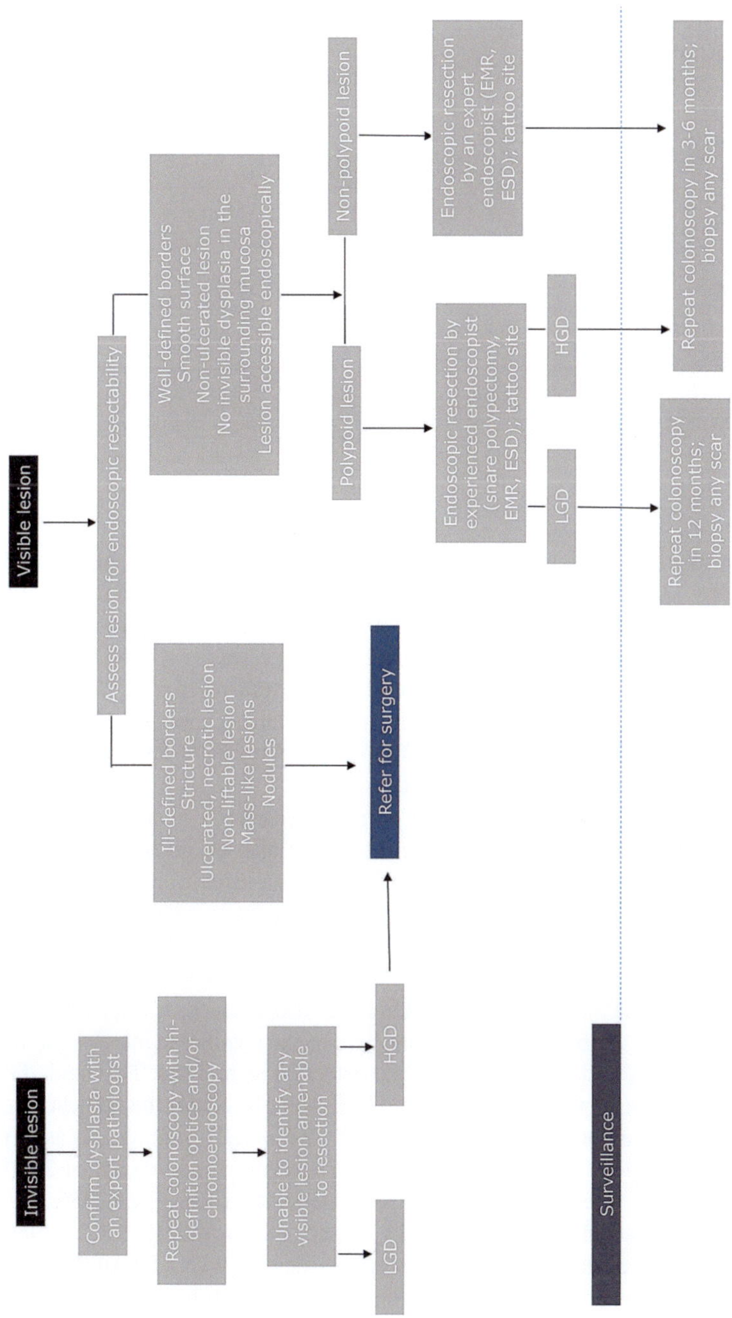

Fig. 5.1 Suggested management of dysplasia in IBD

Table 5.1 Risk factors for dysplasia and/or CRC in IBD colitis

Risk factor [10]	Relative risk (95% confidence intervals, CI) for dysplasia/CRC
Disease extent	
Extensive/pancolitis	14.8 (11.4–18.9)
Left-sided colitis	2.8 (1.6–4.4)
Duration of disease	
10 years	2.4 (0.6–6.0)
20 years	2.8 (1.91–3.97)
Primary sclerosing cholangitis (PSC)	4.8 (3.9–6.4)
Disease activity	
Endoscopic	5.1 (2.7–11.1)
Histologic	3.0 (1.4–6.3)
Family history of CRC	
First-degree relative <50 yo	9.2 (3.7–23.0)
First-degree relative ≥50 yo	2.5 (1.4–4.4)
Stricture	5.7 (1.7–18.9)

scars may compromise the dysplasia surveillance exam. Despite high-definition colonoscopy, chromoendoscopy, and other enhanced detection modalities, 10% of dysplasia is still diagnosed on random biopsy and may relate to the less-experienced eye or suboptimal surveillance milieu. In general, but certainly if "invisible" dysplasia is detected, there should be a low threshold for referral to a gastroenterologist experienced in IBD dysplasia surveillance. If surveillance cannot be adequately performed, such as in the presence of severe pseudopolyposis or an impassable stricture, then colectomy should be discussed.

Although management decisions are primarily guided by endoscopic and histologic characteristics of lesions, consideration must also be given to an individual patient's risk for CRC development according to both disease- and patient-specific factors. Disease-specific factors include disease duration, extent, and activity and/or presence of primary sclerosing cholangitis (PSC), while patient-specific factors include prior history of dysplasia/CRC, family history of CRC, and earlier age of disease onset (Table 5.1). Relative and absolute risks of each of these factors vary, and most numbers are based on older data prior to the significant increase in the use of biologic therapy and enhanced dysplasia detection techniques. That said, disease extent and duration, as well as concomitant PSC, seem to confer the highest disease-related risk for development of dysplasia and/or CRC in IBD. Pancolitis is associated with relative risk (RR) of 14.8 (95% CI 11.4–18.9) compared to a RR of 2.8 (95% CI 1.6–4.4) in left-sided colitis; PSC is associated with a RR of 4.8 (95% CI 3.9–6.4); and UC disease duration of 10 years is associated with a RR of 2.4 (95% CI 0.6–6.0), while disease duration of 20 years is associated with a RR of 2.8 (95% CI 1.91–3.97) for developing dysplasia and/or CRC in IBD. Active disease endoscopically (RR 5.1, 95% CI 2.7–11.1) and/or histologically (RR 3.0, 95% CI 1.4–6.3) also impacts the risk of progression to CRN. Having a first-degree relative with CRC younger than 50 years old confers a RR of 9.2 (95% CI 3.7–23.0) compared to a RR of 2.5 (95% CI 1.4–4.4) if the relative is above 50 years old. If disease onset is before age 15, patients have a 40% absolute risk of dysplasia/CRC compared to 25% in the 15–39-year-old age of onset. The presence of a stricture (RR 5.7, 95% CI 1.7–18.9) is also a risk factor [10]. If several of these factors are present, there should be a lower threshold to recommend definitive total proctocolectomy.

Management of Visible Lesions

The management of visible lesions can be categorized as to whether they are endoscopically resectable or unresectable. Criteria for what constitutes endoscopically resectable lesions are not clearly delineated in published guidelines and depend largely on the comfort level and expertise of the individual endoscopist. In general, endoscopic resectability should follow the same considerations in IBD patients as in non-IBD patients, with the additional note that if dysplasia is found in the surrounding mucosa of an allegedly fully resected lesion, the lesion should be considered unresectable and the patient should be referred for surgery. Similarly, if dysplasia is found in other areas of the colon (multifocal dysplasia), surgery should be considered due to concern for an overall field defect and high risk of synchronous and/or metachronous CRN.

When assessing lesions, distinction should be made between polypoid and nonpolypoid lesions, not only because methods for endoscopic resection vary but because the risk of progression to cancer is higher in the latter [11, 12]. Whether the more benign course of polypoid lesions reflects the underlying biology of the lesions or that polypoid lesions are generally more easily removed endoscopically with less risk of incomplete resection remains to be clarified, but it is likely a combination of these factors. While a larger proportion of nonpolypoid lesions are being detected as a result of improved technology, this may also represent a true shift in the clinical paradigm and natural history of dysplasia in IBD.

Polypoid, well-circumscribed lesions, in principle, should be amenable to en bloc resection by standard snare polypectomy or mucosectomy. The mucosa surrounding the polyp should be biopsied to confirm the absence of dysplasia. Nonpolypoid lesions are more challenging, and several features should be assessed to determine whether endoscopic resection should be pursued or the patient instead referred for surgery. Given the complexity of these decisions, a multidisciplinary team approach is recommended with special attention to not only appropriately characterizing the lesion (Fig. 5.1) but also taking into consideration the patient's age, comorbidities, and preferences. The absence of clearly defined borders precludes endoscopic resection. For lesions in the non-IBD colon, the presence of depressed ulceration, irregular contours, deformity, and mass-like appearance or the inability to elevate the lesion raises concern for the presence of underlying malignancy. In the IBD colon, some of these features may be more difficult to assess. For example, submucosal fibrosis in IBD due to chronic inflammation or prior attempts at removal may lead to inability to elevate the lesion but does not

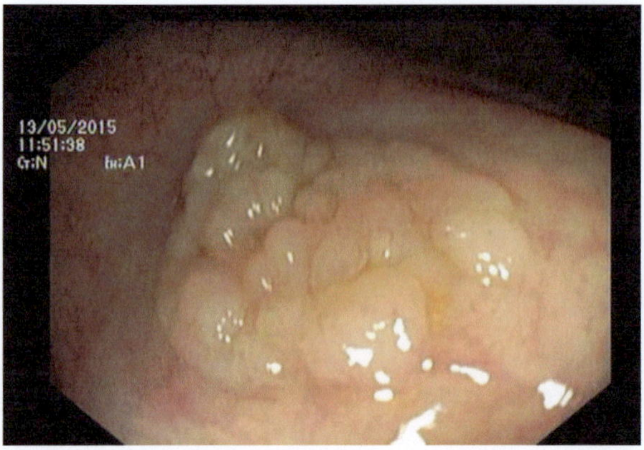

Fig. 5.2 Image of a nonpolypoid lesion, which is superficially elevated (Paris IIa) with well-defined borders and smooth surface within an area of quiescent colitis. After en bloc resection, pathology revealed low-grade dysplasia

necessarily imply underlying malignancy. Well-demarcated, non-multifocal lesions without features suggestive of invasion (Fig. 5.2) should be completely resected by an endoscopist with appropriate expertise regardless of grade of dysplasia. En bloc endoscopic mucosal resection (EMR) is the preferred modality, although the size of some lesions may necessitate piecemeal resection and is therefore at higher risk of recurrence. In those centers with expertise, endoscopic submucosal dissection (ESD) may also be an option and may be associated with even lower risk of recurrence, although evidence is still limited [13]. The folds near the lesion should be tattooed so that this area can be adequately surveyed. Even in the presence of clearly defined lesion borders, biopsies around the lesion should be performed to exclude invisible dysplasia. Biopsies should also be taken regardless of apparent disease activity and submitted in a separate pathology jar [14]. Whether the lesion was found in a background of quiescent disease, active colitis, or other mucosal abnormalities such pseudopolyposis should be noted in the procedure report. If both the resection margins from the lesion and the surrounding mucosa are negative and there is no additional dysplasia detected in the colon, then continued endoscopic surveillance according to a modified schedule may be adequate. If biopsies taken from the mucosa surrounding the original lesion are positive for dysplasia, the patient should be referred for surgical consultation given the high risk for additional synchronous lesions or later development of metachronous lesions, since this dysplasia is thought to represent a "field effect," i.e., the entire colon is at risk for neoplasia if not already present. For lesions located within strictures, poorly circumscribed, with irregular surface, indistinct borders, ulcerated or necrotic center, mass-like appearance, non-liftable, or endoscopically inaccessible, endoscopic resection should be deferred in favor of referring for surgery (Fig. 5.3). In general, there is a much lower threshold for classifying nonpolypoid lesions as endoscopically unresectable given their higher risk of recurrence and higher risk of endoscopically unsuccessful resection with increased CRC risk.

Once dysplasia is found, it signifies that this colon is at increased risk to develop CRC. Thus, the histologic grade—i.e., LGD, HGD, and/or IND—strongly impacts management decisions. Each is associated with a different risk of progression to HGD (if IND or LGD) and/or CRC. The estimated risk of progression is unclear and

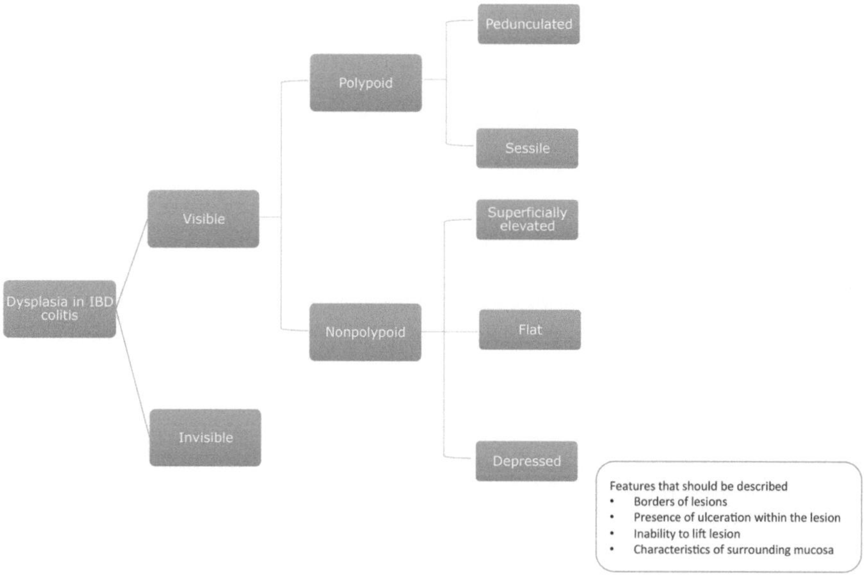

Fig. 5.3 Description and classification of dysplasia in IBD

remains an area of active research. Recently, the group at St. Mark's Hospital, United Kingdom, identified four risk factors associated with progression of LGD to HGD and/or CRC—nonpolypoid lesion (hazard ratio (HR) 8.6, 95% confidence interval (CI) 3–24.8), macroscopically invisible dysplasia (HR 4.1, 95% CI 1.3–13.4), lesion size ≥1 cm (HR, 3.8, 95% CI 1.5–13.4), and prior history of IND (HR 2.8, 95% CI 1.3–13.4) [15]. It is reasonable to consider colectomy in patients with LGD and at least one of these risk factors and certainly if more than one since the authors reported a strongly positive correlation between the number of risk factors and later HGD and/or CRC. It should be noted, though, that this study may have underestimated the true rate of HGD/CRC, as patients with LGD who were referred for colectomy and classified according to their presurgical pathology actually had HGD/CRC on surgical specimen pathology. Whether this represents metachronous lesions versus misclassification is unclear but again underscores the importance of expert review of all pathology. The rate of "surprise" HGD/CRC on colectomies performed for LGD or non-dysplastic indications is unclear and an additional area of investigation. Of 21 patients referred for colectomy for LGD, 7 (33.3%) had CRC, 3 (14.3%) had HGD, 8 (38.1%) had LGD, and 3 (14.3%) had no neoplasia [15].

Dysplasia Not Endoscopically Detected ("Endoscopically Invisible")

As noted above, the vast majority of dysplasia can be seen on endoscopy in the current era of high-definition colonoscopy and/or chromoendoscopy. Indeed, as much as one-third of dysplasia initially considered to be "invisible" is actually visible and may be amenable to endoscopic resection [8, 16, 17]. If no lesions are identified despite careful examination, random biopsies should be taken because there is a small percentage that may still be detected on random biopsies in the absence of a discrete lesion. If a dysplastic lesion is identified by random biopsies (presumably invisible dysplasia), the pathologic diagnosis of dysplasia should first be confirmed by an expert pathologist with particular expertise in IBD. If confirmed, a repeat colonoscopy with enhanced detection capabilities (e.g., high definition, chromoendoscopy) should be performed by an endoscopist with adequate experience in IBD dysplasia surveillance exams. If no lesions are identified despite careful examination, random biopsies should be taken. Subsequent management should also take into consideration the individual patient and disease-related risk factors for CRC as described previously.

If low-grade dysplasia (LGD) is detected on random biopsy, the surveillance interval should be shortened to every 3–6 months. The idea of colectomy should be discussed with the patient, as well as documentation of their understanding that although biopsies revealed LGD, they are at significant risk of progressing to high-grade dysplasia (HGD) and cancer and may even harbor such pathology currently [15]. If HGD is detected on random biopsy, the histological interpretation should be confirmed by an expert GI pathologist. If confirmed, a repeat colonoscopy in expert hands using enhanced imaging techniques should see whether there may have in fact been a visible lesion that could be endoscopically resected. If that is not the case, colectomy should be strongly considered.

In UC, the presence of dysplasia is assumed to be a field effect placing the entire colon at risk of harboring neoplasia, thus justifying total colectomy; whether this is true in the segmentally affected Crohn's colon remains to be clarified. The safest approach would be total proctocolectomy, but this should be thoroughly discussed with the patient, and referral to an experienced IBD gastroenterologist and surgeon with review of all pathology by an expert is recommended. It remains to be clarified, though, whether patients with segmental Crohn's colitis found to have HGD (and/or cancer) in the affected colitic segment have similar outcomes if they undergo segmental resection for localized CRN, as opposed to total colectomy. Current data favor total proctocolectomy in these patients due to the high risk of synchronous dysplasia or even cancer, as well as later development of metachronous neoplasia [18]. A retrospective study of 75 patients with Crohn's disease and localized colon cancer undergoing segmental resection or subtotal colectomy found that 39% had at least one metachronous cancer despite the majority having annual screening colonoscopy; the mean time to new dysplasia and cancer was 5 and 6.8 years, respectively [18]. Total proctocolectomy is therefore the procedure of choice for neoplasia in IBD colitis unless there are special considerations precluding this.

Surveillance Intervals

Management after removal of a dysplastic lesion deemed endoscopically resectable depends on whether the visible lesion was polypoid or nonpolypoid and also assumes that biopsies of the surrounding mucosa were negative for dysplasia.

There is now rather strong evidence to continue endoscopic surveillance rather than surgery following removal of polypoid dysplasia. A recent meta-analysis of 376 patients from ten studies with mean follow-up of 54 months reported an annual incidence of 0.05% for developing CRC after resection of polypoid dysplasia [12]. Based on this study and other smaller studies, guidelines recommend surveillance colonoscopy rather than colectomy following complete resection of polypoid dysplastic lesions [8]. However, the interval at which to perform surveillance exams has not been clearly defined. Suggested intervals are instead extrapolated from the non-IBD literature. Patients with smaller lesions (<1 cm) resected en bloc can safely return for annual surveillance, while larger lesions or those removed piecemeal should have a repeat exam under high definition and chromoendoscopy in 3–6 months with subsequent interval based on findings of that exam. For patients with nonpolypoid dysplastic lesions, guidelines are less clear given their less favorable course. That said, if the lesion is completely resected and there is no dysplasia in the surrounding mucosa, intervals used for polypoid lesions may be applied. The first follow-up surveillance exam should be at 3–6 months and with high definition and chromoendoscopy. If this short-interval exam is negative for dysplasia, patients can typically be followed annually; however, this decision should be made in the context of their overall risk for CRC. On the opposite side of the spectrum, if no dysplasia is detected on repeated surveillance exams, one could argue that the patient is at low risk to develop neoplasia. Whether surveillance intervals can be lengthened in such cases must await further studies given the concern for interval neoplasia, defined as CRN that develops in the interval between appropriate and adequate surveillance colonoscopic exams [19].

Chemoprevention

Patients often want to take some control over their neoplasia risk by taking agents that might be chemopreventive. However, any chemopreventive effect of medications used to treat IBD remains controversial [10, 20]. There are currently no guideline recommendations supporting the use of medications and/or dietary supplements to mitigate the risk of CRN in IBD patients. While there are several cohort and case-control studies on a variety of agents, the significant heterogeneity in terms of study population, study design, and methodology, as well as outcome measures, limits their applicability in the broader sense. While there may be some evidence for direct antineoplastic properties of 5-aminosalicylic acid-based therapies, similar data do not exist for other agents. Nevertheless, the observed decrease in cumulative CRC risk in IBD may be attributable, at least in part, to improved medical therapies achieving more durable and sustained control of mucosal inflammation, coupled with better surveillance programs and techniques. Not only does a healed colon with quiescent disease allow for better endoscopic detection of lesions and better histological distinction between reactive changes and dysplasia [21], but mucosal healing itself may also be associated with lower rates of CRN.

Additional Considerations

The above discussion emphasized management decisions based on patient, disease, endoscopic, and histologic characteristics. However, it must be emphasized that a patient's quality of life factors strongly into any decision in this regard. The decision to undergo surgery represents a balance between cancer prevention on the one hand and quality of life on the other. Surgery for neoplasia in IBD often results in a large change in bowel habit and quality of life, which has to be carefully integrated into the individualized care of the patient.

Conclusion

Thanks to better endoscopic detection and complete removal of dysplastic lesions, and more sophisticated pathological interpretation of dysplasia, we have come a long way from the almost reflexive recommendation for colectomy when dysplasia is detected in IBD colitis. Nonetheless, optimal management of dysplasia in IBD remains an area of ongoing research. Indeed, whether the natural course and progression of dysplasia to CRC in IBD are modified in our current era of improved IBD therapy and increased biologic use, as well as improved endoscopic technology to detect and resect dysplasia, remains to be determined. Ongoing research into ways to risk stratify patients at higher CRC risk speaks to the exciting milieu of ongoing development and progress in the world of cancer biology for the IBD population.

References

1. Zisman TL, Rubin DT. Colorectal cancer and dysplasia in inflammatory bowel disease. World J Gastroenterol. 2008;14:2662–9.
2. Eaden JA, Abrams KR, Mayberry JF. The risk of colorectal cancer in ulcerative colitis: a meta-analysis. Gut. 2001;48:526–35.
3. Andersen NN, Jess T. Has the risk of colorectal cancer in inflammatory bowel disease decreased? World J Gastroenterol. 2013;19:7561–8.
4. Jess T, Simonsen J, Jørgensen KT, Pedersen BV, Nielsen NM, Frisch M. Decreasing risk of colorectal cancer in patients with inflammatory bowel disease over 30 years. Gastroenterology. 2012;143:375–81.e1. quiz e13.
5. Jess T, Rungoe C, Peyrin-Biroulet L. Risk of colorectal cancer in patients with ulcerative colitis: a meta-analysis of population-based cohort studies. Clin Gastroenterol Hepatol. 2012;10:639–45.
6. Lutgens M, Vermeire S, Van Oijen M, et al. A rule for determining risk of colorectal cancer in patients with inflammatory bowel disease. Clin Gastroenterol Hepatol. 2015;13:148–54.e1.
7. Canavan C, Abrams KR, Mayberry J. Meta-analysis: colorectal and small bowel cancer risk in patients with Crohn's disease. Aliment Pharmacol Ther. 2006;23:1097–104.
8. Laine L, Kaltenbach T, Barkun A, et al. SCENIC international consensus statement on surveillance and management of dysplasia in inflammatory bowel disease. Gastrointest Endosc. 2015;81:489–501.e26.

9. Endoscopic Classification Review Group. Update on the Paris classification of superficial neoplastic lesions in the digestive tract. Endoscopy. 2005;37:570–8.
10. Farraye FA, Odze RD, Eaden J, Itzkowitz SH. AGA technical review on the diagnosis and management of colorectal neoplasia in inflammatory bowel disease. Gastroenterology. 2010;138:746–74. 774.e1.
11. Voorham QJ, Rondagh EJ, Knol DL, et al. Tracking the molecular features of nonpolypoid colorectal neoplasms: a systematic review and meta-analysis. Am J Gastroenterol. 2013;108:1042–56.
12. Wanders LK, Dekker E, Pullens B, Bassett P, Travis SP, East JE. Cancer risk after resection of polypoid dysplasia in patients with longstanding ulcerative colitis: a meta-analysis. Clin Gastroenterol Hepatol. 2014;12:756–64.
13. Iacopini F, Saito Y, Yamada M, et al. Curative endoscopic submucosal dissection of large nonpolypoid superficial neoplasms in ulcerative colitis (with videos). Gastrointest Endosc. 2015;82:734–8.
14. Magro F, Langner C, Driessen A, et al. European consensus on the histopathology of inflammatory bowel disease. J Crohns Colitis. 2013;7:827–51.
15. Choi CH, Rutter MD, Askari A, et al. Forty-year analysis of colonoscopic surveillance program for neoplasia in ulcerative colitis: an updated overview. Am J Gastroenterol. 2015;110:1022–34.
16. Kaltenbach T, Leite G, Soetikno R. Colonoscopy surveillance and management of dysplasia in inflammatory bowel disease. Curr Treat Options Gastroenterol. 2016;14(1):103–14. https://doi.org/10.1007/s11938-016-0072-4.
17. Kaltenbach T, McQuaid KR, Soetikno R, Laine L. Improving detection of colorectal dysplasia in inflammatory bowel disease surveillance. Gastrointest Endosc. 2016;83:1013–4.
18. Maser EA, Sachar DB, Kruse D, Harpaz N, Ullman T, Bauer JJ. High rates of metachronous colon cancer or dysplasia after segmental resection or subtotal colectomy in Crohn's colitis. Inflamm Bowel Dis. 2013;19:1827–32.
19. Mooiweer E, Oldenburg B. The debate continues over the best method of endoscopic surveillance for colorectal cancer in patients with colitis. Clin Gastroenterol Hepatol. 2015;13:1782–4.
20. Beaugerie L, Itzkowitz SH. Cancers complicating inflammatory bowel disease. N Engl J Med. 2015;373:195.
21. Chapman CG, Rubin DT. The potential for medical therapy to reduce the risk of colorectal cancer and optimize surveillance in inflammatory bowel disease. Gastrointest Endosc Clin N Am. 2014;24:353–65.

Beyond Piecemeal Polypectomy: EMR and ESD

6

Patrick Vincent Saitta, Krishna C. Gurram, and Stavros N. Stavropoulos

Introduction

Large colon polyps have an increased risk of harboring invasive carcinoma, and while pedunculated polyps have traditionally been removed endoscopically, laterally spreading sessile polyps have frequently been referred to surgery outside of expert centers. Endoscopic mucosal resection (EMR) techniques have evolved for the successful removal of these laterally spreading polyps. However, frequent need for piecemeal resection for polyps >2 cm in size is unacceptable in the setting of early-stage colon cancer as this disrupts interpretation of histologic margins, making it difficult to confirm curative resection while resulting in high recurrence rates and possibly systemic disease. Therefore, endoscopic techniques offering the option of en bloc resection are preferred to assure negative lateral and vertical margins that are essential for a curative (R0) resection. Furthermore, the challenge of removing polyps with excessive submucosal fibrosis, often after prior manipulation, has also prompted the development of new endoscopic dissection techniques.

P.V. Saitta
Department of Internal Medicine, Division of Gastroenterology, Winthrop University Hospital, Mineola, NY, USA
e-mail: psaitta@winthrop.org

K.C. Gurram
Department of Gastroenterology, Winthrop University Hospital, Mineola, NY, USA
e-mail: Kcgurrammd@gmail.com

S.N. Stavropoulos (✉)
Division of Digestive and Liver Diseases, Columbia University Medical Center, New York, NY, USA

Division of Gastroenterology, Hepatology, & Nutrition, NYU Winthrop Hospital, Mineola, NY, USA
e-mail: sns10md@gmail.com

C.M. Schlachta, P. Sylla (eds.), *Current Common Dilemmas in Colorectal Surgery*,
https://doi.org/10.1007/978-3-319-70117-2_6

Endoscopic submucosal dissection (ESD) is a technique that was developed in Asia to facilitate curative endoscopic removal of early-stage gastric cancers, and this has now been implemented for successful en bloc resection of large, laterally spreading colon polyps, early-stage colon cancers, and lesions previously deemed not amenable to endoscopic resection due to extensive fibrosis from prior attempts at removal.

Endoscopic Mucosal Resection (EMR)

Preparation

Preparation for EMR consists of clear liquid diet the day before the procedure and bowel preparation starting the evening before the procedure with a split dosing preparation consisting of taking half the preparation the night before and the other half the morning of the procedure now preferred due to superior prep quality [1]. EMR is considered a high-risk endoscopic procedure in terms of potential bleeding complications [2]. However, it is always imperative to weigh the risk of bleeding against the risks of thromboembolic or cardiac complications before deciding on discontinuation of anticoagulant or antiplatelet agents, and appropriate clearance by the patient's cardiologist or neurologist is typically requested. In patients who are not at high risk for thromboembolic events, it is typically recommended to hold vitamin K antagonists such as warfarin 5 days prior to the procedure with a INR goal <1.5 [3]. Direct factor Xa inhibitors such as dabigatran, rivaroxaban, and apixaban in patients with normal renal function are typically held 1–2 days prior to the procedure due to their short half-lives [4]. Bridge therapy with heparin or Lovenox needs to be considered in all patients who are at high risk for thromboembolic events at the discretion of the physician prescribing the patient's anticoagulant therapy.

The use of aspirin or NSAIDs does not clearly increase the risk of bleeding after high-risk endoscopic procedures and can be continued unless not clinically indicated. If not indicated, it is typically recommended to hold aspirin or NSAIDs 5–7 days prior to the procedure [5]. P2Y12 platelet receptor blockers such as clopidogrel, prasugrel, and ticagrelor block the binding of ADP, inhibiting adenylyl cyclase and platelet aggregation. These agents are associated with increased risk of post-polypectomy bleeding and should be discontinued if the patient is at low risk for thromboembolic or cardiac event [6]. It is recommended to hold clopidogrel for 5 days, ticagrelor for 3–5 days, and prasugrel for 7 days prior to the planned procedure. If the patient is on dual antiplatelet agents, aspirin should be continued, or if the patient is on single-antiplatelet therapy with P2Y12 blocker, aspirin should be added before and after the procedure while the other antiplatelet agent is being held. If the patient has cardiac stents, cardiac clearance is imperative, and it is advised to delay the procedure until the patient has received the minimum duration of required antiplatelet therapy after stent placement, typically 6 weeks for bare metal stents and 6 months for drug-eluting stents [2].

Resection Criteria

When considering a polyp for endoscopic resection, it is important to try to exclude underlying invasive malignancy. Evaluating for a positive "lifting sign" can help determine if a polyp is suitable for endoscopic resection as failure to create a submucosal lift is suggestive of submucosal invasion; however, this is difficult to differentiate from extensive submucosal fibrosis, which can also prevent lifting [7]. Furthermore, it has been shown that this is not always reliable for identifying deep submucosal invasion (sm2) [8]. Therefore, close inspection of the mucosal surface as well as manipulation of the lesion is also important. Clues such as surface friability, induration, and ulceration usually suggest submucosal invasion. Smooth "non-granular" type laterally spreading tumors have also more commonly been found to harbor invasive malignancy as compared to "granular type" polyps, which have a nodular surface contour [9]. Furthermore, nonhomogeneous, mixed granular lesions with large nodules have been more commonly associated with underlying malignancy within the large nodules [10]. Paris classification IIc lesions (Fig. 6.1) [11] (i.e., lesions with an area of pseudo-depression) and polyps with Kudo mucosal pit pattern type V (Fig. 6.2) [12] are also more likely to contain invasive malignancy.

The location of the lesion as well as history of prior manipulation may also impact the decision to proceed with endoscopic resection. Involvement of the ileocecal valve (OR 3.4) and prior attempt at EMR (OR 3.8) have been identified as negative predictors for successful endoscopic resection [13]. Moreover, polyps taking up one third of the circumference of the colon, polyps straddling two haustral folds, polyps arising inside a colonic diverticulum, and polyps arising from the base of the appendiceal orifice have also been reasons to consider surgical referral. If a

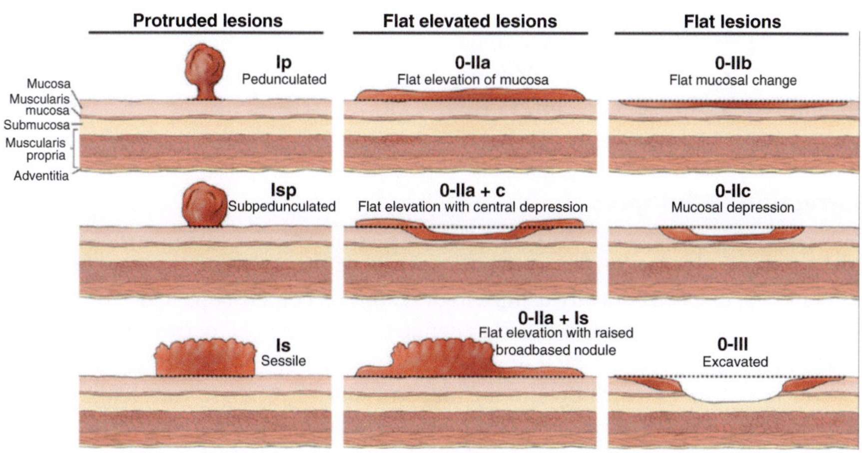

Fig. 6.1 Paris classification of colorectal neoplasms. Reproduced with permission from: Holt B, Bourke M. Wide Field Endoscopic Resection for Advanced Colonic Mucosal Neoplasia: Current Status and Future Directions, In: Clinical Gastroenterology and Hepatology, 9/2012. Elsevier. AGA institute. Copyright © 2012

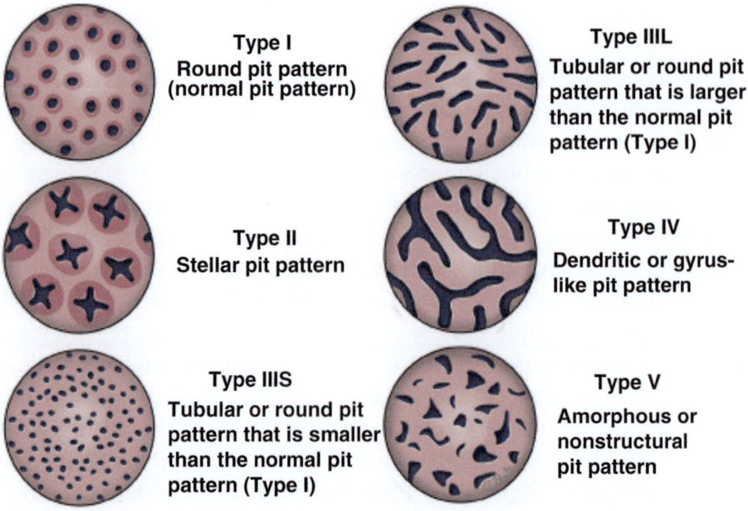

Fig. 6.2 Kudo pit pattern classification of colonic mucosal lesions. Reproduced with permission from: Canto MI. Chromoendoscopy. In: UpToDate, Post TW (Ed), UpToDate, Waltham, MA. (Accessed on 2017.) Copyright © 2017 UpToDate, Inc. For more information visit www.uptodate.com

polyp demonstrates mucosal surface or pit pattern features concerning for submucosal invasion, further evaluation with endoscopic ultrasound using a 20 MHz mini probe (diameter 2.5 mm, working length 2050 mm, Olympus America Center Valley, PA) may also be considered to better assess depth of invasion as this can easily be advanced through all commercially available colonoscopies. However, this has not clearly been shown to improve accurate assessment of depth of invasion beyond the accuracy of a detailed inspection of the mucosal pit pattern utilizing magnification chromoendoscopy [14].

Resection Techniques

EMR typically begins by delineating the margins of the lesion of interest. The margins are first inspected ideally using a high-definition colonoscope under white light imaging. If the margins are difficult to define with white light, narrowband imaging (NBI) can be employed which applies blue (wavelength 440–460 nm) and green (wavelength 540–560 nm) light to the mucosal surface. At these wavelengths, light is maximally absorbed by hemoglobin causing vascular structures to appear dark, which helps to better define subtle surface characteristics including mucosal pit pattern to better distinguish normal mucosa from adenomatous or neoplastic mucosa. The margins may further be defined using chromoendoscopy which consists of spraying diluted indigo carmine or methylene blue over the area of the lesion under evaluation to provide better contrast against the red mucosa allowing the operator to appreciate subtle surface abnormalities. These agents are also routinely added to submucosal lifting agents mainly to help distinguish the muscularis propria (which is not stained by these dyes and remains white) from the submucosa (which appears as a blue layer as it is readily stained by these dyes). A secondary beneficial effect, however, of using these blue dyes in the submucosal injectate is that they can help better define the borders of subtle lesions such as serrated adenomas since the blue hue of the submucosal injection is visible through the thin normal mucosa surrounding a lesion but not through the thicker mucosa of the adenoma. After the lesion's margin is defined, particularly if this proved challenging, markers can be applied surrounding the lesion of interest to help confirm that a clean margin of resection is achieved. The APC (argon plasma coagulation) device is typically used to apply these marks, which result in superficial mucosal blanching using a low cautery setting. One can also use the less costly technique of applying the marks with the tip of the snare using a soft coagulation setting. However, this technique requires more skill than the APC technique to avoid deep wall injury. The lesion is then raised by applying a lifting solution to the submucosal plane to create a fluid cushion which will separate the lesion of interest in the mucosal layer from the underlying muscularis propria layer. Normal saline is typically used for lifting combined with methylene blue or indigo carmine as described above. This is applied to the submucosal layer using a 23 or 25 gauge needle. More viscous solutions have also been employed including hyaluronic acid, hydroxypropyl methyl cellulose, 10% glycerol and 5% fructose mixture, and hetastarch, which prolong the duration of the lift to allow more time for resection while creating a more vertical lift to facilitate tissue capture by the snare. Such viscous solutions have been shown to potentially reduce procedure time and improve the likelihood of successful endoscopic resection when compared to normal saline [15, 16]. Dilute 1:10,000 epinephrine can also be added to the lifting solution to help prevent post-polypectomy bleeding; however, there are conflicting data on whether this provides any significant benefit in preventing early or delayed bleeding when compared to normal saline alone [17, 18].

Typically, the lesion of interest is injected along the periphery rather than in the central portion of the lesion given a theoretical concern for "seeding" of the needle track if underlying malignancy is suspected. Also, it is typically beneficial to inject the part of the lesion that is located farthest from the endoscope (usually the proximal/oral part of the lesion unless a retroflexed approach is employed) first. This part of the lesion may be partially located behind a fold limiting visualization and may be further obscured by injecting and lifting first the portion of the lesion closest to the endoscope (usually the distal/aboral/anal portion of the lesion again unless a retroflexed approach is employed). For piecemeal EMR of larger lesions, segmental lifting is often employed for each section targeted with the snare rather than lifting the entire lesion prior to initiating the resection. Again, this ensures optimal positioning and visualization of each area targeted for capture within the snare. The tissue targeted should be positioned if possible in the 6 o'clock position by torqueing the endoscope if necessary. This orientation lines up the tissue with the instrument channel of the colonoscope. Polyps <2 cm can potentially be removed en bloc; however, polyps larger than 2 cm typically need to be removed in a piecemeal fashion. A snare device is used to resect the polyp. Snares are available with variable stiffness and shape designs with oval-shaped or hexagonal-shaped snares most commonly used for polypectomy. The width of the snare typically ranges from 1 cm to 3 cm; however, a stiff, medium-sized (approximately 1.5–2.0 cm width) snare is optimal for endoscopic mucosal resection as this can allow for en bloc resection of lesions <2 cm while allowing good control for piecemeal resection of larger lesions. Although there is no firm consensus among experts with regard to snare shape, it is widely accepted that a stiff snare is essential. A pure coagulation setting (e.g., forced coagulation effect 2, 25 W on the ERBE electrosurgical device VIO300D) or a blended setting combining coagulation and cutting (e.g., Endo Cut Q, effect 3, cut duration 1, cut interval 6) is typically employed. There are limited data to guide optimal current selection, but generally, a blended setting is used in most polyps at average risk of intraprocedural bleeding since it may minimize heat injury to the wall of the colon (which may place the patient at risk of "post-polypectomy" syndrome or even delayed perforation) and to the specimen (which may interfere with proper histologic assessment of any invasive lesions within the specimen due to the resultant cautery artifact). During EMR, "tenting" of the tissue away from the colon wall is employed once the tissue is ensnared during application of thermal energy to limit risk of thermal injury to the wall. If piecemeal resection is required, it is best to start at one border of the polyp (usually the most challenging one) and then proceed with contiguous resection taking care to avoid leaving islands of residual tissue in the central portion of the polypectomy site, which may later be difficult to resect. If residual tissue remains after snare polypectomy, which cannot be removed with a smaller diameter snare, this can be removed utilizing hot biopsy forceps (Endo Cut I, effect 3, cut interval 1, cut duration 3) with an avulsion technique where a short burst of pure cutting current is applied to the tissue as it is being tented away from the resection site, which allows for the residual tissue to be peeled away after the initial cutis applied. This technique again limits transmission of thermal energy and risk of transmural burn [19]. If this is not successful, APC can be applied using a setting of 20–40 W and 0.5–1 L of argon flow per minute, or the snare tip can be utilized (soft coag effect 4–6, 80 W) for ablation of residual tissue; however, this limits complete histologic evaluation of the lesion and has been associated with increased risk of polyp recurrence. After polypectomy is completed, the polypectomy site is closely inspected for active bleeding or injuries to the muscularis propria which can range from exposure of the muscle to partial burns to the muscle and full-thickness perforations [20]. Prophylactic clip placement can be utilized to close polypectomy sites if deep muscle injury to the muscularis propria is identified, if the patient needs to resume antiplatelet or anticoagulation therapy, or in the setting of known bleeding diathesis. Interestingly, previous studies have demonstrated conflicting results regarding the cost-effectiveness of this technique [21, 22]. Some operators have also employed prophylactic coagulation of non-bleeding exposed vessels within the resection crater. However, in a recent randomized study of this intervention, even though delayed bleeding was seen in 5% of the patients that received prophylactic coagulation versus 8% in the control group, this difference was not statistically significant [23].

Outcomes: Efficacy and Adverse Events

EMR has a technical success rate of approximately 95% in high-volume centers [24, 25]. Recurrence of adenomatous tissue at 4–16 months after resection of lesions ≥2 cm, which generally cannot be reliably resected en bloc via EMR, has been reported in approximately 20% of patients. In most studies from expert centers, recurrences can be managed endoscopically in about 90% of these patients, but this requires follow-up endoscopic interventions with expert resection, avulsion, and/or ablation techniques within the area of the prior EMR scar. Furthermore, complete remission is documented in these patients with treated recurrence only up to 1 year post-intervention [25–29]. Identified risk factors for recurrence are polyp size >40 mm, APC treatment of residual adenomatous tissue not successfully removed by snare polypectomy, intraprocedural bleeding, and piecemeal resection [25, 28, 29]. The most common complication associated with EMR is delayed bleeding which can occur in up to 6% of cases. Proximal colonic location (OR 3.7), intraprocedural bleeding (OR 2.2), lesion size >30 mm (OR 2.5), presence of a major comorbidity (OR 1.5), and lack of epinephrine in injection solution were identified as risk factors for delayed bleeding [17, 24, 30–32]. Delayed bleeding does not necessarily require repeat colonoscopy and can be often managed conservatively in over half of the patients while reserving colonoscopy with hemostasis for those with severe, continuing hematochezia and/or hemodynamic instability. Perforation is the most serious complication after EMR but is rare occurring in less than 1% of cases and in the vast majority of cases can be managed nonsurgically with endoscopic closure using endoscopic clips or with endoscopic suturing which may be more secure [20, 33, 34].

Endoscopic Submucosal Dissection (ESD)

Endoscopic submucosal dissection (ESD) is a technique developed in Japan in the 1990s. It utilizes electrosurgical knives to remove early GI neoplasms en bloc irrespective of their size, thus achieving demonstrably negative lateral and deep margins with negligible risk of recurrence and allowing optimal histologic assessment of the specimen including detailed assessment of any submucosal invasion, which represents the major determinant of the risk of lymph node metastasis. ESD was developed to offer oncologically appropriate, organ-preserving, margin-negative en bloc resection for early gastric cancer, a highly prevalent condition in Asia. Prior to the advent of ESD, early gastric cancers were referred for morbid gastrectomy and lymphadenectomy. However, careful examination of these specimens revealed that using criteria such as depth and extent of submucosal invasion, degree of tumor differentiation, and presence of lymphovascular invasion (LVI), one could select certain T1 carcinomas for which the risk of lymph node metastasis was negligible and could thus be amenable to curative endoscopic resection via ESD [35]. Gradually, ESD indications expanded to include early esophageal neoplasms (mainly of squamous histology which is highly prevalent in Asia) and finally, tentatively, to colonic neoplasms given the challenges of ESD in the colon and the uncertainty of the degree of ESD benefit over EMR for adenomas without advanced histology. Even though colonic ESD was only certified by the Japanese national healthcare system in 2012, colonic ESD outcome data from Japan have rapidly expanded. ESD adoption in the USA has lagged due to its technical difficulty and the low prevalence in the West of early gastric cancers which present easier and safer targets for ESD than colonic lesions. Adoption is further hindered by the difficult pathway in the USA to obtain fair reimbursement for novel procedures such as ESD that require a significant time commitment to learn and perform competently.

Resection Criteria

There are certain shortcomings to EMR for colonic lesions compared to ESD:

1. EMR often results in incomplete resection of adenomas. In a recent authoritative study from Europe, EMR for even smaller adenomas, 10–20 mm in size, resulted in incomplete resection in 17%, and, for serrated adenomas in particular, incomplete resection was seen in 31% [36]. In comparison, ESD, which is generally applied for more challenging and larger lesions >2 cm, based on multiple studies and meta-analyses, mainly from Japan, delivers complete resection in close to 100% of lesions with en bloc, one piece resection in over 90% of lesions [37].
2. Recurrence after piecemeal EMR of lesions ≥2 cm is 18–34% within 1–2 years [13, 29, 38–40]. In contrast, recurrence after ESD is 0–2% [37, 40–42].
3. Advanced histology is present in as many as 30% of polyps over 10 mm resected endoscopically [43]. Even more alarmingly, as many as 5–15% of colon lesions resected via EMR or ESD can harbor cancer invading the submucosa [29, 40]. Such advanced histology lesions require detailed histologic analysis of the resection specimen with regard to margins (to ensure complete resection) and depth of invasion if carcinoma is present (in order to estimate the risk of lymph node metastasis and ensure that the endoscopic resection could be considered curative). However, for larger polyps, particularly ≥2 cm, EMR results in "piecemeal" resection, which hinders reliable histologic assessment of the resection specimen margins and depth of invasion. Piecemeal EMR often results in indeterminate or positive lateral and deep margins in these lesions which leave the patient in a state of uncertainty as to whether a "curative" endoscopic resection has been achieved. ESD provides assessable lateral and deep margin and maximizes the chance for en bloc margin-negative R0 resection, and ESD facilitates precise pathologic assessment of depth of invasion (an important predictor for lymph node metastasis). Finally, we should note that ESD can also allow definitive curative resection in lesions at challenging locations such as circumferential lesions at the ileocecal valve where EMR may not be possible or even if attempted may result in residual or recurrent lesional tissue that cannot be definitively treated (Fig. 6.3).

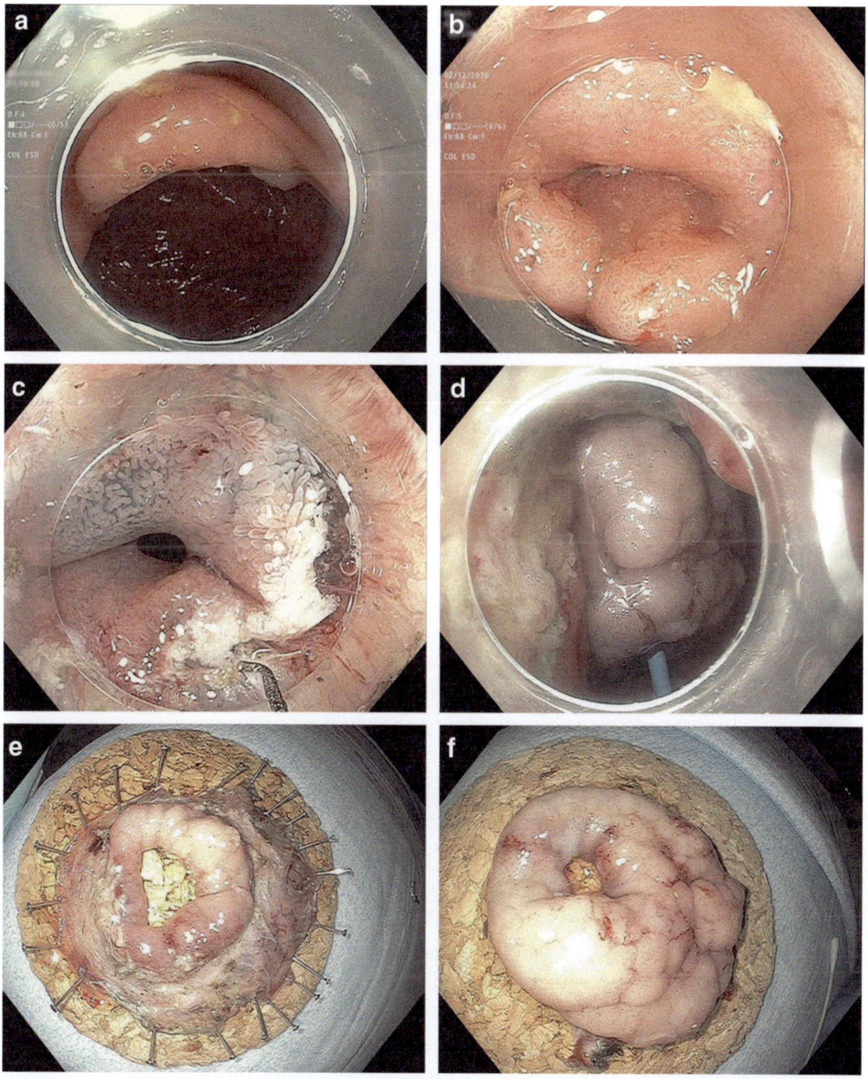

Fig. 6.3 ESD “doughnut” en bloc resection of large circumferential ileocecal valve adenoma. (**a**) Aboral view of lesion circumferentially involving the ICV. En face view of the entire lesion is not possible given its tangential hidden location. (**b**) En face view of the valve showing the lesion extending few mm into terminal ileal mucosa. (**c**) Circumferential incision at the ileal border of the lesion (Olympus Hook knife is used). (**d**) Completion of the resection with en bloc excision of the lesion which is doughnut shaped (with the inner circle representing the ileal border and the outer circle the cecal border). Here it is seen surrounding a stent placed through the ileocecal valve to facilitate orientation during the dissection. (**e**) The pinned specimen was approximately 6 cm in diameter. The specimen was pinned with the cecal side facing the cork. This picture clearly demonstrates the circumferential ileal border of the resection at the center of the specimen with “curled” ileal mucosa. (**f**) The resected specimen seen from the cecal side prior to pinning. The valve orifice can be seen at the center of the specimen

Table 6.1 European Society of Gastrointestinal Endoscopy ESD guidelines [44]

European Society of Gastrointestinal Endoscopy (ESGE) guidelines for colon ESD
Lesions with high suspicion of harboring carcinoma with superficial submucosal invasion (e.g. lesions with depressed morphology such as Paris classification IIc lesions and lesions with non-granular surface pattern), particularly if the lesions are larger than 20 mm
Lesions that cannot be optimally and radically removed by snare-based techniques (such as lesions with poor lifting and extensive submucosal fibrosis due to prior endoscopic manipulation, inflammatory disorders or other reasons)

Table 6.2 Japanese Gastrointestinal Endoscopy Society (JGES) [45]

Japanese Gastrointestinal Endoscopy Society (JGES) guidelines for colon ESD
>20 mm lesion—difficult to remove en-bloc with EMR technique
Non granular >20 mm spreading tumors
Kudo Pit pattern V (indicative of invasive carcinoma)
T1 Carcinoma with submucosal invasion (SM1)
Large (>2 cm) depressed-type lesions (Paris IIc component)
Large elevated lesions suspected of being carcinoma (nodular mixed subtype)
Mucosal lesions with submucosal fibrosis (secondary to prolapse from peristalsis or prior manipulation)
Sporadic localized tumors in the presence of chronic inflammation (Inflammatory bowel disease)
Local residual or recurrent early carcinoma after prior endoscopic resection

The above data have informed recent European and Japanese guidelines attempting to define the subset of colon lesions for which ESD is recommended. Current guidelines from the European Society of Gastrointestinal Endoscopy (ESGE) and from the Japanese Gastrointestinal Endoscopy Society (JGES) defining current indications for colorectal ESD are detailed in Tables 6.1 and 6.2 [44, 45].

Lesions in the colon with submucosal invasion limited to less than 1000 μm (sm1) without LVI or poorly differentiated component have been shown to have negligible risk of lymph node metastases [46]. However, T1 lesions with invasion of the deep submucosa >1000 μm (sm2) have a 6–12% risk of lymph node metastases [46–48]. Therefore, it is important to estimate the depth of submucosal invasion prior to resection. Kudo pit pattern type V (Fig. 6.2) has been associated with deep submucosal invasion [49]. The mucosal pit pattern can be examined utilizing a technique called chromoendoscopy where 3–5 cm^3 of 0.4% indigo carmine is sprayed along with 15 cm^3 of air using a 20 cm^3 syringe over the lesion of interest. The lesion is then inspected using a high-definition colonoscope. Magnification chromoendoscopy can also be employed using magnifying colonoscopies, which are not commercially available in the West. These endoscopes magnify the image up to 80–100 times. Utilizing this technique to assess the pit pattern, it is possible to differentiate mucosal cancer or sm 1 invasion from sm 2–3 invasion with sensitivity,

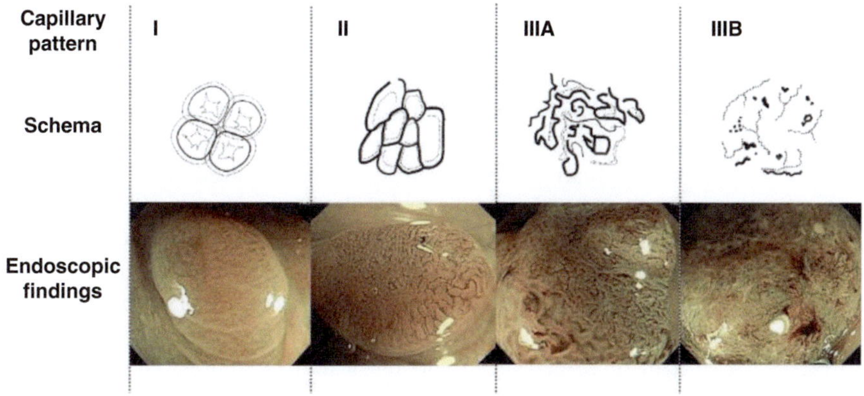

Fig. 6.4 Sano capillary pattern

specificity, and accuracy of 86%, 99%, and 99%, respectively [49]. With current high-definition endoscopes, these pit patterns can also be readily appreciated using magnifying techniques available in the West such as digital zoom and near-focus examination augmented by further magnification achieved by underwater examination along with the addition of "virtual chromoendoscopy" systems available in most current generation endoscopes. "Virtual chromoendoscopy" is achieved by various technologies including a blue light filter technology to exclude longer wavelengths (e.g., narrowband imaging, NBI), blue laser illumination, or digital, post-processing image enhancement technology. Virtual chromoendoscopy permits detailed inspection of the mucosal capillary networks and surface pit morphology which can help differentiate nonneoplastic lesions and lesions with superficial versus deep submucosal invasion. A number of classifications based mainly on the NBI virtual chromoendoscopy system have been proposed in Japan such as the Sano system. As an example, a Sano capillary pattern IIIB characterized by nearly avascular or loose micro-capillary networks as compared to the high-density, nonuniform, branching, blind-ending capillary networks seen with IIIA (Fig. 6.4) can differentiate deep versus superficial submucosal invasion (sensitivity 85%, specificity 89%, NPV 94%, PPV 72%) [50]. Recently, these various NBI classifications have coalesced into a somewhat simpler "consensus" classification, the "Narrow-band imaging International Colorectal Endoscopic" (NICE), which can be readily learned and applied by Western operators [51]. Endoscopic ultrasound (EUS) can also be utilized to exclude underlying invasion of the muscularis propria layer or the presence of suspicious lymph nodes that would preclude the possibility of a curative endoscopic resection and confirm the need for surgical resection. EUS when used in this fashion, particularly when high-frequency EUS probes are used that can be inserted through the colonoscope channel, is quick and reasonably accurate [52]. However, it is doubtful that this modest accuracy has a major clinical impact in this era of superb high-definition endoscopes with advanced imaging systems such as those described for virtual chromoendoscopy.

Technique

A high-definition colonoscope with water jet capability fitted with a 4 mm transparent cap is typically utilized for colonic ESD; however, a gastroscope can be more effective for lesions in the left colon and rectum. A pediatric colonoscope is usually preferred in situations where retroflexion is required in the right colon given its more narrow diameter and increased flexibility. Carbon dioxide (CO_2) is preferred for air insufflation as it has previously been shown with other forms of ESD to reduce post-procedural abdominal discomfort and procedural analgesia requirements [53]. The margins of the lesion of interest are first defined utilizing high-definition white light or narrowband imaging as previously described for EMR. A margin of resection around the lesion of interest can further be delineated utilizing the APC device at a low power setting or the tip of the ESD knife at a low power soft coagulation setting. The lesion is then typically lifted by injecting close to the margins using a viscous solution that some operators combine with epinephrine at 1:100,000 dilution and indigo carmine or methylene blue to give the solution a light-blue hue. ESD is then carried out utilizing an electrosurgical knife.

There are multiple knives currently available in the USA for colon ESD (Fig. 6.5). The Dual knife (Olympus Optical Co, Tokyo, Japan) is most commonly used in the colon followed by the Hook knife (Olympus Optical Co, Tokyo, Japan), often used in difficult resections involving submucosal fibrosis or resections perpendicular to the wall of the colon (Fig. 6.5). In certain occasions, the newer smaller insulated tip knife, the IT-nano (Olympus Optical Co, Tokyo, Japan), is used in lesions where a large and unwieldy mucosal flap is obstructing the view of the dissection plane (Fig. 6.5). Alternatively, a multifunctional knife can be used

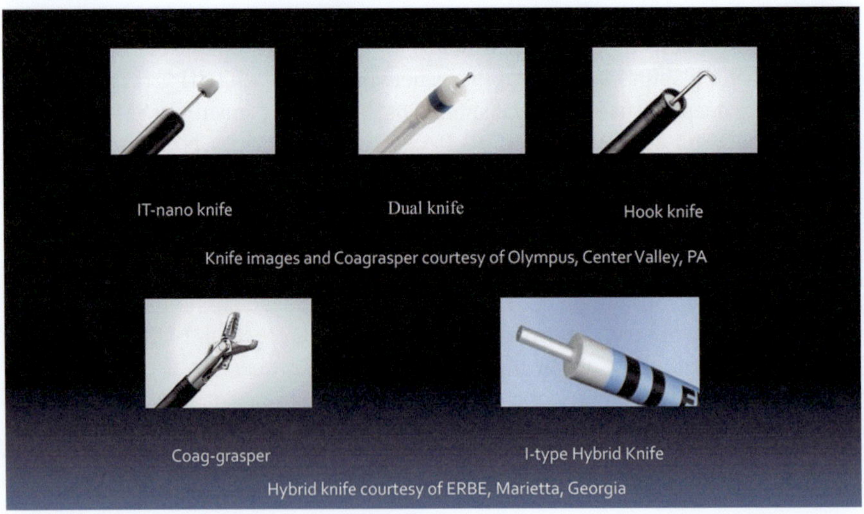

Fig. 6.5 ESD knives and hemostatic accessories

with a combined submucosal injection and dissection capability (HybridKnife-ERBE, Tubingen, Germany) (Fig. 6.5). Due to the longer length and diameter of this knife as well as its somewhat rigid catheter, it is most often used in rectal lesions. In the rectum, this particular knife is essential for a technique of "submucosal tunneling" or "submucosal pocket." This technique consists of not completing the circumferential mucosal incision until the final stages of the submucosal dissection. A submucosal operating space is then created under a stretched partially fixed mucosal flap held by the residual uncut mucosa which greatly facilitates the submucosal dissection. Unfortunately, this is usually only feasible in the esophagus, distal stomach, and rectum.

The three electrosurgical steps of ESD include mucosal incision, submucosal dissection, and vessel coagulation. It should be noted that the suggested electrosurgical currents provided for each of these steps may vary among expert operators based on their personal preferences and according to tissue conductance, tissue vascularity, and electrode characteristics (such as knife thickness and tip morphology) [54–56]. We should also note that the terminology used for electrosurgical currents refers to the VIO generator by ERBE which is used by the vast majority of ESD operators.

Discussion of the three electrosurgical steps of ESD follows:

1. Mucosal incision—Incision created around the lesion of interest through the muscularis mucosal layer to enter the submucosal plane typically using Dry Cut, effect 3, 30–80 W, or Endo Cut Q or I at various settings (ERBE VIO300D generator).
2. Submucosal dissection—Dissection through the submucosal plane is carried out until the lesion of interest is completely excised. This is typically performed using Swift coagulation, effect 2, 40–100 W, or for less vascular areas Endo Cut Q with some operators occasionally utilizing forced coagulation or Dry Cut currents.
3. Vessel coagulation—As submucosal vessels are encountered, they are typically coagulated to maintain hemostasis and to keep a clean field of view for dissection. All of the knives described previously can be used for coagulation of vessels using a forced coagulation setting, effect 2, 40 W, or less commonly a spray coagulation setting [54–56]. The knife is lightly applied to the vessel (avoiding compression or tenting of the vessel that may result in disruption of the vessel prior to "heat sealing" of its lumen with resultant hemorrhage) followed by application of coagulation current until full desiccation of the vessel is achieved. Larger vessels are typically managed with coagraspers using Soft coagulation current, effect 5–6, 80–100 W. This is the electrosurgical setting with broadest consensus among expert operators [54–56]. The coagraspers are used to clamp the lumen of the vessel before providing coagulation current to seal the vessel. The soft coagulation current, which is the lowest voltage program in the VIO generator, delivers a low amount of energy that slowly denatures the tissue and desiccates it eliminating its ability to conduct current and thus preventing deeper injury to the GI wall as is the case with high-voltage coagulation currents (e.g., spray coagulation) or cutting currents such as Endocut.

ESD resection results in the formation of a large mucosal defect and possibly significant thermal injury of the muscularis propria layer with associated risks of delayed bleeding, symptomatic transmural burn injury (post-polypectomy syndrome), or delayed perforation. Therefore, some operators have advocated endoscopic closure of the mucosal defect to mitigate these potential complications. Endoscopic hemoclip placement has been shown to significantly accelerate complete mucosal healing as compared to non-closure 4 weeks post resection [57]. Mucosal defect closure has also been shown to significantly decrease postoperative pain, local inflammatory response, post-polypectomy syndrome, and delayed bleeding with a trend toward decreased hospital length of stay [21, 58, 59]. Nevertheless, concerns remain about the costs associated with hemoclip closure as large defects can require multiple clips at an approximate cost of $150 per clip in the USA. Currently, data and opinions remain conflicting regarding the cost-effectiveness of this practice [60].

The ability to appose the edges of a wide defect for tight closure may also be limited by the use of hemoclips. The endoscopic suturing device (OverStitch; Apollo Endosurgery, Austin, TX) which is compatible with a double-channel gastroscope (Olympus GIF-2TH180) has recently been demonstrated to be an efficient and effective tool for post ESD endoscopic closure, and it can possibly reduce costs compared to hemoclip closure while possibly preventing the need for hospitalization [61]. The endoscopic suturing device has also been shown to perform better than hemoclip placement in the setting of intraprocedural perforation, which can occur in approximately 5% of ESD cases, greatly reducing the need for subsequent surgical intervention and possible segmental colectomy [37, 62]. This is attributed to superior full-thickness colon tissue approximation with the suturing device compared to inadequate mucosal tissue approximation achieved with hemoclip placement. However, it should be noted that advancement of the double-channel gastroscope to the right colon can be technically challenging due to its shorter length and looping of the endoscope during advancement. A complete pictographic list of steps for ESD is displayed in Fig. 6.6.

Efficacy and Complications

Most of the data for colorectal ESD comes from Asia, as this procedure has not been universally accepted as standard of care in the West, with most patients still being treated by EMR or referred for surgery. Efficacy and complications reported for this technique from the largest studies published to date are detailed in Table 6.3 at the conclusion of this chapter.

Combined Endoscopic Laparoscopic Surgery (CELS)

Collaborative laparo-endoscopic approaches have been described for the management of gastric subepithelial tumors and to allow for lymph node resection after endoscopic resection of gastric cancers with poorly differentiated histology, LVI,

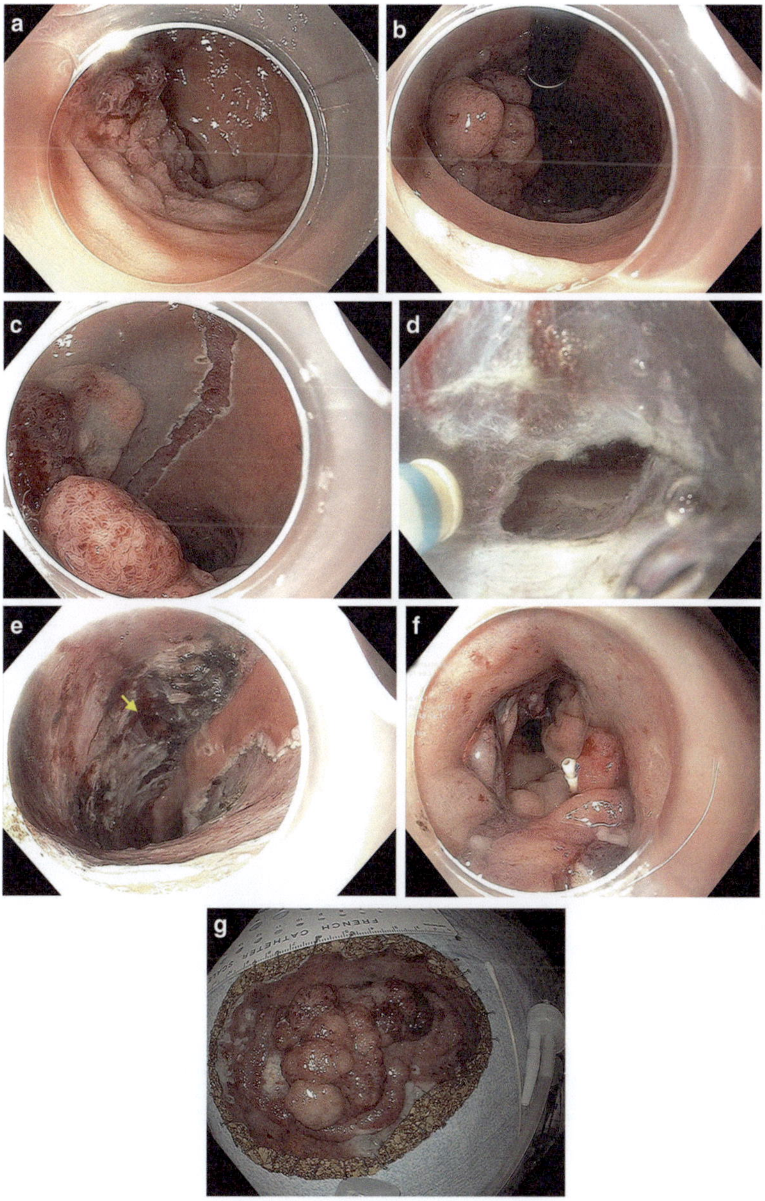

Fig. 6.6 Steps in ESD. (**a**) Ascending colon, granular, laterally spreading lesion, Paris classification (IIa+1s), Kudo pit pattern (type IV). (**b**) Retroflexed view revealing mixed nodularity with large nodules possibly suggestive of focal superficial carcinoma. (**c**) Mucosal incision. (**d**) Submucosal dissection (tunnel approach). (**e**) Status post ESD resection with evidence of possible deep penetration injury to the muscularis propria (indicated by arrow). (**f**) Status post closure of resection site with endoscopic suturing device. (**g**) Specimen status post resection pinned on cork to facilitate histologic assessment of lateral margins. Note the ample normal lateral margin afforded by ESD that can be readily assessed by the pathologist

Table 6.3 Efficacy and complications associated with ESD

References	Patients (%Rectal)	Study design	Lesion size (mm)	Time (min)	En bloc/RO (%)	Perforation/ Bleeding	Follow up
Fujishiro et al. [63]	35(100)	Prospective	32.8	Not specified	88.6/62.9	5.7/28.6	Mean 36 months, 96.8% recurrence free at 3 year
Tamegai et al. [64]	71(23.9)	Not specified	32.7	61.1	98.6/95.6	Not specified/1.4	Mean 12.2 months, recurrences 0%
Hurlstone et al. [65]	42(33.3)	Prospective	31	48	78.6/73.8	2.4/2.4	Median 6 months, recurrences 11%
Fujishiro et al. [66]	200(26)	Not specified	29.9	Not specified	91.5/70.5	6/0.5	Median 18 months, recurrences 1.8%
Saito et al. [67]	200(30.5)	Not specified	35	90	84/70	5/2	Median 7 months, recurrences 0.5%
Tanaka et al. [68]	70(48.6)	Not specified	28	70.5	80/Not specified	10/1.4	Not specified
Zhou et al. [69]	74(56.7)	Not specified	32.6	110	93.2/89.2	8.1/1.4	Median 14.3 months, recurrences 0%
Isomoto et al. [70]	292(26.7)	Not specified	26.8	Not specified	90.1/79.8	7.9/0.7	Median 33 months in RO, 36 months in non RO, 0% recurrence in RO, 1 recurrence in non RO
Saito et al. [71]	405(27.4)	Not specified	40	90	86.9/Not specified	3.5/1	Mean 20 months, recurrences 2%
Iizuka et al. [72]	44(59)	Retrospective	39	110	61/58	8/Not specified	Not specified
Nimi et al. [42]	310(26.1)	Retrospective	28.9	Not specified	90.3/74.5	4.8/1.3	Median 38.7 months, recurrences 2%, disease free survival at 3 and 5 year-100%
Yoshida et al. [73]	250(31.6)	Not specified	29.6	106	86.8/81.2	6/2.4	Not specified
Saito et al. [32]	145(50.3)	Retrospective	37	108	84/Not specified	6.2/1.4	Median 20 months, recurrences 2%

Hotta et al. [74]	120(27.5)	Not specified	30	141	93.3/85	7.5/Not specified	Not specified
Saito et al. [75]	1111(30.3)	Prospective	35	116	88/89	5.3/1.5	Not specified
Toyonaga et al. [76]	268(25.7)	Retrospective	40.3	64.5	99.2/98.1	2.2/0.37	Median 32.2 months, curative resections-94.2%, recurrences 0%
Matsumoto et al. [77]	203(Not specified)	Not specified	33	Not specified	85.7/Not specified	6.9/Not specified	Not specified
Uraoka et al. [78]	202(32.7)	Not specified	40	Not specified	91.6/87.1	2.4/0.5	Median 11.4 months, 0% disease specified mortality
Shono et al. [79]	137(26.2)	Not specified	29.2	79.2	89.1/85.41	3.6/3.6	0% recurrences
Kim et al. [80]	108(44)	Retrospective	27.6	61.9	Not specified/78.7	20.4/Not specified	Not specified
Lee et al. [81]	314(19.1)	Retrospective	28.9	54.7	92.7/87.6	8/0.64	Not specified
Lee et al. [82]	499(18.1)	Retrospective	28.9	61.3	95/Not specified	7.4/Not specified	Not specified
Hisabe et al. [83]	200(30)	Not specified	32.7	108.9	86/Not specified	7/1	Not specified
Saito et al. [84]	1321(25.6)	Not specified	34.2	90	95.4/87.2	2.9/2.5	Not specified
Okamoto et al. [85]	30(50)	Not specified	36	61	Not specified/100	0/0	Not specified
Lee et al. [41]	874(20.7)	Retrospective	26.5	53.8	97.1/90.5	6.1/0.5	Not specified
Nakajima et al. [86]	816(36.3)	Prospective	39.4	96	94.5/90.6	2/2.2	Not specified

(continued)

Table 6.3 (continued)

References	Patients (%Rectal)	Study design	Lesion size (mm)	Time (min)	En bloc/RO (%)	Perforation/ Bleeding	Follow up
Nawata et al. [87]	150(20.6)	Retrospective, 2 groups: A < 50 mm/B > 50 mm	26(59)	38/86	98.7/97.3	0/0	Not specified
Sakamoto et al. [88]	164(38)	Retrospective	30	95	95/92	4/3	Not specified
Saito et al. [89]	900(Not specified)	Not specified	40	100	91/87	2.7/1.7	Not specified
Lee et al. [90]	173(24.3)	Retrospective	25.95	Not specified	88.4/81.5	11/3.4	Not specified
Rahmi et al. [91]	28(25)	Retrospective	17.5	63	96.4/92.9	3.5/0	Not specified

and submucosal invasion [92–94]. This combined approach often termed combined endoscopic laparoscopic surgery (CELS) has also been used to remove "challenging" colon polyps [95–97]. Laparoscopic guidance during removal of complex colon polyps allows manipulation of the colon to facilitate polyp removal. This also allows for extraluminal observation of colonic wall integrity during resection and facilitates seromuscular suturing if deep transmural burn injury is visualized or if a perforation occurs. This approach also allows for concurrent sentinel node removal in the setting of suspected deep submucosal invasion. However, it should be noted that CELS represents a significantly more invasive approach than purely endoscopic resection; therefore, it should be reserved for lesions that cannot be safely and effectively removed by a purely endoscopic approach (whether piecemeal EMR or ESD) by experienced endoscopists. CELS should not be used as a "substitute" for expert endoscopic resection.

ESD Versus EMR

Performance of ESD has been compared prospectively to EMR in a large study of 1845 patients with lesions greater than 20mm revealing a significant increase in en bloc resection rate (ESD vs EMR: 94.5 vs 56.9%, $p < 0.01$) and a significant increase in the perforation rate (1.6 vs 0.8%, $p < 0.05$) in the ESD group, but no significant increase in the incidence of delayed bleeding, which was approximately 2% in both groups. Of note, the procedure time was significantly longer in the ESD vs EMR group (96 ± 69 vs 18 ± 23 min). This increased even more substantially in lesions >40 mm (129 ± 83 min) [41].

Another study from the National Cancer Center Hospital in Tokyo compared retrospectively ESD versus EMR removal of 373 colorectal tumors >20 mm in size with histologically confirmed curative resections. The ESD group included larger lesions (37 ± 14 vs 28 ± 8 mm, $p = 0.0006$), and again, en bloc resection rate was significantly higher (ESD vs EMR: 84 vs 33%, $p < 0.0001$), which resulted in lower tumor recurrence rate at follow-up colonoscopy (ESD vs EMR: 2 vs 14%, $p < 0.0001$). However, ESD was again associated with significantly longer procedure times (108 ± 71 vs 29 ± 25 min, $p < 0.0001$) and increased perforation rate (6.2 vs 1.3%, p = NS) [32]. Additional studies from Japan and South Korea have demonstrated consistent results of increased en bloc and R0 resection with lower follow-up recurrence rates at the expense of increased procedure time and perforation rate when comparing ESD versus EMR [32, 41, 98–101]. It should be noted, however, that ESD-associated perforations are uniformly small and easily manageable by endoscopic closure without significant morbidity or need for surgical intervention. These findings have also been confirmed by several recent meta-analyses comparing ESD and EMR for colorectal lesions [102–104].

Treatment of recurrent or residual adenomas after initial attempt at endoscopic resection is a separate dilemma due to increased submucosal fibrosis, which hinders the ability to create a submucosal cushion with lifting agents to facilitate removal by ESD or EMR technique. The best treatment strategy for managing these lesions is controversial as various studies have demonstrated conflicting results. Expert groups have demonstrated high success rates of managing recurrent adenomas after EMR with greater than 90% successfully treated with subsequent endoscopic therapies [29]. In a retrospective Japanese study looking at the management of recurrent adenomas, 60 patients had 69 recurrent lesions with 58/60 patients treated endoscopically while the remaining 2 (3%) required surgery. In the patients that were treated with endoscopy, 58 of 67 lesions (87%) were resected by EMR and the remaining 13% by ESD. Technique selection apparently was based on operator preference. En bloc resection rate was 39% (23/58) in the EMR group and 56% (5/9) in the ESD group which suggests that even in these challenging previously manipulated lesions, en bloc resection by ESD may be feasible [105]. In fact, even better outcomes were reported in a more recent study focusing on the use of ESD to treat patients referred to an expert ESD center for treatment of recurrent or residual lesions after prior EMR. This study demonstrated en bloc resection rate of 96% with a 93% curative resection rate and 0% recurrence rate [91]. The studies reviewed suggest that both EMR and ESD can be successfully employed for the management of recurrent adenomas after prior endoscopic resection with avoidance of surgery in the majority of patients if submucosal invasive malignancy is not present. However, again, as in de novo lesions, ESD may have a significant advantage in achieving complete en bloc resection of recurrent lesions particularly in cases with extensive fibrosis from the prior resection attempts (Fig. 6.7).

ESD Versus Minimally Invasive Surgery

The two minimally invasive surgical options for the management of large colonic adenomas or early colon cancer include laparoscopic-assisted colorectal surgery (LACS) also known as combined endoscopic laparoscopic surgery (CELS) and transanal endoscopic microsurgery (TEM). Recent studies have started to compare ESD with these surgical modalities. A retrospective study at the National Cancer Center of Tokyo compared ESD with CELS for removal of early colorectal carcinoma. ESD was only attempted in those patients with mucosal (T1m) or superficial submucosal (T1sm1) involvement, while CELS was utilized for those patients with deep submucosal involvement (T1sm2), in patients with non-curative prior EMR, and in those deemed not amenable to purely endoscopic resection. ESD resulted in shorter procedure time (106 vs 206 min, $p < 0.001$), shorter hospital stay (5 vs 13 days, $p < 0.001$), and lower complication rates (6.4 vs 13.6%), with perforation (4.7%) and wound infection (10.6%) representing the most common complications in the ESD and CELS groups, respectively. Nevertheless, en bloc and curative resection rates were lower in the ESD group (87.2 and 80.4%, respectively) compared to 100% for surgical patients. Of note, stomas were necessary for 93% of the patients undergoing CELS for resection of rectal cancers located below the peritoneal reflection [106]. Another retrospective study comparing ESD to CELS revealed shorter procedure time (90 vs 185 min, $p < 0.001$), shorter hospital stay (5 vs 10 days, $p < 0.001$), and lower complication rates (7 vs 15%, $p = 0.005$) with ESD compared

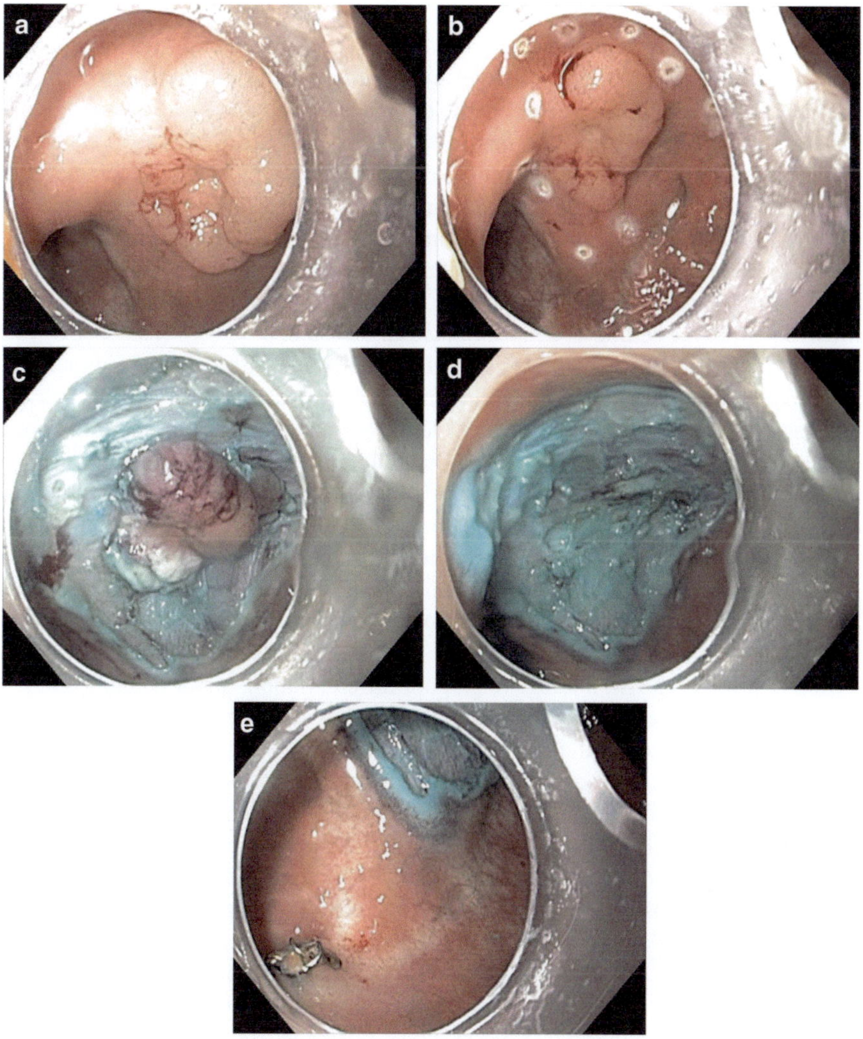

Fig. 6.7 ESD procedure in extensive fibrosis. (**a**) Recurrent adenoma after segmental sigmoid resection at the site of the surgical anastomosis. A challenging lesion due to extensive fibrosis (seen as white scar tissue at the right upper border of the lesion; the border of the lesion closest to the surgical anastomosis). The lesion was not amenable to submucosal lifting and EMR due to the extensive fibrosis. (**b**) Coagulation marks are placed using soft coagulation current to mark the perimeter of the resection in order to achieve en bloc resection with negative lateral margins (R0 resection). (**c**) ESD in progress with margination of the lesion having been achieved. Very scant submucosal layer is visible due to the extensive fibrosis from prior surgical resection. (**d**) Completed en bloc resection. (**e**) The proximity of the resection to the surgical anastomosis is evident with protruding staples apparent. Reproduced with permission from von Renteln D, Schmidt A, Vassiliou MC, Rudolph H-C, Caca K. Endoscopic fullthickness resection and defect closure in the colon. Gastrointestinal Endoscopy. Elsevier. 2010

to CELS. There were also statistically significant differences favoring ESD over CELS in postoperative analgesia requirements, in transfusion requirements, as well as in the amount of time required to resume full diet and ambulation. Furthermore, a high en bloc and curative resection rate of approximately 91% was reported in the ESD group. However, it is important to keep in mind that CELS was reserved for patients with evidence of deep submucosal invasion based on results of non-curative endoscopic resection or based on initial endoscopic impression as determined by pit pattern analysis by magnification chromoendoscopy with narrowband imaging [107]. In this setting, CELS offers a definitive en bloc and curative resection with concurrent lymph node dissection due to increased likelihood of lymph node involvement in the setting of deep submucosal invasion.

A recent systematic review confirmed the utility of CELS as a technique that represents a viable alternative to segmental colon resection with a trend toward decreased operative times and hospital length of stay when endoscopic methods alone do not suffice [96]. Therefore, ESD should be considered as the primary therapy in centers of expertise for resection of T1m/sm1 cancers due to high en bloc and curative resection rates with improved postoperative recovery time, hospital length of stay, and complication rates compared to CELS. On the other hand, CELS should be considered when ESD expertise is not available, after failed attempt at endoscopic resection, or after successful en bloc endoscopic resection where final histopathologic assessment reveals a positive deep margin, deep submucosal invasion (sm2), or other high-risk findings (e.g., poor differentiation, tumor budding, etc.).

Transanal endoscopic microsurgery (TEM) has become one of the standard approaches for early rectal cancer (T1N0) [108]. Prior studies have demonstrated lower rate of positive resection margins, fragmented specimens, and recurrence rates with this technique as compared to traditional transanal excisions for early rectal cancer [109–111]. Transanal minimally invasive surgery (TAMIS) has also recently been introduced as a technique for removal of early rectal cancers with low reported rates of positive margins and postoperative complications; however, very limited data is available comparing this technique to TEM [112]. TEM and ESD have been compared for the management of early rectal cancers. A South Korean study demonstrated no significant difference in en bloc and R0 resection rates between these two techniques (ESD vs TEM, 96.7% vs 100% and 96.7 vs 97.0%, respectively), with no statistically significant difference in adverse event rates but a trend for higher adverse events after TEM (ESD vs TEM, 3.3 vs 6.1%). Furthermore, ESD resulted in significantly shorter procedure time (84 min vs 116 min) and hospital length of stay (3.6 vs 6.6 days). Of note, local recurrence or metastatic progression was not noted in either group during long-term follow-up [113]. A smaller study from Brazil also demonstrated no significant difference in en bloc resection rates with tumor-free margins (ESD vs TEM, 81.8 vs 84.6%, $p = 0.040$). Differences in procedure time (ESD vs TEM, 133 ± 99.8 vs 150 ± 66.3 min, $p = 0.69$) and hospital stay (ESD vs TEM, 3.8 ± 3.3 days vs 4.08 ± 1.7, $p = 0.81$) favored ESD but did not reach statistical significance in this small study [114]. In a recent meta-analysis of studies comparing ESD to transanal surgical local excision (LE) including TEM (notably only four such studies were identified in this 2016 meta-analysis), there were no significant differences in en bloc resection rate, R0 resection rate, overall complication rate, and tumor size between ESD and LE. When adopting the fixed effect model which takes into account the study size, ESD was associated with a lower recurrence rate than LE (OR 0.15; 95% CI 0.03–0.87; $p = 0.03$), while with the random effects model, the difference was not significant (OR 0.18; 95% CI 0.02–2.04; $p = 0.17$) [115]. A larger systematic review comparing pooled estimates of outcomes from single technique ESD studies and TEM studies reported improved en bloc and R0 resection rates with TEM as compared to ESD (98.7 vs 87.8%, $p < 0.001$ and 88.5 vs 74.6%, $p < 0.001$). Interestingly, in contrast to other studies, procedure time was found to be significantly shorter in the TEM group (67 vs 96 min, $p = 0.003$). There was no significant difference in adverse event rates (ESD vs TEM, 8 vs 8.4%, $p = 0.874$) [116]. We should note here, however, that the adverse events for ESD only included delayed rectal bleeding (3.5%) and small perforations (3.7%) which were easily managed endoscopically with minimal or no morbidity. In contrast, most of the adverse events of TEM (occurring in 3.7%) included suture leaks (3.2%) and fistulas (0.5%). We should also note that it is unclear whether subacute adverse events such as temporary incontinence caused by the 4 cm rectoscope used in TEM were assessed. Furthermore, despite the reported improved en bloc and R0 resection rate with TEM, adenoma recurrence rate was higher in the TEM group (5.2 vs 2.6%, $p = 0.068$). Another important finding that was not addressed and may greatly limit the validity of the findings of this meta-analysis involves the target lesions for each technique. Perplexingly, in the pooled ESD series, 68% of the lesions were carcinomas compared to only 11% of the lesions targeted by TEM being carcinomas. This suggests that the lesions in the ESD series were significantly more challenging than those targeted by TEM. These unusual findings raise significant methodological concerns regarding this comparison of pooled estimates of ESD series to those of TEM series. Therefore, the results of the much smaller meta-analysis mentioned above looking at studies comparing the two techniques directly appear to be more reliable than the larger systemic review. It is clear that at this point prospective randomized trials comparing ESD and TEM for rectal adenomas and T1 N0 carcinomas are necessary.

Conclusion

Current colorectal screening programs have increased detection of early neoplastic lesions suitable for endoscopic resection. EMR has traditionally been used for removal of large colon polyps and has a technical success rate of approximately 95% in high-volume centers with acceptable delayed bleeding and perforation rates [24, 25]. Currently, this remains the primary technique utilized by endoscopists to manage these lesions in Western countries. However, en bloc resection rate with this technique is low as polyps >2 cm frequently require piecemeal resection. This subsequently interferes with histologic assessment for negative margins, which is imperative if early-stage (T1) colonic adenocarcinoma is present. Furthermore, this technique results in higher recurrence rates.

Recently, ESD has become widely utilized in Asia for removal of large colon polyps, lesions with prior manipulation resulting in extensive submucosal fibrosis, and for lesions with suspected early adenocarcinoma. Numerous studies have demonstrated high en bloc and R0 resection rates with low recurrence and acceptable complication rates. This technique has also been shown to compare favorably to more invasive surgical techniques such as CELS and TEM while potentially reducing hospital length of stay and healthcare costs. However, ESD has not yet been widely accepted in Western countries due to longer procedure times, lack of reimbursement, long learning curve, and lack of access to training. In Asian countries, ESD training typically follows a progression from gastric to rectal to proximal colonic lesions; however, lower prevalence of gastric dysplasia and early gastric cancer as well as lack of ESD expertise in the West prevents this training approach necessitating more self-directed learning and reliance on animal models. Furthermore, Western trainees are often required to progress early in their training to colorectal ESD to gain experience, which may result in poorer outcomes and higher complications rates as compared to the results demonstrated by our Asian colleagues.

Reimbursement is hampered by the lack of a specific CPT code for ESD requiring the procedure to be billed as either an unlisted code or using colon EMR coding (CPT 45390), which yields 6.04 work RVUs and $878 facility fee according to 2017 National Medicare Averages. Therefore, the substantially higher time commitment to complete these procedures as compared to EMR is not compensated accordingly. Furthermore, reimbursement pales in comparison to surgical alternatives such as laparoscopic hemicolectomy (CPT code 44205) which yields 22.95 work RVUs and $1393 facility fee. Unfortunately, reimbursement and training challenges will likely continue to hinder the widespread adoption of ESD in the West. Nevertheless, ESD should be considered as a minimally invasive surgical alternative in expert centers, and standardized training programs and guidelines should be created to further advance expertise and implementation of this technique.

References

1. Bucci C, Rotondano G, Hassan C, et al. Optimal bowel cleansing for colonoscopy: split the dose! A series of meta-analyses of controlled studies. Gastrointest Endosc. 2014;80:566–76 e2.
2. Committee ASoP, Acosta RD, Abraham NS, et al. The management of antithrombotic agents for patients undergoing GI endoscopy. Gastrointest Endosc. 2016;83:3–16.
3. Baron TH, Kamath PS, McBane RD. Management of antithrombotic therapy in patients undergoing invasive procedures. N Engl J Med. 2013;368:2113–24.
4. Desai J, Granger CB, Weitz JI, Aisenberg J. Novel oral anticoagulants in gastroenterology practice. Gastrointest Endosc. 2013;78:227–39.
5. Manocha D, Singh M, Mehta N, Murthy UK. Bleeding risk after invasive procedures in aspirin/NSAID users: polypectomy study in veterans. Am J Med. 2012;125:1222–7.
6. Gandhi S, Narula N, Mosleh W, Marshall JK, Farkouh M. Meta-analysis: colonoscopic post-polypectomy bleeding in patients on continued clopidogrel therapy. Aliment Pharmacol Ther. 2013;37:947–52.

7. Uno Y, Munakata A. The non-lifting sign of invasive colon cancer. Gastrointest Endosc. 1994;40:485–9.
8. Kobayashi N, Saito Y, Sano Y, et al. Determining the treatment strategy for colorectal neoplastic lesions: endoscopic assessment or the non-lifting sign for diagnosing invasion depth? Endoscopy. 2007;39:701–5.
9. Uraoka T, Saito Y, Matsuda T, et al. Endoscopic indications for endoscopic mucosal resection of laterally spreading tumours in the colorectum. Gut. 2006;55:1592–7.
10. Kim BC, Chang HJ, Han KS, et al. Clinicopathological differences of laterally spreading tumors of the colorectum according to gross appearance. Endoscopy. 2011;43:100–7.
11. Holt BA, Bourke MJ. Wide field endoscopic resection for advanced colonic mucosal neoplasia: current status and future directions. Clin Gastroenterol Hepatol. 2012;10:969–79.
12. Tanaka S, Kaltenbach T, Chayama K, Soetikno R. High-magnification colonoscopy (with videos). Gastrointest Endosc. 2006;64:604–13.
13. Moss A, Bourke MJ, Williams SJ, et al. Endoscopic mucosal resection outcomes and prediction of submucosal cancer from advanced colonic mucosal neoplasia. Gastroenterology. 2011;140:1909–18.
14. Fu KI, Kato S, Sano Y, et al. Staging of early colorectal cancers: magnifying colonoscopy versus endoscopic ultrasonography for estimation of depth of invasion. Dig Dis Sci. 2008;53:1886–92.
15. Fasoulas K, Lazaraki G, Chatzimavroudis G, et al. Endoscopic mucosal resection of giant laterally spreading tumors with submucosal injection of hydroxyethyl starch: comparative study with normal saline solution. Surg Laparosc Endosc Percutan Tech. 2012;22:272–8.
16. Yoshida N, Naito Y, Inada Y, et al. Endoscopic mucosal resection with 0.13% hyaluronic acid solution for colorectal polyps less than 20 mm: a randomized controlled trial. J Gastroenterol Hepatol. 2012;27:1377–83.
17. Bahin FF, Rasouli KN, Byth K, et al. Prediction of clinically significant bleeding following wide-field endoscopic resection of large sessile and laterally spreading colorectal lesions: a clinical risk score. Am J Gastroenterol. 2016;111:1115–22.
18. Lee SH, Chung IK, Kim SJ, et al. Comparison of postpolypectomy bleeding between epinephrine and saline submucosal injection for large colon polyps by conventional polypectomy: a prospective randomized, multicenter study. World J Gastroenterol. 2007;13:2973–7.
19. Veerappan SG, Ormonde D, Yusoff IF, Raftopoulos SC. Hot avulsion: a modification of an existing technique for management of nonlifting areas of a polyp (with video). Gastrointest Endosc. 2014;80:884–8.
20. Burgess NG, Bassan MS, McLeod D, Williams SJ, Byth K, Bourke MJ. Deep mural injury and perforation after colonic endoscopic mucosal resection: a new classification and analysis of risk factors. Gut. 2016;66(10):1779–89.
21. Liaquat H, Rohn E, Rex DK. Prophylactic clip closure reduced the risk of delayed postpolypectomy hemorrhage: experience in 277 clipped large sessile or flat colorectal lesions and 247 control lesions. Gastrointest Endosc. 2013;77:401–7.
22. Dokoshi T, Fujiya M, Tanaka K, et al. A randomized study on the effectiveness of prophylactic clipping during endoscopic resection of colon polyps for the prevention of delayed bleeding. Biomed Res Int. 2015;2015:490272.
23. Bahin FF, Naidoo M, Williams SJ, et al. Prophylactic endoscopic coagulation to prevent bleeding after wide-field endoscopic mucosal resection of large sessile colon polyps. Clin Gastroenterol Hepatol. 2015;13:724–30 e1-2.
24. Arebi N, Swain D, Suzuki N, Fraser C, Price A, Saunders BP. Endoscopic mucosal resection of 161 cases of large sessile or flat colorectal polyps. Scand J Gastroenterol. 2007;42:859–66.
25. Swan MP, Bourke MJ, Alexander S, Moss A, Williams SJ. Large refractory colonic polyps: is it time to change our practice? A prospective study of the clinical and economic impact of a tertiary referral colonic mucosal resection and polypectomy service (with videos). Gastrointest Endosc. 2009;70:1128–36.

26. Doniec JM, Lohnert MS, Schniewind B, Bokelmann F, Kremer B, Grimm H. Endoscopic removal of large colorectal polyps: prevention of unnecessary surgery? Dis Colon Rectum. 2003;46:340–8.
27. Khashab M, Eid E, Rusche M, Rex DK. Incidence and predictors of "late" recurrences after endoscopic piecemeal resection of large sessile adenomas. Gastrointest Endosc. 2009;70:344–9.
28. Luigiano C, Consolo P, Scaffidi MG, et al. Endoscopic mucosal resection for large and giant sessile and flat colorectal polyps: a single-center experience with long-term follow-up. Endoscopy. 2009;41:829–35.
29. Moss A, Williams SJ, Hourigan LF, et al. Long-term adenoma recurrence following wide-field endoscopic mucosal resection (WF-EMR) for advanced colonic mucosal neoplasia is infrequent: results and risk factors in 1000 cases from the Australian Colonic EMR (ACE) study. Gut. 2015;64:57–65.
30. Burgess NG, Metz AJ, Williams SJ, et al. Risk factors for intraprocedural and clinically significant delayed bleeding after wide-field endoscopic mucosal resection of large colonic lesions. Clin Gastroenterol Hepatol. 2014;12:651–61 e1-3.
31. Conio M, Repici A, Demarquay JF, Blanchi S, Dumas R, Filiberti R. EMR of large sessile colorectal polyps. Gastrointest Endosc. 2004;60:234–41.
32. Saito Y, Fukuzawa M, Matsuda T, et al. Clinical outcome of endoscopic submucosal dissection versus endoscopic mucosal resection of large colorectal tumors as determined by curative resection. Surg Endosc. 2010;24:343–52.
33. Kantsevoy SV, Bitner M, Piskun G. New endoscopic platform for endoluminal en bloc tissue resection in the gastrointestinal tract (with videos). Surg Endosc. 2016;30:3145–51.
34. Stavropoulos SN, Modayil R, Friedel D. Current applications of endoscopic suturing. World J Gastrointest Endosc. 2015;7:777–89.
35. Gotoda T, Yanagisawa A, Sasako M, et al. Incidence of lymph node metastasis from early gastric cancer: estimation with a large number of cases at two large centers. Gastric Cancer. 2000;3:219–25.
36. Pohl H, Srivastava A, Bensen SP, et al. Incomplete polyp resection during colonoscopy-results of the complete adenoma resection (CARE) study. Gastroenterology. 2013;144:74–80 e1.
37. Fujiya M, Tanaka K, Dokoshi T, et al. Efficacy and adverse events of EMR and endoscopic submucosal dissection for the treatment of colon neoplasms: a meta-analysis of studies comparing EMR and endoscopic submucosal dissection. Gastrointest Endosc. 2015;81:583–95.
38. Akintoye E, Kumar N, Aihara H, Nas H, Thompson CC. Colorectal endoscopic submucosal dissection: a systematic review and meta-analysis. Endosc Int Open. 2016;4:E1030–E44.
39. Buchner AM, Guarner-Argente C, Ginsberg GG. Outcomes of EMR of defiant colorectal lesions directed to an endoscopy referral center. Gastrointest Endosc. 2012;76:255–63.
40. Oka S, Tanaka S, Saito Y, et al. Local recurrence after endoscopic resection for large colorectal neoplasia: a multicenter prospective study in Japan. Am J Gastroenterol. 2015;110:697–707.
41. Lee EJ, Lee JB, Lee SH, et al. Endoscopic submucosal dissection for colorectal tumors--1,000 colorectal ESD cases: one specialized institute's experiences. Surg Endosc. 2013;27:31–9.
42. Niimi K, Fujishiro M, Kodashima S, et al. Long-term outcomes of endoscopic submucosal dissection for colorectal epithelial neoplasms. Endoscopy. 2010;42:723–9.
43. Lieberman D, Moravec M, Holub J, Michaels L, Eisen G. Polyp size and advanced histology in patients undergoing colonoscopy screening: implications for CT colonography. Gastroenterology. 2008;135:1100–5.
44. Pimentel-Nunes P, Dinis-Ribeiro M, Ponchon T, et al. Endoscopic submucosal dissection: European Society of Gastrointestinal Endoscopy (ESGE) Guideline. Endoscopy. 2015;47:829–54.
45. Tanaka S, Kashida H, Saito Y, et al. JGES guidelines for colorectal endoscopic submucosal dissection/endoscopic mucosal resection. Dig Endosc. 2015;27:417–34.
46. Inoue H, Kashida H, Kudo S, Sasako M, Shimoda T, Watanabe H, Yoshida S, Guelrud M, Lightdale CJ, Wang K, Riddell RH. The Paris endoscopic classification of superficial neoplas-

tic lesions: esophagus, stomach, and colon: November 30 to December 1, 2002. Gastrointest Endosc. 2003;58:S3–43.
47. Kitajima K, Fujimori T, Fujii S, et al. Correlations between lymph node metastasis and depth of submucosal invasion in submucosal invasive colorectal carcinoma: a Japanese collaborative study. J Gastroenterol. 2004;39:534–43.
48. Morson BC, Whiteway JE, Jones EA, Macrae FA, Williams CB. Histopathology and prognosis of malignant colorectal polyps treated by endoscopic polypectomy. Gut. 1984;25:437–44.
49. Matsuda T, Fujii T, Saito Y, et al. Efficacy of the invasive/non-invasive pattern by magnifying chromoendoscopy to estimate the depth of invasion of early colorectal neoplasms. Am J Gastroenterol. 2008;103:2700–6.
50. Ikematsu H, Matsuda T, Emura F, et al. Efficacy of capillary pattern type IIIA/IIIB by magnifying narrow band imaging for estimating depth of invasion of early colorectal neoplasms. BMC Gastroenterol. 2010;10:33.
51. Hayashi N, Tanaka S, Hewett DG, et al. Endoscopic prediction of deep submucosal invasive carcinoma: validation of the narrow-band imaging international colorectal endoscopic (NICE) classification. Gastrointest Endosc. 2013;78:625–32.
52. Matsumoto T, Hizawa K, Esaki M, et al. Comparison of EUS and magnifying colonoscopy for assessment of small colorectal cancers. Gastrointest Endosc. 2002;56:354–60.
53. Kim SY, Chung JW, Park DK, Kwon KA, Kim KO, Kim YJ. Efficacy of carbon dioxide insufflation during gastric endoscopic submucosal dissection: a randomized, double-blind, controlled, prospective study. Gastrointest Endosc. 2015;82:1018–24.
54. Mönkemüller KWC, Muñoz-Navas M. Interventional and therapeutic gastrointestinal endoscopy. Front Gastrointest Res. 2010;27:287–95.
55. Morita Y. Electrocautery for ESD: settings of the electrical surgical unit VIO300D. Gastrointest Endosc Clin N Am. 2014;24:183–9.
56. Yamamoto H. Technology insight: endoscopic submucosal dissection of gastrointestinal neoplasms. Nat Clin Pract Gastroenterol Hepatol. 2007;4:511–20.
57. Osada T, Sakamoto N, Ritsuno H, et al. Closure with clips to accelerate healing of mucosal defects caused by colorectal endoscopic submucosal dissection. Surg Endosc. 2016;30:4438–44.
58. Fujihara S, Mori H, Kobara H, et al. The efficacy and safety of prophylactic closure for a large mucosal defect after colorectal endoscopic submucosal dissection. Oncol Rep. 2013;30:85–90.
59. Zhang QS, Han B, JH X, Gao P, Shen YC. Clip closure of defect after endoscopic resection in patients with larger colorectal tumors decreased the adverse events. Gastrointest Endosc. 2015;82:904–9.
60. Burgess NG, Bourke MJ. Mucosal colonic defect post EMR or ESD: to close or not? Endosc Int Open. 2016;4:E1073–E4.
61. Kantsevoy SV, Bitner M, Mitrakov AA, Thuluvath PJ. Endoscopic suturing closure of large mucosal defects after endoscopic submucosal dissection is technically feasible, fast, and eliminates the need for hospitalization (with videos). Gastrointest Endosc. 2014;79:503–7.
62. Kantsevoy SV, Bitner M, Hajiyeva G, et al. Endoscopic management of colonic perforations: clips versus suturing closure (with videos). Gastrointest Endosc. 2016;84:487–93.
63. Fujishiro M, Yahagi N, Nakamura M, et al. Endoscopic submucosal dissection for rectal epithelial neoplasia. Endoscopy. 2006;38:493–7.
64. Tamegai Y, Saito Y, Masaki N, et al. Endoscopic submucosal dissection: a safe technique for colorectal tumors. Endoscopy. 2007;39:418–22.
65. Hurlstone DP, Atkinson R, Sanders DS, Thomson M, Cross SS, Brown S. Achieving R0 resection in the colorectum using endoscopic submucosal dissection. Br J Surg. 2007;94:1536–42.
66. Fujishiro M, Yahagi N, Kakushima N, et al. Outcomes of endoscopic submucosal dissection for colorectal epithelial neoplasms in 200 consecutive cases. Clin Gastroenterol Hepatol. 2007;5:678–83. quiz 45

67. Saito Y, Uraoka T, Matsuda T, et al. Endoscopic treatment of large superficial colorectal tumors: a case series of 200 endoscopic submucosal dissections (with video). Gastrointest Endosc. 2007;66:966–73.
68. Tanaka S, Oka S, Kaneko I, et al. Endoscopic submucosal dissection for colorectal neoplasia: possibility of standardization. Gastrointest Endosc. 2007;66:100–7.
69. Zhou PH, Yao LQ, Qin XY. Endoscopic submucosal dissection for colorectal epithelial neoplasm. Surg Endosc. 2009;23:1546–51.
70. Isomoto H, Nishiyama H, Yamaguchi N, et al. Clinicopathological factors associated with clinical outcomes of endoscopic submucosal dissection for colorectal epithelial neoplasms. Endoscopy. 2009;41:679–83.
71. Saito Y, Sakamoto T, Fukunaga S, Nakajima T, Kiriyama S, Matsuda T. Endoscopic submucosal dissection (ESD) for colorectal tumors. Dig Endosc. 2009;21(Suppl 1):S7–12.
72. Iizuka H, Okamura S, Onozato Y, Ishihara H, Kakizaki S, Mori M. Endoscopic submucosal dissection for colorectal tumors. Gastroenterol Clin Biol. 2009;33:1004–11.
73. Yoshida N, Naito Y, Kugai M, et al. Efficient hemostatic method for endoscopic submucosal dissection of colorectal tumors. World J Gastroenterol. 2010;16:4180–6.
74. Hotta K, Oyama T, Shinohara T, et al. Learning curve for endoscopic submucosal dissection of large colorectal tumors. Dig Endosc. 2010;22:302–6.
75. Saito Y, Uraoka T, Yamaguchi Y, et al. A prospective, multicenter study of 1111 colorectal endoscopic submucosal dissections (with video). Gastrointest Endosc. 2010;72:1217–25.
76. Toyonaga T, Man-i M, Fujita T, et al. Retrospective study of technical aspects and complications of endoscopic submucosal dissection for laterally spreading tumors of the colorectum. Endoscopy. 2010;42:714–22.
77. Matsumoto A, Tanaka S, Oba S, et al. Outcome of endoscopic submucosal dissection for colorectal tumors accompanied by fibrosis. Scand J Gastroenterol. 2010;45:1329–37.
78. Uraoka T, Higashi R, Kato J, et al. Colorectal endoscopic submucosal dissection for elderly patients at least 80 years of age. Surg Endosc. 2011;25:3000–7.
79. Shono T, Ishikawa K, Ochiai Y, et al. Feasibility of endoscopic submucosal dissection: a new technique for en bloc resection of a large superficial tumor in the colon and rectum. Int J Surg Oncol. 2011;2011:948293.
80. Kim ES, Cho KB, Park KS, et al. Factors predictive of perforation during endoscopic submucosal dissection for the treatment of colorectal tumors. Endoscopy. 2011;43:573–8.
81. Lee EJ, Lee JB, Lee SH, Youk EG. Endoscopic treatment of large colorectal tumors: comparison of endoscopic mucosal resection, endoscopic mucosal resection-precutting, and endoscopic submucosal dissection. Surg Endosc. 2012;26:2220–30.
82. Lee EJ, Lee JB, Choi YS, et al. Clinical risk factors for perforation during endoscopic submucosal dissection (ESD) for large-sized, nonpedunculated colorectal tumors. Surg Endosc. 2012;26:1587–94.
83. Hisabe T, Nagahama T, Hirai F, Matsui T, Iwashita A. Clinical outcomes of 200 colorectal endoscopic submucosal dissections. Dig Endosc. 2012;24(Suppl 1):105–9.
84. Saito Y, Kawano H, Takeuchi Y, et al. Current status of colorectal endoscopic submucosal dissection in Japan and other Asian countries: progressing towards technical standardization. Dig Endosc. 2012;24(Suppl 1):67–72.
85. Okamoto K, Kitamura S, Muguruma N, et al. Mucosectom2-short blade for safe and efficient endoscopic submucosal dissection of colorectal tumors. Endoscopy. 2013;45:928–30.
86. Nakajima T, Saito Y, Tanaka S, et al. Current status of endoscopic resection strategy for large, early colorectal neoplasia in Japan. Surg Endosc. 2013;27:3262–70.
87. Nawata Y, Homma K, Suzuki Y. Retrospective study of technical aspects and complications of endoscopic submucosal dissection for large superficial colorectal tumors. Dig Endosc. 2014;26:552–5.
88. Sakamoto T, Sato C, Makazu M, et al. Short-term outcomes of colorectal endoscopic submucosal dissection performed by trainees. Digestion. 2014;89:37–42.

89. Saito Y, Yamada M, So E, et al. Colorectal endoscopic submucosal dissection: Technical advantages compared to endoscopic mucosal resection and minimally invasive surgery. Dig Endosc. 2014;26(Suppl 1):52–61.
90. Lee SP, Kim JH, Sung IK, et al. Effect of submucosal fibrosis on endoscopic submucosal dissection of colorectal tumors: pathologic review of 173 cases. J Gastroenterol Hepatol. 2015;30:872–8.
91. Rahmi G, Tanaka S, Ohara Y, et al. Efficacy of endoscopic submucosal dissection for residual or recurrent superficial colorectal tumors after endoscopic mucosal resection. J Dig Dis. 2015;16:14–21.
92. Abe N, Takeuchi H, Ohki A, et al. Long-term outcomes of combination of endoscopic submucosal dissection and laparoscopic lymph node dissection without gastrectomy for early gastric cancer patients who have a potential risk of lymph node metastasis. Gastrointest Endosc. 2011;74:792–7.
93. Abe N, Takeuchi H, Yanagida O, et al. Endoscopic full-thickness resection with laparoscopic assistance as hybrid NOTES for gastric submucosal tumor. Surg Endosc. 2009;23:1908–13.
94. Hiki N, Yamamoto Y, Fukunaga T, et al. Laparoscopic and endoscopic cooperative surgery for gastrointestinal stromal tumor dissection. Surg Endosc. 2008;22:1729–35.
95. Franklin ME Jr, Portillo G. Laparoscopic monitored colonoscopic polypectomy: long-term follow-up. World J Surg. 2009;33:1306–9.
96. Nakajima K, Sharma SK, Lee SW, Milsom JW. Avoiding colorectal resection for polyps: is CELS the best method? Surg Endosc. 2016;30:807–18.
97. Wilhelm D, von Delius S, Weber L, et al. Combined laparoscopic-endoscopic resections of colorectal polyps: 10-year experience and follow-up. Surg Endosc. 2009;23:688–93.
98. Kim YJ, Kim ES, Cho KB, et al. Comparison of clinical outcomes among different endoscopic resection methods for treating colorectal neoplasia. Dig Dis Sci. 2013;58:1727–36.
99. Kobayashi N, Yoshitake N, Hirahara Y, et al. Matched case-control study comparing endoscopic submucosal dissection and endoscopic mucosal resection for colorectal tumors. J Gastroenterol Hepatol. 2012;27:728–33.
100. Tajika M, Niwa Y, Bhatia V, et al. Comparison of endoscopic submucosal dissection and endoscopic mucosal resection for large colorectal tumors. Eur J Gastroenterol Hepatol. 2011;23:1042–9.
101. Terasaki M, Tanaka S, Oka S, et al. Clinical outcomes of endoscopic submucosal dissection and endoscopic mucosal resection for laterally spreading tumors larger than 20 mm. J Gastroenterol Hepatol. 2012;27:734–40.
102. Arezzo A, Passera R, Marchese N, Galloro G, Manta R, Cirocchi R. Systematic review and meta-analysis of endoscopic submucosal dissection vs endoscopic mucosal resection for colorectal lesions. United European Gastroenterol J. 2016;4:18–29.
103. Cao Y, Liao C, Tan A, Gao Y, Mo Z, Gao F. Meta-analysis of endoscopic submucosal dissection versus endoscopic mucosal resection for tumors of the gastrointestinal tract. Endoscopy. 2009;41:751–7.
104. Wang J, Zhang XH, Ge J, Yang CM, Liu JY, Zhao SL. Endoscopic submucosal dissection vs endoscopic mucosal resection for colorectal tumors: a meta-analysis. World J Gastroenterol. 2014;20:8282–7.
105. Sakamoto T, Saito Y, Matsuda T, Fukunaga S, Nakajima T, Fujii T. Treatment strategy for recurrent or residual colorectal tumors after endoscopic resection. Surg Endosc. 2011;25:255–60.
106. Kiriyama S, Saito Y, Yamamoto S, et al. Comparison of endoscopic submucosal dissection with laparoscopic-assisted colorectal surgery for early-stage colorectal cancer: a retrospective analysis. Endoscopy. 2012;44:1024–30.
107. Nakamura F, Saito Y, Sakamoto T, et al. Potential perioperative advantage of colorectal endoscopic submucosal dissection versus laparoscopy-assisted colectomy. Surg Endosc. 2015;29:596–606.
108. Morino M, Risio M, Bach S, et al. Early rectal cancer: the European Association for Endoscopic Surgery (EAES) clinical consensus conference. Surg Endosc. 2015;29:755–73.

109. Christoforidis D, Cho HM, Dixon MR, Mellgren AF, Madoff RD, Finne CO. Transanal endoscopic microsurgery versus conventional transanal excision for patients with early rectal cancer. Ann Surg. 2009;249:776–82.
110. de Graaf EJ, Burger JW, van Ijsseldijk AL, Tetteroo GW, Dawson I, Hop WC. Transanal endoscopic microsurgery is superior to transanal excision of rectal adenomas. Colorectal Dis. 2011;13(7):762.
111. Moore JS, Cataldo PA, Osler T, Hyman NH. Transanal endoscopic microsurgery is more effective than traditional transanal excision for resection of rectal masses. Dis Colon Rectum. 2008;51:1026–30. discussion 30-1.
112. Albert MR, Atallah SB, deBeche-Adams TC, Izfar S, Larach SW. Transanal minimally invasive surgery (TAMIS) for local excision of benign neoplasms and early-stage rectal cancer: efficacy and outcomes in the first 50 patients. Dis Colon Rectum. 2013;56:301–7.
113. Park SU, Min YW, Shin JU, et al. Endoscopic submucosal dissection or transanal endoscopic microsurgery for nonpolypoid rectal high grade dysplasia and submucosa-invading rectal cancer. Endoscopy. 2012;44:1031–6.
114. Kawaguti FS, Nahas CS, Marques CF, et al. Endoscopic submucosal dissection versus transanal endoscopic microsurgery for the treatment of early rectal cancer. Surg Endosc. 2014;28:1173–9.
115. Wang S, Gao S, Yang W, Guo S, Li Y. Endoscopic submucosal dissection versus local excision for early rectal cancer: a systematic review and meta-analysis. Tech Coloproctol. 2016;20:1–9.
116. Arezzo A, Passera R, Saito Y, et al. Systematic review and meta-analysis of endoscopic submucosal dissection versus transanal endoscopic microsurgery for large noninvasive rectal lesions. Surg Endosc. 2014;28:427–38.

Transanal Endoscopic Surgery (TES)

7

Susana Wu and Elisabeth C. McLemore

Introduction

Transanal excision (TAE) was introduced by Dr. Parks in the 1950s [1]. In comparison to transabdominal surgery, transanal excision offered an organ sparing approach with decreased morbidity and expedited recovery time. The initial concept of local excision has evolved to more advanced techniques incorporating new technologies to overcome some of the limitations of TAE. Transanal endoscopic surgery (TES) is a generalized term which encompasses various similar endoluminal techniques: transanal endoscopic microsurgery (TEM), transanal minimally invasive surgery (TAMIS), robotic assisted transanal minimally invasive surgery (RATS), and transanal endoscopic operation (TEO).

The introduction of transanal endoscopic microsurgery (TEM) in 1983 in Germany by Dr. Buess created a new arena for transanal endoluminal surgical resection [2]. The TEM technique incorporated the use of an endoscope and pneumorectum which led to significant improvements in visualization and proximal reach compared to TAE. The TEM technique facilitated increased accuracy of resection margins as well as the preservation of intact, un-fragmented specimens. It offered similar functional outcomes with improved outcomes such as lower recurrence rates. However, TEM was slow to gain international interest due to the technical skill set necessary in a pre-laparoscopic proficiency era upon its birth in the 1980s, as well as the capital investment in specialized equipment with unknown projections on annual case volume. At the turn of the century, TEM gained increasing interest and implementation worldwide with improved minimally invasive training and experience, as well as a rise in the interest in natural orifice surgery. The development of TAMIS and disposable transanal access platforms followed shortly thereafter and led to an exponential rise in the implementation of the TES technique into surgical practice.

S. Wu • E.C. McLemore (✉)
General Surgery, Kaiser Permanente, Los Angeles Medical Center, Los Angeles, CA, USA
e-mail: Susana.Wu@kp.org; Elisabeth.C.McLemore@kp.org

C.M. Schlachta, P. Sylla (eds.), *Current Common Dilemmas in Colorectal Surgery*,
https://doi.org/10.1007/978-3-319-70117-2_7

Table 7.1 Local recurrence rates (%) for well or moderately differentiated tumors locally excised using TEM

Depth of invasion	Lymphatic invasion	Maximum invasive component tumor diameter (cm)					
		<1	1.1–2	2.1–3	3.1–4	4.1–5	>5.1
pT1 sm1	No	3.0	3.6	4.4	5.4	6.6	8.1
	Yes	5.2	6.4	7.7	9.4	11.4	13.7
pT1 sm2–3	No	10.5	12.7	15.3	18.5	22.1	26.4
	Yes	17.8	21.4	25.5	30.3	35.7	41.8
pT2	No	9.8	11.9	14.3	17.3	20.7	24.7
	Yes	16.7	20.0	23.9	28.5	33.7	39.5
pT3	No	19.7	23.6	28.0	32.2	39.0	45.4
	Yes	32.2	37.9	44.1	51.0	58.3	65.7

Values are percentages. *pT* pathological tumor stage, *sm* Kikuchi submucosal stage
Prospective National TEM database, 487 subjects with rectal cancer. Association of Coloproctology of Great Britain and Ireland TEM Collaboration (Adapted from data from Table 7 [3])

Indications

The predominant indication for TES is resection of benign and malignant rectal neoplasms including adenomatous polyps, intraepithelial neoplasia, carcinoid tumors, and early-stage rectal cancers (T1 lesions with favorable histology, Table 7.1) [3]. TES is frequently used for lesions that are not deemed to be endoscopically resectable [4]. TES has also became an appealing treatment option for patients who may be unable to tolerate radical proctectomy with total mesorectal excision due to advanced and higher-risk medical comorbidities.

There are distinct advantages of TES over traditional TAE, including the ability to resect more complex and proximal lesions. TAE is often limited to tumors less than 3–4 cm in size, located within 6–8 cm from the anal verge, and occupying less than 30% of the bowel circumference [5, 6]. In comparison, TES using the long channel transanal platforms can provide access to lesions up to 25 cm from the anal verge [7] as well as the ability to remove lesions greater than 4 cm [8]. Darwood et al. reported success in resection of complex lesions with minimal morbidity, including lesions beyond 15 cm from anal verge, lesions greater than 8 cm in size, lesions in previously dissected areas, and lesions involving two or more quadrants of the anal canal. In this study, the median hospital stay was 2 days, mean duration of surgery was 60 min, and the majority were benign (T0) lesions on final pathology [9].

Technique

Prior to undergoing TES, patients should undergo complete workup to establish the anatomic location of the lesion, technical feasibility, and appropriate clinical staging and application of TES. This includes endoscopy, endorectal ultrasound and/or rectal cancer protocol magnetic resonance imaging (MRI), and chest, abdomen, and pelvis cross-sectional imaging staging with computed tomography (CT) when indicated. A polyethylene glycol preoperative bowel preparation is recommended. The principal technique of TES involves three steps: (1) margin outline of the lesion (Fig. 7.1), (2) full-thickness versus submucosal resection with the goal of an intact specimen (Fig. 7.2), and (3) closure of the resultant defect (Fig. 7.3).

The patient is placed in lithotomy, prone, or lateral position depending on the location of the tumor for the TEM and TEO platforms. The lithotomy position can frequently be employed when using the disposable transanal access platforms. However, some tumor locations (especially the low anterior lesions) may be more easily removed in the prone position regardless of the transanal platform utilized. With TEM and TEO, the patient is positioned so the tumor is in the right lower quarter of the cross-sectional area of the proctoscope for optimal tissue handling and technical reach of the equipment. A 40 mm angled proctoscope (with various lengths from 12 to 25 cm) is attached to the faceplate with four ports. A 50° angled stereoscope is applied through one port, and the additional ports accommodate the suction, irrigation, insufflator, and working instruments. Most operating instruments are 5 mm with a downward deflection [4]. Pneumorectum starting at 15 mmHg is achieved through continuous insufflation, and the rectal pressure is monitored. The pressure may be increased to 20 mmHg pressure to optimize visualization.

The lesion is outlined with electrocautery with the goal of a 1 cm margin. The decision for a full-thickness versus a submucosal excision depends on the initial

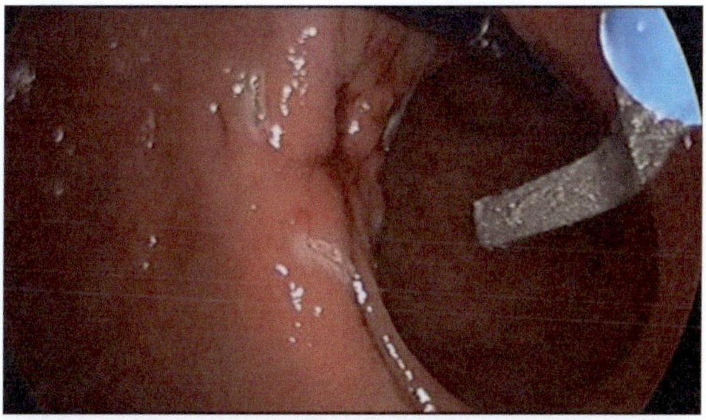

Fig. 7.1 Transanal endoluminal surgical resection of a rectal lesion—margin outline

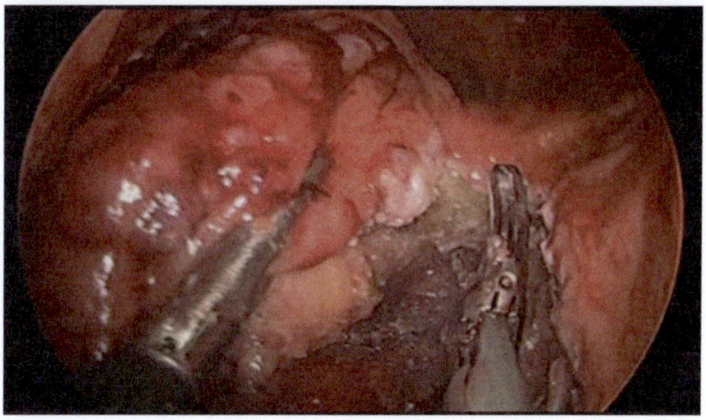

Fig. 7.2 Transanal endoluminal surgical resection of a rectal lesion—endoluminal resection

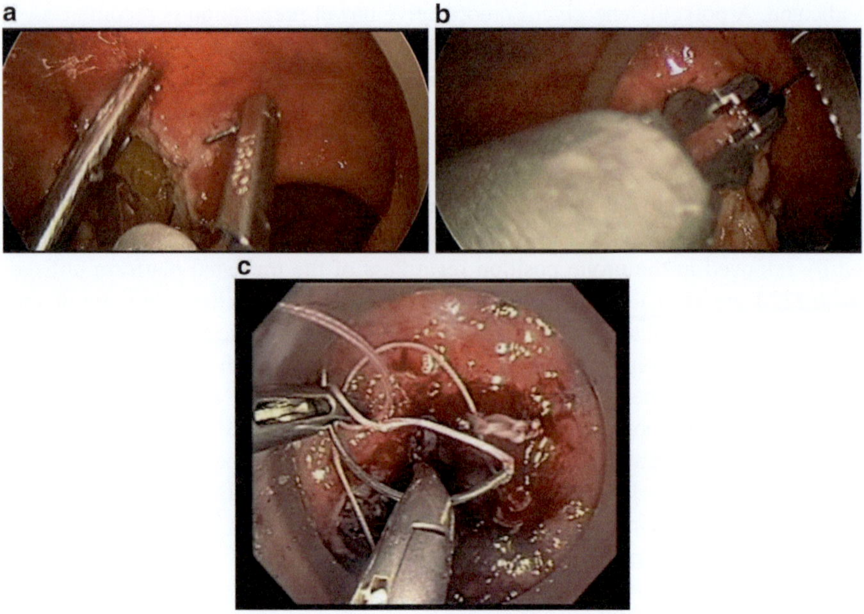

Fig. 7.3 Transanal endoluminal surgical resection of a rectal lesion—defect closure. (**a**) Laparoscopic suture assist device. (**b**) Laparoscopic knot assist device. (**c**) Laparoscopic suture closure

pathologic diagnosis and clinical findings. A full-thickness excision is recommended for malignant or potentially malignant lesions. The lesion is typically dissected from the distal to proximal edge, with a grasper used to elevate the lesion as dissection proceeds. Submucosal dissection may be appropriate for benign lesions or more proximal lesions at high risk for intraperitoneal entry with full-thickness resection. It is generally recommended to close the defect in order to become facile with the closure technique and be prepared for a peritoneal entry defect closure. With the TEM technique, metal beads act as suture knot surrogates as it can be difficult to tie a knot endoluminally, given the limited working space. Additional surgical suturing and knot devices exist for the TAMIS platforms as well.

Different equipment is utilized for the various TES techniques. The initial TAMIS technique was performed using a single-port laparoscopic device (SILS™, Covidien/Medtronic). Many other disposable platforms have been developed in order to facilitate the TAMIS technique. With the TAMIS technique, a transanal access disposable platform is utilized, and instrumentation includes readily available laparoscopic equipment including a 30 or 45° laparoscope with right-angle light cord adaptor for visualization and standard laparoscopic instruments and suction irrigation to work with. The patient can be positioned in lithotomy rather than a tumor-dependent position for most cases due to the flexibility of the disposable transanal access platforms and 360 degree view. TEM is limited to a 220° view provided by the proctoscope [6]. The advantage of the 30 or 45 degree laparoscope is that it allows better visualization of proximal lesions. Some surgeons may opt to use an endoscope rather than a laparoscope for visualization as the lens can be readily cleaned, as well as the submucosal injection and retraction with biopsy forceps capabilities of the endoscope [10, 11]. The learning curve is less steep for TES in the modern era as more surgeons are comfortable with conventional laparoscopic equipment and basic laparoscopic skillsets [12].

Postoperative care varies according to lesion size, lesion location, medical comorbidities, and surgical practice. Oral intake is generally resumed on the same day of the procedure. A majority of patients will stay for at least 24 h observation. However, same day discharge is also a common practice for small lesions removed with TES in young, healthy patients who reside locally.

Complications

The complication rates for TES are variable, ranging from 7.2 to 29% [13–16]. Common postoperative complications include bleeding, suture line dehiscence, rectal pain, and/or spasm. Late complications include anal stricture, rectourethral fistula, rectovaginal fistula, and local recurrence. Pelvic nerve injury can lead to functional complications such as urinary retention, fecal incontinence, and impotence. Anal dysfunction is of particular interest due to its negative impact on quality of life for patients. Jin et al. performed postoperative anal manometry on patients at 1 week, 2 weeks, 3 months, and 6 months after TEM for benign and malignant rectal tumors. The authors found an initial decrease in anal resting pressure from preoperative levels. However, resting pressures eventually returned to preoperative levels, and anal function was well preserved [17]. Platz et al. suggest the risk factors that may be associated with anal dysfunction are tumor location greater than 8 cm from anal verge, large tumor size (greater than 2–4 cm), and prolonged duration of surgery (greater than 2 h) [18].

Results

Although local excision is favorable for reduced operative morbidity compared to radical proctectomy with total mesorectal excision, high recurrence rates after transanal excision (TAE) precluded its standardization as the preferred oncologic treatment of early-stage rectal neoplastic lesions [1]. Nash et al. compared TAE and radical resection for patients with T1 rectal cancer limited to the distal 12 cm of the rectum and found a higher recurrence rate for transanal excision: 13.2% compared to 2.7% [19]. However, TEM has demonstrated lower local recurrence rates compared to TAE for benign disease and favorable T1 rectal cancers. A retrospective review of patients with early-stage rectal cancers treated with TAE or TEM demonstrated high estimated 5-year local recurrence rate with TAE (29.1%) and TEM (15.4%). Sixteen percent of patients who underwent TAE had positive margins compared to 2% of patients who underwent TEM. The authors also noted that patients with low tumors, within 5 cm of the anal verge, tended to have decreased disease-free survival compared to tumors above 5 cm from the anal verge [13]. Caution should be employed when using TES for malignant rectal lesions.

Long-term follow-up after TEM also demonstrates fewer local recurrences when compared to TAE. Junginger et al. evaluated 133 patients who underwent TEM for low-risk rectal carcinoma. The median follow-up was 8.6 years. The local recurrence rates after complete resection, as defined by resection margins >1 mm, were 6.6% and 11.6% at 5 and 10 years, respectively. For patients with high-risk or incompletely resected carcinomas, the local recurrence rates at 5 and 10 years were 32.5% and 35%, respectively. The authors report cure rates by TEM alone to be 93% for the low-risk rectal cancer group and 78% for the high-risk rectal cancer group [20]. Again, caution should be employed when using TES for malignant rectal lesions as these oncologic outcomes are less favorable than that achieved with radical proctectomy and total mesorectal excision for early-stage rectal cancers.

The current recommendation for TES management of rectal cancer is caution, careful selection of favorable T1 rectal cancers, and informed consent. With increasing T stage, the likelihood of nodal disease increases, and higher recurrence rates are noted. Therefore, T1 tumors without nodal involvement may be the most appropriate for TES [3]. However, if the final pathology demonstrates a positive margin, higher-risk histologic features such as lymphovascular invasion, tumor budding, high grade, or ≥T2 lesions, the patient should proceed with completion radical proctectomy with total mesorectal excision typically performed 8–12 weeks after TES in order to minimize rectal retraction perforation during salvage radical proctectomy. This will allow adequate staging and will guide the recommendation for systemic therapy if indicated [21–23].

TEM alone for advanced stage rectal neoplasms is inadequate. Local excision alone for T2 and T3 disease each has greater than 20% recurrence rate and significantly decreased survival compared to radical resection. Rullier et al. conducted a retrospective series, identifying a marked decrease in recurrence rate for T2 and T3 disease after neoadjuvant therapy and local excision, 7%, compared to local excision and adjuvant therapy, 15–20%. The authors maintain that neoadjuvant therapy and local excision should only be offered to very select T2 and T3 rectal cancer patients, namely, those greater than 75 years old with a mortality rate >10% and potentially for younger patients with major comorbidities [24].

TES vs EMR and ESD

The significant advantages of TES compared to radical resection are organ preservation, reduced morbidity, and reduced hospitalization. This thinking led to studies evaluating whether endoscopic mucosal resection offers reduced morbidity, operative costs, and length of hospital stay compared to TES, while maintaining similar outcomes. Van Den Broek et al. suggest piecemeal endoscopic mucosal resection is equally as effective as TES, with decreased length of hospital stay and fewer complications. The postoperative complication rate for TES was 28% compared to 9.8%

for EMR. While initial recurrence rates were higher for EMR compared to TES (16% vs 2.9%), no difference was found in late recurrence rate after endoscopic resection of the remnant lesion (10.5% vs 9.3% for EMR and TEM, respectively) [25]. It is difficult to determine if two or more outpatient endoscopic procedures are associated with a lower cost than one surgical procedure. In addition, patients lost to follow-up will be at risk for untreated local recurrence. Patients managed with EMR should be followed with a stringent protocol and safety net to ensure appropriate follow-up and screening.

Endoscopic submucosal dissection (ESD) offers similar decreased hospital length of stay and morbidity comparable to EMR with a greater likelihood of achieving an en bloc resection. However, the ESD technique has a steep learning curve and requires a prolonged endoscopic procedure time as well as specialized equipment and training. In experienced hands, endoscopic submucosal dissection achieves comparable en bloc resection rates and outcomes as TES [26, 27]. However, these studies were limited by small sample size [26, 27]. A meta-analysis which included 2077 patients from 11 ESD to 10 TEM studies demonstrated a higher rate of en bloc resection with TEM (98.7%) compared to ESD (87.8%) and higher R0 resection rate for TEM (88.5%) compared to ESD (74.6%) [28]. At this time, ESD may be an adequate alternative to TES in well-selected lesions and experienced hands, especially in more proximal lesions of the colon where TES is not feasible and an organ sparing approach is preferred.

Beyond Endoluminal Resection

Increasing experience and comfort with TES have led to additional applications of the technique. Case reports have demonstrated successful use of TES for treatment of pelvic abscesses, anorectal fistulas, rectourethral fistulas, rectovaginal fistulas, control of gastrointestinal hemorrhage, low pelvic anastomotic leak, anastomotic strictures, and foreign body retrieval [29–32].

References

1. Albert M, et al. Minimally invasive anorectal surgery: from parks local excision to transanal endoscopic microsurgery to transanal minimally invasive surgery. Sem Colon Rectal Surg. 2013;24(1):42–9.
2. Buess BF. Local surgical treatment of rectal cancer. Eur J Cancer. 1995;31A:1233–7.
3. Bach SP, Jill J, Monson JRT, Simson JNL, Lane L, Merrie A, Warren B, Mortensen NJ. A predictive model for local recurrence after transanal endoscopic microsurgery for rectal cancer. Br J Surg. 2009;96:280–90.
4. Cataldo PA. Transanal endoscopic microsurgery. Surg Clin North Am. 2006;86:915–25.
5. Rai V, Mishra N. Transanal approach to rectal polyps and cancer. Clin Colon Rectal Surg. 2016; 29(1):65–70.
6. Althumairi A, Gearhart SL. Local excision for early rectal cancer: transanal endoscopic microsurgery and beyond. J Gastrointest Oncol. 2015;6(3):296–306.
7. Whiteford M. Transanal endoscopic microsurgery (TEM) resection of rectal tumors. J Gastrointest Surg. 2007;11(2):155–7.

8. Khoury R, Duek SD, Issa N, Khoury W. Transanal endoscopic microsurgery for large benign rectal tumors; where are the limits? Int J Surg. 2016;29:128–31.
9. Darwood RJ, Wheeler JM, Borley NR. Transanal endoscopic microsurgery is a safe and reliable technique even for complex rectal lesions. Br J Surg. 2008;95(7):915–8.
10. McLemore EC, Weston LA, Coker AM, Jacobsen GR, Talamini MA, Horgan S, Ramamoorthy SL. Transanal minimally invasive surgery for benign and malignant rectal neoplasia. Am J Surg. 2014;208(3):372–81.
11. McLemore EC, Coker A, Jacobsen G, Talamini MA, Horgan S. eTAMIS: endoscopic visualization for transanal minimally invasive surgery. Surg Endosc. 2013;27(5):1842–5.
12. Seva-Pereira G, Tomagnolo L, Filho J, Bolzam-Nascimiento R, Pedroso de Moraes S, Ribeiro G. Transanal minimally invasive surgery (TAMIS) for local excision of selected rectal neoplasms: efficacy and outcomes in the first 11 patients. J Coloproctol. 2014;34(3):148–53.
13. Christoforidis D, Cho HM, Dixon MR, Mellgren AF, Madoff RD, Finne CO. Transanal endoscopic microsurgery versus conventional transanal excision for patients with early rectal cancer. Ann Surg. 2009;249(5):776–8.
14. Ganai S, Kanumuri P, Rao RS, Alexander AI. Local recurrence after transanal endoscopic microsurgery for rectal polyps and early cancers. Ann Surg Oncol. 2006;13(4):547–56.
15. van Vledder MG, et al. Transanal excision of benign rectal polyps: indications, technique, and outcomes. Sem Colon Rectal Surg. 2015;26(1):9–14.
16. Moraes Rda S, Malafaia O, Telles JE, Trippia MA, Buess GF, Coelho JC. Transanal endoscopic microsurgery in the treatment of rectal tumors: a prospective study in 50 patients. Arq Gastroenterol. 2008;45(4):268–74.
17. Jin Z, Yin L, Xue L, Lin M, Zheng Q. Anorectal functional results after transanal endoscopic microsurgery in benign and early malignant tumors. World J Surg. 2010;34(5):1128–32.
18. Platz J, Cataldo P. Functional outcomes following transanal rectal surgery. Sem Colon Rectal Surg. 2015;26(1):41–4.
19. Nash GM, Weiser MR, Guillem JG, et al. Long-term survival after transanal excision of T1 rectal cancer. Dis Colon Rectum. 2009;52:577–82.
20. Junginger T, Goenner U, Hitzler M, Trinh TT, Heintz A, Wollschlaeger D, Blettner M. Long-term oncologic outcome after transanal endoscopic microsurgery for rectal carcinoma. Dis Colon Rectum. 2016;59(1):8–15.
21. Chow O, Smith J, Gollub M, Garcia-Aguilar J. Transanal surgery for cT1 rectal cancer: patient selection, technique, and outcomes. Sem Colon Rectal Surg. 2015;26(1):20–5.
22. Perez RO, Habr-Gama A, São Julião GP, Proscurshim I, Fernandez LM, de Azevedo RU, Vailati BB, Fernandes FA, Gama-Rodrigues J. Transanal endoscopic microsurgery (TEM) following neoadjuvant chemoradiation for rectal cancer: outcomes of salvage resection for local recurrence. Ann Surg Oncol. 2016;23(4):1143–8.
23. Borstlap W, Coeymans T, Tanis P, MArijnen C, Cunningham C, Bemelman W, Tuynman J. Meta-analysis of oncologic outcomes after local excision of pT1-T2 rectal cancer requiring adjuvant (chemo)radiotherapy or completion surgery. Br J Surg. 2016. https://doi.org/10.1002/bjs.10163.
24. Rullier E, Denost Q. Transanal surgery for cT2T3 rectal cancer: patient selection, adjuvant therapy, and outcomes. Sem Colon Rectal Surg. 2015;26(1):26–31.
25. Den Broek V, Frank J, et al. Endoscopic mucosal resection appears equally effective, but is associated with less morbidity than transanal endoscopic microsurgery for the treatment of large rectal adenomas. Gastrointest Endosc. 2009;69(5):AB288.
26. Park S, Min Y, Park Y, Chang D, Kim Y, Kim J, Kim J, Lee W, Yun S, Kim H, Cho Y, Chun H. Comparison of clinical outcomes between the endoscopic submucosal dissection and the transanal endoscopic microsurgery for early rectal cancers. Gastrointest Endosc. 2012;73(4):AB305.
27. Kawaguti F, Nahas CS, Marques CF, Martins BC, Retes FA, Medeiros RS, Hayashi T, Wada Y, de Lima MS, Uemura RS, Nahas SC, Kudo SE, Maluf-Filho F. Endoscopic submucosal dissection versus transanal endoscopic microsurgery for the treatment of early rectal cancer. Surg Endosc. 2014;28(4):1173–9.

28. Arezzo A, Passera R, Saito Y, Sakamoto T, Kobayashi N, Sakamoto N, Yoshida N, Naito Y, Fujishiro M, Niimi K, Ohya T, Ohata K, Okamura S, Iizuka S, Takeuchi Y, Uedo N, Fusaroli P, Bonino MA, Verra M, Morino M. Systematic review and meta-analysis of endoscopic submucosal dissection versus transanal endoscopic microsurgery for large noninvasive rectal lesions. Surg Endosc. 2014;28(2):427–38.
29. Sneider E, Maykel J. Management of anastomotic leak after low anterior resection with transanal endoscopic microsurgical (TEM) debridement and repair. J Surg Case Rep. 2012;2012(9):1.
30. Kato K, Saito T, Matsuda M, Imai M, Kasai S, Mito M. Successful treatment of a rectal anastomotic stenosis by transanal endoscopic microsurgery (TEM) using the contact Nd:YAG laser. Surg Endosc. 1997;11(5):485–7.
31. Fichera A, Zoccali M. Transanal endoscopic microsurgery for recurrent lower gastrointestinal bleeding. SAGES. 2012; Session Number: VidTV2; Program Number: V101.
32. Szczepkowski M, Przywózka A, Zieliński T. Removal of gallstone from mesorectum after laparoscopic cholecystectomy – new indication for transanal endoscopic microsurgery technique. Videosurg Min Tech. 2015;10(4):580–3. https://doi.org/10.5114/wiitm.2015.56494.

Part III

Emergency Bowel Surgery

The 3 A.M. Laparoscopic Bowel Surgery: Selection, Preparation and Techniques

8

O.N.M. Panton

Introduction

Laparoscopic management of acute colorectal diseases and trauma is slowly evolving despite the fact that scheduled laparoscopic surgery has become the gold standard for many procedures such as cholecystectomy and anti-reflux surgery [1, 2]. Laparoscopic colorectal surgery is not inferior to open surgery for curable cancer [3]. Surgeons have been slow to adopt emergency colorectal surgical techniques because of the learning curve, technical challenges with access, adhesiolysis, purulent abdominal contamination, loss of domain related to inflammation and bowel distension and lack of evidence to support adoption. Organizing after-hours laparoscopic surgery poses challenges with operating room access, team composition and equipment especially in rural hospitals. Team composition has been demonstrated to influence operative performance [4].

Advances in technology have facilitated performance of more difficult advanced laparoscopic surgery. Hand ports were introduced in the 1990s, and hand-assisted emergency colectomy is an alternative to open colectomy [5]. The availability of ultrasonic and bipolar energy sources facilitates safe efficient dissection and vessel sealing.

Patient Selection

Patient selection is key to the successful management of patients with acute colorectal disease. Relative contraindications include obesity, extensive adhesions due to multiple prior abdominal operations, bleeding dyscrasias and inability to tolerate the carbon dioxide pneumoperitoneum. Haemodynamic instability secondary to

O.N.M. Panton (✉)
Division of General Surgery, Vancouver General Hospital, Vancouver, BC, Canada
e-mail: neely.panton@vch.ca

C.M. Schlachta, P. Sylla (eds.), *Current Common Dilemmas in Colorectal Surgery*,
https://doi.org/10.1007/978-3-319-70117-2_8

haemorrhagic shock or sepsis is a contraindication for laparoscopic management [1]. Emergency colectomy is associated with a higher mortality in immunosuppressed patients [6]. Distended small and large bowels due to ileus or mechanical obstruction may compromise abdominal domain and are relative contraindications.

Preparation

With respect to preoperative management, the standard approach to performing emergency abdominal surgery is applicable when considering a laparoscopic approach. Anaesthetic consultation and a strategic plan discussion with the operative nursing team are vital. Preparation of the operating room is second only to patient selection in the priority order. Modern laparoscopic towers, high-resolution videolaparoscopy (VL), trocars to permit insertion of all required instruments, needle drivers, retrieval bags, haemostatic clips, efficient suction and irrigation devices, advanced instrumentation including angled scopes, hand ports (HP), vessel-sealing devices, endoscopic staplers and smoke evacuation devices are essential. The patient must be secured to the operating table to permit extremes of positioning. Lithotomy position is key for trans-anal stapling.

Specific Applications

Emergency laparoscopic colectomy is currently performed for lower GI bleeding, colonic obstruction including cancer, iatrogenic perforation, complicated diverticulitis and inflammatory bowel disease [1, 2, 5, 7].

Diverticular Perforation

In the pre-laparoscopic era, exteriorization or resection with colostomy was recommended for perforated diverticulitis [8, 9]. The surgical approach to the management of diverticulitis has changed radically in the past decade [1]. Twenty years ago laparoscopic peritoneal lavage in combination with intravenous antibiotics was introduced as an alternative to resection with stoma formation in Hinchey III diverticulitis [10]. In most patients with perforated diverticulitis and generalized peritonitis, there is no evidence of faecal contamination. At the time of surgery, the perforation has sealed or cannot be found [11].

Nineteen articles were published between 1996 and 2013 addressing laparoscopic peritoneal lavage. Ten were cohort studies, eight case series and one controlled clinical trial reporting a success rate of 24.3%. The overall conversion rate for Hinchey III and IV was 1% and 45%, respectively. The 30-day mortality was 2.9% [2]. The first results from the randomized controlled trial DIverticulitis-LAparoscopic LAvage versus resection (DILALA) comparing peritoneal lavage versus Hartmann resection demonstrated no difference in morbidity and mortality

[12]. The Ladies trial was split into two arms: the LOLA arm comparing laparoscopic lavage with sigmoidectomy and the DIVA arm comparing Hartmann resection with sigmoidectomy plus primary anastomosis. Between July 1, 2010 and February 22, 2013, 90 patients were randomly assigned in the LOLA arm of the trial. The study was terminated by the data and safety monitoring board because of an increased event rate in the lavage group. By 12 months four patients had died after lavage and six after sigmoidectomy ($p = 0.43$) [13]. Because the safety of laparoscopic lavage for purulent or faecal peritonitis remains to be proven, these patients require close monitoring for postoperative complications [14]. This approach will be further elaborated in a subsequent chapter.

Hinchey II classification patients with planned intravenous antibiotics and percutaneous drainage management are potentially candidates for laparoscopic drainage if the percutaneous drainage fails or is not feasible (Fig. 8.1).

Complicated sigmoid diverticulitis can be managed with laparoscopic resection (LR) or hand-assisted laparoscopic surgical (HALS) resection with primary anastomosis. Ureteric stents aid identification and preservation of the ureters. HALS facilitates exposure, retraction and dissection. Port placement is optional. The author's preference is to place the hand port in a lower epigastric midline incision. A 5 mm trocar is inserted in a right lateral position for the VL, and a 12 mm trocar is placed in the right lower quadrant for dissecting and stapling and a 5 mm suprapubic trocar for smoke evacuation, dissection and retraction (Fig. 8.2).

Current evidence indicates that HALS reduces operating time and conversion rates [16]. Surgeons who prefer LR have the established options of Veress needle technique, Hasson technique or optical trocar entry for access and establishing the pneumoperitoneum. Trocar size and placement are similar to scheduled colectomy. Additional ports may be required for visualization, retraction and dissection (Fig. 8.3). Port placement for complicated right-sided diverticulitis is shown in Fig. 8.4 and can be configured according to surgeon preference.

Laparoscopic Hartmann resection remains an option if anastomosis is deemed unsafe by the surgeon. Hartmann colostomy closure is associated with significant morbidity and mortality. A significant percentage of these patients do not have colostomy reversal [2, 15, 16].

Obstructing Cancers

Obstructing right colon cancer can be managed with LR or HALS techniques. Comparative studies have reported smaller incisions, less blood loss and earlier recovery in comparison to open right hemicolectomy [17, 18]. The author places the HP in a midline sub-umbilical position, a 5 mm trocar adjacent to the HP for dissecting and a 5 mm left subcoastal trocar for the VL. Five millimeter right upper and right lateral abdominal ports are necessary for insufflation and smoke evacuation when using 5 mm instruments but not essential if 10 mm trocars are used (Fig. 8.5). The VL and instruments can be repositioned to facilitate visibility and surgical performance. Port placement for LR is discussed above.

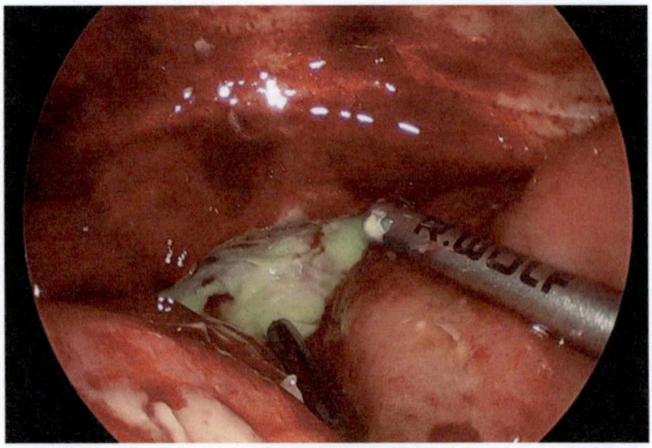

Fig. 8.1 Laparoscopic drainage of sigmoid diverticular abscess

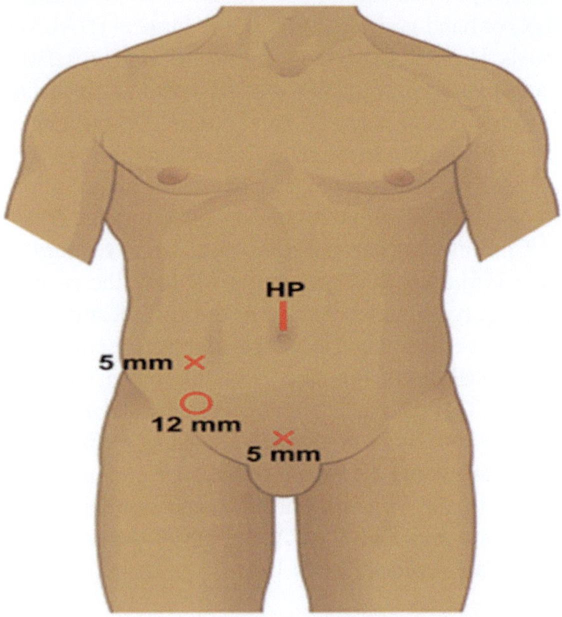

Fig. 8.2 Hand-port and trocar placement for HALS sigmoid resection

Emergency left colon resections can also be managed by LR or HALS. Trocar placement was previously described. Stenting of these tumours is an option allowing decompression, mechanical preparation and scheduled surgery [19]. A prospective multicentre trial from Japan reported clinical and technical success rates of 95.5% and 97.9%, respectively, in 513 cases. Of these 71.8% were left colon tumours [20]. Another Japanese prospective multicentre study on stents as a bridge to surgery reported technical and clinical success rates of 98 and 92%, respectively; elective surgery was performed in 297 patients and emergency surgery in eight patients for complications. Open and laparoscopic surgery was performed in 121 and 184 patients, respectively [21].

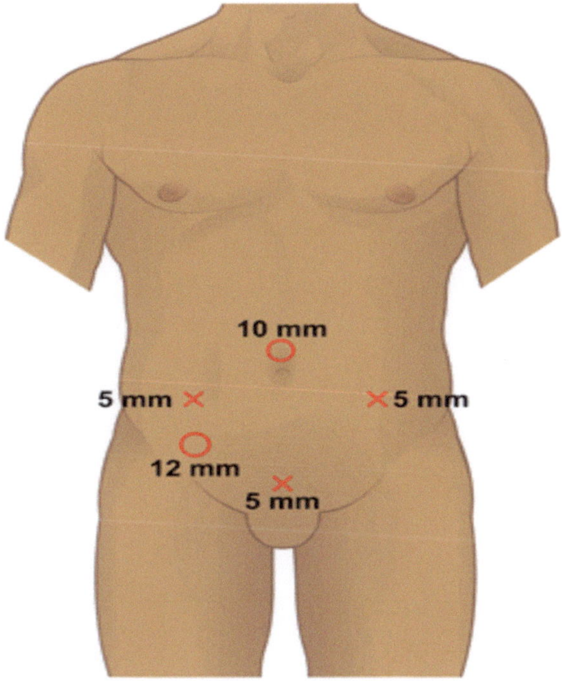

Fig. 8.3 Port placement for laparoscopic sigmoid and left colon resection

Inflammatory Bowel Disease

In the elective setting, laparoscopic surgery has been shown to be a safe alternative to open resection for Crohn's disease and ulcerative colitis with faster recovery and shorter length of stay. Laparoscopic colon surgery in the emergency setting for inflammatory bowel disease has been reported, but there is a lack of high-level data. Most studies reporting management of Crohn's disease and inflammatory bowel disease are case-matched. Published data reports shorter hospital stay, increased operating room time and morbidity which is equivalent or better than open surgery [19].

Colonoscopic Perforations

Colonoscopic perforations are fortunately rare but can result in serious complications. The incidence for diagnostic colonoscopy is between 0.03–0.8% and 0.15–3% for therapeutic interventions. Laparoscopic management has been reported since the 1990s. Surgical techniques include primary sutured or stapled repairs, segmental resection and resection with diversion in contaminated cases. Enhanced recovery, smaller incisions and reduction in morbidity are reported outcome improvements in comparison to open surgery [22, 23]. A large retrospective Korean study reviewed 48,088 colonoscopies with 28 (0.06%) perforations. Thirteen patients from other centres were enrolled. Fourteen patients had diagnostic and 27

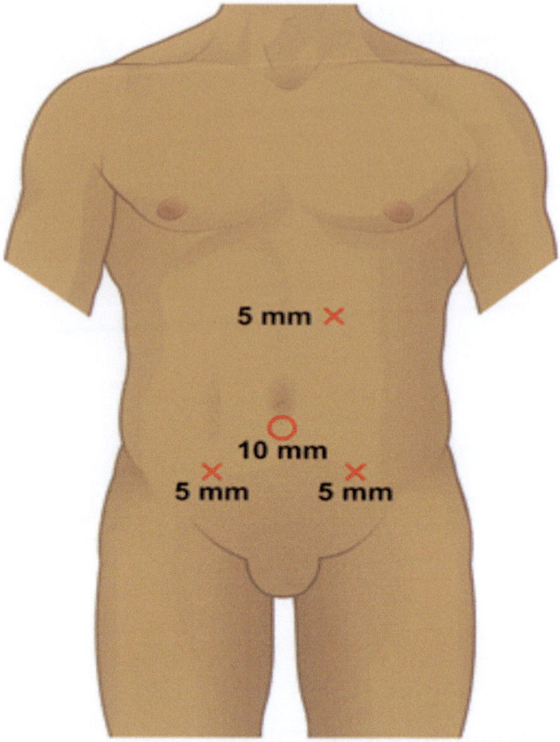

Fig. 8.4 Port placement for right hemicolectomy

therapeutic colonoscopy. Conservative management was attempted in 20 patients and successful in 90%. Endoscopic clipping was done in nine patients with a success rate of 78%. Twenty-one patients underwent surgery plus two failures after conservative therapy. Eight patients were managed laparoscopically, five had primary closure and three had segmental colectomy. One patient in the laparotomy group required a second laparotomy for leakage. Fifty-six percent of perforations were in the rectum and sigmoid colon. The laparoscopic group had faster recovery and fewer adverse events [24].

Small Bowel Obstruction

Laparoscopic adhesiolysis for mechanical small bowel obstruction is a well-established option in selected patients. Safe abdominal access can be challenging in the patient with multiple prior laparotomies; loss of domain due to the distended bowel can make visibility and dissection difficult. Mechanical intestinal obstruction is associated with intra-abdominal hypertension and compartment syndrome. Correa-Martin et al. conducted a mechanical obstruction study in a porcine model similar to the human pathophysiology. Systemic vascular resistance, central venous pressure, pulse pressure variation, airway resistance and lactate increased within 2 h

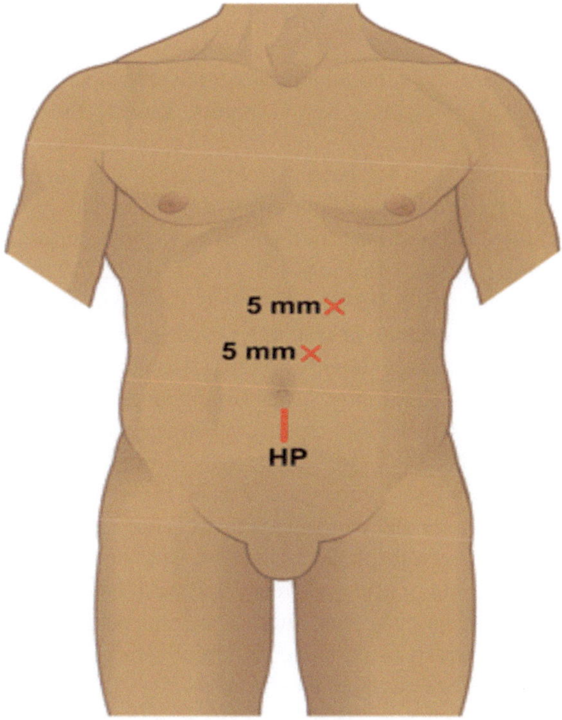

Fig. 8.5 Hand-port and trocar placement for HALS right hemicolectomy

from starting intra-abdominal hypertension [26]. Theoretically the pneumoperitoneum could aggravate intra-abdominal hypertension and lead to gut ischaemia.

Okamoto et al. reported 28 patients undergoing laparoscopic adhesiolysis comparing outcomes with 25 patients undergoing conventional laparotomy [27]. Laparoscopic adhesiolysis was completed in 89% of patients; operating time was 112 min in the laparoscopic group and 79 in the open group. Patients in the laparoscopic group resumed oral intake at 3 days versus 6.5 in the open group, and length of stay was shorter for the laparoscopic group. Complications were higher in the open group.

Kelly et al. reported a large series of small bowel obstruction cases selected from the ACS National Surgical Quality Improvement Program [28]. There were 9619 cases included in the analysis; 14.9% had laparoscopic adhesiolysis. Patients in the laparoscopic group had shorter operating times and decreased postoperative length of stay. After controlling for comorbidities and surgical factors, the laparoscopic group was less likely to develop major complications and incision complications. The 30-day mortality was 1.3% in the laparoscopic group versus 4.7% in the open group.

Byrne et al. reported a cohort of 269 patients with mechanical small bowel obstruction [29]. One hundred and eighty six had open and 83 laparoscopic adhesiolysis. 38.65% of the laparoscopic group were converted to open surgery. Recovery was faster and complications lower in the laparoscopic group.

Conclusions

In the last 25 years, surgeons have adopted laparoscopic techniques for the management of emergency bowel surgery. Despite the fact that advanced laparoscopic scheduled surgery was introduced in the 1990s, the management of acute bowel conditions has not been disseminated to the same extent as scheduled colorectal surgery. The increased numbers of patients undergoing screening colonoscopy had resulted in increased numbers of iatrogenic perforations [24]. A national population-based study from the USA reviewed 22,719 non-elective colectomies between 2008 and 2011. 95.8% of patients had open management. Most cases were performed at urban non-teaching hospitals by general surgeons. Colorectal surgeons were more likely to perform laparoscopic surgery. Laparoscopic cases had significantly better mortality, lower complication rates, reduced length of stay and lower costs. Less than 5% of urgent and emergent colectomies in the USA were performed laparoscopically [25].

Adhesiolysis for mechanical small bowel resection is being reported with increasing frequency, but there are no prospective randomized series reported to date.

Surgeons must make a global effort to disseminate and incorporate laparoscopic management of acute colorectal and small bowel conditions in an attempt to provide better patient outcomes. Surgical training programmes will have to continue to train general laparoscopic surgeons to deliver optimal care for patients requiring interventions for colorectal emergencies.

References

1. Mandrioll M, Inaba K, Piccinini A, Biscardi A, Sartelli M, Agresta F, Catena F, Cirocchi R, Jovine E, Tugnoli G, Di Saverio S. Advances in laparoscopy for acute care surgery and trauma. World J of. Gastroenterology. 2016;22(2):668–80. https://doi.org/10.3748/wjg.v22.12.668.
2. Agresta F, Arezzo A, Allaix ME, Arolfo S, Anania G. Current status of laparoscopic colorectal surgery in the emergency setting. Updat Surg. 2016;68(1):47–52. https://doi.org/10.1007/s13304-016-0356-1.
3. Morneau M, Boulanger J, Charlebois P, Latulippe J-F, Lougnarath R, Thibault C, Gervais N. Laparoscopic versus open surgery for the treatment of colorectal cancer: a literature review and recommendations from the Comite de l'evolution des pratiques en oncologie. Can J Surg. 2013;56(5):297–310. https://doi.org/10.1503/cjs.005512.
4. Zheng B, Panton ON, Al-Tayeb TA. Operative length independently affected by surgical team size: data from 2 Canadian hospitals. Can J Surg. 2012;55(6):371–6. https://doi.org/10.1503/cjs.011311.
5. Watanabe K, Funayama Y, Fukushima K, Shibata C, Takahashi K, Sasaki I. Hand-assisted laparoscopic vs. open subtotal colectomy for severe ulcerative colitis. Dis Colon Rectum. 2009;52(4):640–5. https://doi.org/10.1007/DCR.0b013e1819d47b5.
6. Al-Khamis A, Abou Khalil J, Demian M, Morin N, Vasilevsky C, Gordon P, Boutros M. Sigmoid colectomy for acute diverticulitis in immunosuppressed vs immunocompetent patients: outcomes from the ACS-NSQIP database. Dis Colon Rectum. 2016;59(2):101–9. https://doi.org/10.1097/DCR.0000000000000513.
7. Koh F, Tan K, Tsang C, Koh D. Laparoscopic versus open colectomy in an emergency setting: a case-controlled study. Ann Coloproctol. 2013;29(1):12–6. https://doi.org/10.3393/ac.2013.29.1.12.

8. Hinchey E, Schaal P, Richards G. Treatment of perforated diverticular disease of the colon. Adv Surg. 1978;12:85–109.
9. Bell G, Panton ON. Hartmann resection for perforated sigmoid diverticulitis. A retrospective study of the Vancouver general hospital experience. Dis Colon Rectum. 1984;27(4):253–6.
10. O'Sullivan G, Murphy D, O'Brien M, Ireland A. Laparoscopic management of generalized peritonitis due to perforated colonic diverticula. Am J Surg. 1996;171(4):432–4.
11. Matheson KZ. Acute diverticulitis. Rec Adv Surg. 1988;13:125–41.
12. Angenete E, Thornell A, Burcharth J, Pommergaard H-C, Skullman S, Bisgaard T, Jess P, Lackberg Z, Matthiessen P, Heath J, Rosenberg J, Haglind E. Laparoscopic lavage is feasible and safe for the treatment of perforated diverticulitis with purulent peritonitis. The first results from the randomized controlled trial DILALA. Ann Surg. 2016;263(1):117–22. https://doi.org/10.1097/SLA.0000000000001061.
13. Vennix S, Musters G, Mulder I, Swank H, Consten E, Belgers E, van Geloven A, Gerhards M, Govaert M, van Grevenstein W, Hoofwijk A, Kruty P, Nienhuijs S, Boermeester M, Vermuelen J, van Dieren S, Lange J, Bemelman W, Ladies trial collaborators. Laparoscopic peritoneal lavage or sigmoidectomy for perforated diverticulitis with purulent peritonitis: a multicentre, parallel-group, randomised, open-label trial. Lancet. 2015;386(10000):1269–77. https://doi.org/10.1016/S0140-6736(15)61668-0.
14. Feingold D, Steele S, Lee S, Boushey R, Buie W, Rafferty J. Practice parameters for the treatment of sigmoid diverticulitis. Dis Colon Rectum. 2014;57(3):284–94. https://doi.org/10.1097/DCR.0000000000000075.
15. McDermott F, Collins D, Heeney A, Winter D. Minimally invasive and surgical management strategies tailored to the severity of acute diverticulitis. Br J Surg. 2014;101(1):e90–9. https://doi.org/10.1002/bjs2014.101.issue-1/issuetoc.
16. Aalbers A, Biere S, van Berge Henegouwen M, Bamelman W. Hand-assisted or laparoscopic approach in colorectal surgery: a systematic review and meta-analysis. Surg Endosc. 2008;22(8):1769–80. https://doi.org/10.1007/s00464-008-9857-4.
17. Ng S, Lee J, Yiu R, Leung W, Leung K. Emergency laparoscopic-assisted versus open right hemicolectomy for obstructing right-sided colonic carcinoma: a comparative study of short-term clinical outcomes. World J Surg. 2008;32(3):454–8. https://doi.org/10.1007/s00268-007-9400-0.
18. Li Z, Li D, Jie Z, Zhang G, Liu Y. Comparative study on therapeutic efficacy between hand-assisted laparoscopic surgery and conventional laparotomy for acute obstructive right-sided colon cancer. J Laparoendosc Adv Surg Tech. 2015;25(7):548–54. https://doi.org/10.1089/lap.2014.0645.
19. Chand M, Siddiqui M, Gupta A, Rasheed S, Tekkis P, Parvaiz A, Mirnezami A, Qureshi T. Systematic review of emergent laparoscopic colorectal surgery for benign and malignant disease. World J Gastroenterol. 2014;20(45):16956–63. https://doi.org/10.3748/wjg.v20.i45.16956.
20. Matsuzawa T, Ishida H, Yoshida S, Isayama H, Kuwai T, Maetani I, Shimada M, Yamada T, Saito S, Tomita M, Koizumi K, Hirata N, Sasaki T, Enomoto T, Saida YA. Japanese prospective multicentre study of self-expandable metal stent placement for malignant colorectal obstruction: short-term safety and efficacy within 7 days of stent procedure in 513 cases. Gastrointest Endosc. 2015;82(4):697–707. 10.10161/j.gie.2015.03.1978. Epub 2015 May 12
21. Saito S, Yoshida S, Isayama H, Matsuzawa T, Kuwai T, Maetani I, Shimada M, Yamada T, Tomita M, Koizumi K, Hirata N, Kanazawa H, Enomoto T, Sekido H, Saida Y. A prospective multicentre study on self-expandable metallic stents as a bridge to surgery for malignant colorectal obstruction in Japan: efficacy and safety in 312 patients. Surg Endosc. 2015;30(9):3976–86.
22. Makarawo T, Damadi A, Mittal V, Itawi E, Rana G. Colonoscopic perforation managed by laparoendoscopy: an algorithm. JSLS. 2014;18(1):20–7. https://doi.org/10.4293/108680813x13693422518759.
23. Bleier J, Moon V, Feingold D, Whelan R, Arnell T, Sonoda T, Milsom J, Lee S. Initial repair of iatrogenic colon perforation using laparoscopic methods. Surg Endosc. 2008;22(3):646–9.

24. Shin D, Shin S, Park C, Jin S, Cho Y, Kim W, Kwon C, Ko K, Hahm K, Park P, Kim J, Hong S. Optimal methods for the management of iatrogenic colonoscopic perforation. Clin Endosc. 2016;49(3):282–8. https://doi.org/10.5946/ce.2015.046.
25. Keller D, Pedraza R, Flores-Gonzales J, LeFave J, Mahmood A, Haas E. The current status of emergent laparoscopic colectomy: a population-based study of clinical and financial outcomes. Surg Endosc. 2015;30(8):3321–6.
26. Correa–Martin I, Parraga E, Sanchez-Margallo FM, Latorre R, Lopez-Albors O, Wise R, Malbrain M, Castellanos G. Mechanical intestinal obstruction in a porcine model: effects of intra-abdominal hypertension. A preliminary study. PLoS One. 2016;11(2):e0148058. https://doi.org/10.1371/journal.pone.0148058.
27. Okamoto H, Wakana H, Kawashima K, Fukasawa T, Fujii H. Clinical outcomes of laparoscopic adhesiolysis for mechanical small bowel obstruction. Asian J Endosc Surg. 2012;5(2):53–8. https://doi.org/10.1111/j. 1758-5910.2011.0011.OOTT/.x.
28. Kelly K, Innauzzi J, Rickles A, Garimella V, Monson J, Fleming F. Laparotomy for small bowel obstruction: first choice or last resort for adhesiolysis? A laparoscopic approach for small bowel obstruction reduces 30-day complications. Surg Endosc. 2014;28(1):65–73. https://doi.org/10.1007/s00464-013-3162-6.
29. Byrne J, Saleh F, Ambrosini L, Quereshy F, Jackson T, Okrainec A. Laparoscopic versus open surgical management of adhesive small bowel obstruction: a comparison of outcomes. Surg Endosc. 2015;29(9):2525–32. https://doi.org/10.1007/s00464-014-4015-7.

Fulminant *Clostridium difficile* Colitis: Indications and Extent of Surgery

9

Nawar A. Alkhamesi

Introduction

Since its first isolation from the meconium of normal infants in 1935 [1], *Clostridium difficile* has become the focus of researchers and clinicians all over the world. *C. difficile* is an obligate Gram-positive, anaerobic, spore-forming, toxin-producing bacillus. It is the most common cause of nosocomial infection contributing to about 15–25% of all cases of antibiotic-associated diarrhea. Its incidence and associated morbidity and mortality are steadily rising in the Western communities with huge impact on human health outcomes and high economic burden [2–4]. However, 3–6% of the population are asymptomatic carriers, an incidence that could be even higher in people living in long-term care institutions [5].

Despite early isolation and successful characterization and culturing of *C. difficile* [6, 7], its identification as a cause of human infection was very late [8, 9]. It became clear that there is a direct correlation between antibiotic usage and the rate of *Pseudomembranous colitis* caused by *C. difficile* especially in surgical patients [10]. In the subsequent years, the term *C. difficile*-associated diarrhea (CDAD) was used, and most recently the term *C. difficile* infection (CDI) is preferred and became widely accepted [11].

Pathophysiology

C. difficile is transmitted via the oral-fecal route. Spores are dormant cells that are highly resistant to environmental conditions [11]. Once it reaches the human intestine, *C. difficile* spores can germinate into its vegetative state aided by the presence

N.A. Alkhamesi (✉)
Department of Surgery, University Hospital, London Health Sciences Centre, London, ON, Canada
e-mail: nalkham2@uwo.ca

C.M. Schlachta, P. Sylla (eds.), *Current Common Dilemmas in Colorectal Surgery*,
https://doi.org/10.1007/978-3-319-70117-2_9

of glycine and cholate derivatives. Normally, cholate derivatives are metabolized by the intestine normal flora; however, in patients receiving antibiotics, the natural microflora are either killed or disrupted which in turn reduce cholate metabolism and increase its availability for *C. difficile* spores to grow and germinate [4]. *C. difficile* pathogenicity is mediated by two exotoxins: toxin A (TcdA) and toxin B (TcdB). The introduction of these toxins to the host cells occurs in seven main steps that start by toxin binding to the cell surface receptors and then toxin internalization and subsequent inactivation of the cell enzymes resulting in toxin-induced cytopathic and cytotoxic effects leading to fulminant CDI [4].

Clinical Manifestation

In addition to antibiotic consumption, other risk factors associated with CDI include advanced age, immunosuppression, chronic renal disease, diabetes, malnutrition, and posttransplant patients. However, in the community-acquired CDI, proton pump inhibitor usage has been attributed to about 31% of *C. difficile* infection with no exposure to antibiotics [12]. The clinical symptoms associated with CDI range from asymptomatic carrier to mild, self-limiting diarrhea to fulminant colitis leading to toxic megacolon and perforation. Three or more watery non-bloody stools per 24-h period are the hallmark of symptomatic illness [13, 14]. This variation in symptoms and presentation resulted in possible disparity in severity assessment of this disease, which led to different criteria used in guidelines [11]. Recent guidelines by the American College of Gastroenterology and the European Society of Clinical Microbiology and Infectious Diseases defined mild CDI as *C. difficile* infection with diarrhea as the only clinical manifestation. Moderate CDI was characterized as *C. difficile* with diarrhea in addition to other symptoms/signs that do not meet the definition of severe CDI. The definition of severe CDI is *C. difficile* infection with any of the following: white cell count $\geq 15 \times 10^9$/L, hypoalbuminemia <30 g/L, or abdominal tenderness. Complicated or fulminant CDI is defined as *C. difficile* infection which presents with development during the course of CDI with at least one of the following: admission to ICU, hypotension with or without the use of vasopressors, temperature ≥ 38.5 °C, ileus or substantial abdominal distension, changes in the mental status, white cell count $\geq 35 \times 10^9$/L, serum lactate >2.2 mmol/L, or any evidence of end-organ failure [15, 16]. Although these criteria have not been validated yet, they could be used to direct patients' care in particular cases with severe and complicated CDI because the specificity of this index increases with each criterion [17–19].

Diagnosis

Accurate and quick diagnosis of CDI is challenging yet important in order to promptly implement therapeutic strategies to reduce morbidity and prevent mortality. The pillar of CDI diagnosis depends on the presence of clinical symptoms in addition to well-chosen laboratory assay to confirm the presence of toxin-producing *C. difficile* in the stool. Several unique assays are available, and these vary in cost, ease of performance, turnout time, and sensitivity and specificity [20]. The diagnostic tests for *C. difficile* can be classified into test for *C. difficile* products (toxins), culture methods (toxigenic culture), and nucleic acid amplification tests for *C. difficile* genes. The test selection is vital to distinguish between patients with CDI and asymptomatic carriers [11]. It is also vital to exclude other viral and bacterial causes of diarrhea particularly in high-risk communities [21]. Table 9.1 summarizes the diagnostic tests for C. *difficile*; however, accurate diagnosis requires an algorithm bundle of 2–3 tests in most cases.

Endoscopic confirmation of CDI is indicated when there is a high index of clinic suspicion of CDI with the absence of laboratory confirmation or there is a suspicion of other causes for the patient's symptoms or colitis. The finding of *Pseudomembranous colitis* on flexible sigmoidoscopy or colonoscopy is pathognomonic for *C. difficile* colitis. This can be confirmed with histopathological examination. The pseudomembranous appear as elevated yellowish-white plaques measuring 2–12 mm in diameter over and erythematous and edematous mucosa [22].

Radiological tests in CDI are neither sensitive nor specific for *C. difficile* colitis. X-ray findings include mucosal thickening, haustral fold thickening, and colonic distension. Computed tomography scan (CT scan) may show low-attenuation colonic mural thickening consistent with mucosal and submucosal edema, pancolitis, pericolonic fat stranding, pneumatosis coli, and free air and fluid in cases of perforation [23]. However, radiological test can be of value in monitoring patients' progress and response to treatment and may aid in surgical decision-making if non-operative strategies are failing.

Table 9.1 Summary of diagnostic tests for *Clostridium difficile*

Test	Indication	Turnaround time	Sensitivity/specificity
GDH-EIA	Initial screening test. Positive patients must undergo confirmation test for toxigenic infection	Less than 2 h	95–99%/80–90%
Toxin A and B—EIA	Confirmation test for GDH-positive patients	Less than 2 h	90–95%/94–98%
CTNA	Standard test for evidence of toxin in stool	24–48 h	98–100%/98–100%
NAAT of toxin genes	Confirmation test for toxigenic infection	15 min to 4 h	94–98%/80–90%
Anaerobic toxigenic culture	Gold standard for confirmation of toxigenic infection	3–5 days	100%/100%

GDH glutamate dehydrogenase, *EIA* enzyme immunoassay, *CTNA* cytotoxin neutralization assay, *NAAT* nucleic acid amplification test

Management

The management of CDI generally speaking can be divided into nonoperative and operative approaches. It requires a multidisciplinary approach that involves many specialties. In addition to the admitting physician, colorectal/general surgery, microbiology and infectious diseases, gastroenterology, intensive care, and pharmacy should be involved in the patient's care. In this chapter, we will be concentrating on the operative approach. The nonoperative and colon-preserving management will be discussed in a subsequent chapter.

Due to the high mortality associated with fulminant CDI that can be as high as 80% in spite of surgical intervention, early surgical intervention has been advocated in severe and complicated cases. However, the role and timing of surgery in the management of CDI management remain controversial. This is partly due to the lack of a consensus by the surgeons on the indications of when to operate, with other factors being the delay in surgical consultation as most of these patients will be under the care of other specialists. The only clear and absolute indications for operative interventions are peritonitis and colonic perforation. Nonetheless, the latter occurs very late in the disease process, and by this time patients' outcome might be extremely compromised. It is important to understand that colonic ischemia and perforation are not inherent to the infection process and are the result of low blood flow caused by severe dehydration and the use of vasopressors or due to abdominal compartment syndrome. Other indications for surgery include failure of nonoperative therapy and clinical deterioration of critically ill patients, multiple organ failure, and toxic megacolon [17, 24]. What is clear from all the published data is that early surgical consultation and possible intervention are associated with lower morbidity and mortality and improved patients' outcomes [25]. This recommendation is mainly based on retrospective and observational studies due to the lack of randomized trials in this field caused by the difficulties in recruiting patients and subjecting them to potential harm caused by delaying surgical intervention.

Based on the disease process that usually involves the entire colon and the difficulty in macroscopically assessing the colon intraoperatively, the standard surgical intervention is total colectomy with end ileostomy. The procedure is usually performed via midline laparotomy owing to the urgent nature of the intervention and the clinical status of the sick patients. However, when the circumstances are favorable and the patient's clinical condition permits, laparoscopic total colectomy can be performed safely in the experienced hands. In both approaches, the author recommends leaving a rectal tube to drain the rectal stump and prevent blowout, which can lead to increased morbidity and mortality. Moreover, the tube can be used to deliver local therapies into the rectum in the very sick patients.

Another surgical approach that was developed in recent years is to perform loop ileostomy accompanied by intraoperative colonic lavage with glycol 3350/balanced electrolyte solution followed by regular antegrade colonic vancomycin flushes through the ileostomy [17]. The aim of this approach is to minimize surgical trauma in sick patients and preserve the colon. The procedure can be performed open or laparoscopic in a very short period. This technique is only recommended in moderate-to-severe cases with no signs or symptoms of perforation, peritonitis, ischemic bowel, or multi-organ failure and will be discussed in more details in Chap. 10. The treating physician should have a very low threshold in adopting the more traditional total colectomy approach if the patient is not responding in a timely manner or shows any signs of deterioration.

Conclusion

In spite of all the advances in screening, preventing, and management of *Clostridium difficile* infection, there has been a steady increase in the incidence, severity, and mortality rate, which could be correlated with the identification of newer strains of *Clostridium difficile* associated with more toxin production and increase cytotoxic activities. Medical treatment is still the gold standard in treating mild-to-moderate cases and occasionally severe infection; however, early surgical consultation and intervention, particularly in severe and complicated infection, have been shown to decrease morbidity and mortality and improve outcomes.

References

1. Hall I, O'Toole E. Intestinal flora in new-born infants with a description of a new pathogenic anaerobe, *Bacillus difficilis*. Am J Dis Child. 1935;49:390–402.
2. Poli A, Di Matteo S, Bruno GM, Fornai E, Valentino MC, Colombo GL. Economic burden of Clostridium difficile in five hospitals of the Florence health care system in Italy. Risk Manag Healthc Policy. 2015;8:207–13.
3. Li X, Wilson M, Nylander W, Smith T, Lynn M, Gunnar W. Analysis of morbidity and mortality outcomes in postoperative clostridium difficile infection in the veterans health administration. JAMA Surg. 2016;151(4):314–22.
4. Di Bella S, Ascenzi P, Siarakas S, Petrosillo N, di Masi A. Clostridium difficile toxins A and B: insights into pathogenic properties and extraintestinal effects. Toxins. 2016;8(5):134.
5. Clabots CR, Johnson S, Olson MM, Peterson LR, Gerding DN. Acquisition of Clostridium difficile by hospitalized patients: evidence for colonized new admissions as a source of infection. J Infect Dis. 1992;166(3):561–7.
6. Smith LD, King EO. Occurrence of Clostridium difficile in infections of man. J Bacteriol. 1962;84:65–7.
7. Hafiz S, Oakley CL. Clostridium difficile: isolation and characteristics. J Med Microbiol. 1976;9(2):129–36.
8. George RH, Symonds JM, Dimock F, Brown JD, Arabi Y, Shinagawa N, et al. Identification of clostridium difficile as a cause of pseudomembranous colitis. Br Med J. 1978;1(6114):695.
9. Kappas A, Shinagawa N, Arabi Y, Thompson H, Burdon D, Dimock F, et al. Diagnosis of pseudomembranous colitis. Br Med J. 1978;1(6114):675–8.
10. Talbot RW, Walker RC, Beart RW. Changing epidemiology, diagnosis, and treatment of Clostridium difficile toxin-associated colitis. Br J Surg. 1986;73(6):457–60.
11. Smits WK, Lyras D, Lacy DB, Wilcox MH, Kuijper EJ. Clostridium difficile infection. Nat Rev Dis Primers. 2016;2:16020.
12. Chitnis AS, Holzbauer SM, Belflower RM, Winston LG, Bamberg WM, Lyons C, et al. Epidemiology of community-associated Clostridium difficile infection, 2009 through 2011. JAMA Intern Med. 2013;173(14):1359–67.

13. Burnham CA, Carroll KC. Diagnosis of Clostridium difficile infection: an ongoing conundrum for clinicians and for clinical laboratories. Clin Microbiol Rev. 2013;26(3):604–30.
14. Burnham CA, Dubberke ER, Kociolek LK, Polage CR, Riley TV. Clostridium difficile-diagnostic and clinical challenges. Clin Chem. 2016;62(2):310–4.
15. Surawicz CM, Brandt LJ, Binion DG, Ananthakrishnan AN, Curry SR, Gilligan PH, et al. Guidelines for diagnosis, treatment, and prevention of Clostridium difficile infections. Am J Gastroenterol. 2013;108(4):478–98. quiz 99
16. Debast SB, Bauer MP, Kuijper EJ. Diseases ESoCMaI. European Society of Clinical Microbiology and Infectious Diseases: update of the treatment guidance document for Clostridium difficile infection. Clin Microbiol Infect. 2014;20(Suppl 2):1–26.
17. Kautza B, Zuckerbraun BS. The surgical management of complicated clostridium difficile infection: alternatives to colectomy. Surg Infect. 2016;17(3):337–42.
18. Ogielska M, Lanotte P, Le Brun C, Valentin AS, Garot D, Tellier AC, et al. Emergence of community-acquired Clostridium difficile infection: the experience of a French hospital and review of the literature. Int J Infect Dis. 2015;37:36–41.
19. Keller PM, Weber MH. Rational therapy of clostridium difficile infections. Viszeralmedizin. 2014;30(5):304–9.
20. Kociolek LK, Bovee M, Carter D, Ciolino JD, Patel R, O'Donnell A, et al. Impact of a health-care provider educational intervention on frequency of clostridium difficile polymerase chain reaction testing in children: a segmented regression analysis. J Pediatric Infect Dis Soc. 2016; 6(2):142–8.
21. Lübbert C. Antimicrobial therapy of acute diarrhoea: a clinical review. Expert Rev Anti-Infect Ther. 2016;14(2):193–206.
22. Ofosu A. Clostridium difficile infection: a review of current and emerging therapies. Ann Gastroenterol. 2016;29(2):147–54.
23. Ash L, Baker ME, O'Malley CM, Gordon SM, Delaney CP, Obuchowski NA. Colonic abnormalities on CT in adult hospitalized patients with Clostridium difficile colitis: prevalence and significance of findings. AJR Am J Roentgenol. 2006;186(5):1393–400.
24. Lübbert C, John E, von Müller L. Clostridium difficile infection: guideline-based diagnosis and treatment. Dtsch Arztebl Int. 2014;111(43):723–31.
25. Luciano JA, Zuckerbraun BS. Clostridium difficile infection: prevention, treatment, and surgical management. Surg Clin North Am. 2014;94(6):1335–49.

Fulminant *Clostridium difficile* Colitis: Colon-Preserving Therapies

10

Maria Abou Khalil and Marylise Boutros

Introduction

Clostridium difficile infection (CDI) can progress to a grave form of the disease characterized by severe colitis and multi-organ system failure referred to as fulminant *Clostridium difficile* colitis (FCDC). The current standard of care for FCDC is a timely total abdominal colectomy with end ileostomy (TAC). However, despite this early intervention, mortality rates remain high ranging from 34 to 57% in the literature [1–4]. Notwithstanding the high mortality associated with this procedure, a recent systematic review confirmed that TAC still offers a survival advantage compared to medical management alone [5]. Patients who survive a TAC for FCDC are often faced with a difficult and long recovery, with significant morbidity [6]. Furthermore, for the majority of patients, the ileostomy remains permanent as is described by low gastrointestinal restoration rates following TAC for FCDC in the literature [6, 7].

In the absence of absolute indications for surgery such as the rare events of colonic ischemia and perforation, no clear guidelines exist on the optimal timing of surgical intervention for FCDC. Thus, with its high associated morbidity and mortality, TAC is usually reserved as a measure of last resort in many patients. Although limited by retrospective designs, many studies have reported improved mortality for patients with FCDC who underwent early operative intervention [1, 8, 9]. In addition, a recent study by Stokes et al. reported a significantly decreased mortality in

M. Abou Khalil
Division of General Surgery, McGill University, Montréal, QC, Canada
e-mail: maria.aboukhalil@mail.mcgill.ca

M. Boutros (✉)
Division of Colon & Rectal Surgery, Jewish General Hospital, McGill University, Montreal, QC, Canada
e-mail: mboutros@jgh.mcgill.ca

C.M. Schlachta, P. Sylla (eds.), *Current Common Dilemmas in Colorectal Surgery*,
https://doi.org/10.1007/978-3-319-70117-2_10

patients with CDI admitted under the care of gastrointestinal surgeons compared to patients admitted under general medical services [10]. Focusing on patients with FCDC, Sailhamer et al. similarly reported a decreased mortality rate in patients admitted under the care of the surgical department compared to medical departments, with a shorter time from admission to operation and a trend toward a higher rate of operation [2]. Thus, it appears that expedient surgical intervention before the development of multi-organ system failure improves survival, and recent evidence places early surgical team involvement and management by surgeons at the center of improved outcomes for patients with CDI.

In view of the high morbidity and mortality associated with TAC and the emergence of evidence to emphasize the importance of early surgical intervention, colon-preserving operative strategies have emerged as attractive alternatives. The option of a minimally invasive yet successful operative intervention for FCDC may encourage appropriate early surgical management. In this chapter, we discuss the available colon-preserving minimally invasive strategies for FCDC outlined in Fig. 10.1 and the optimal timing for intervention.

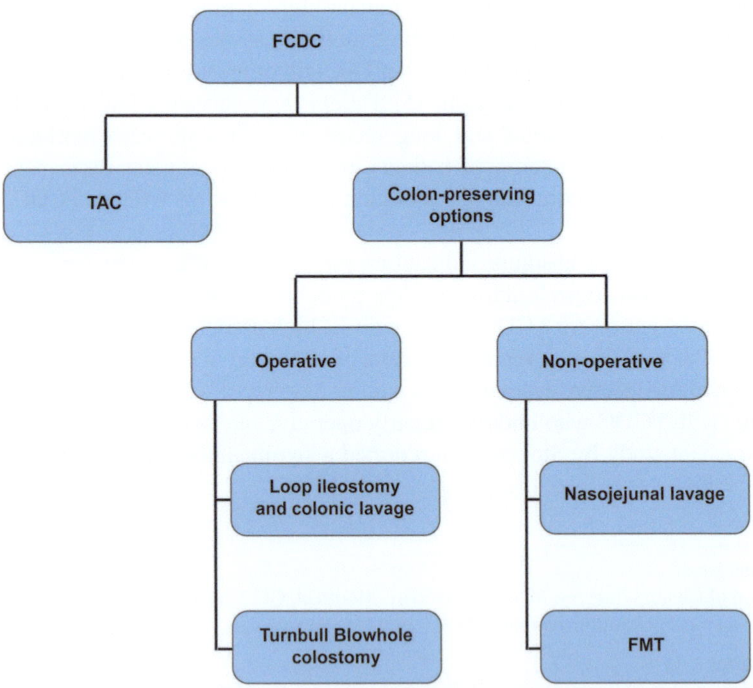

Fig. 10.1 Available operative and non-operative colon-preserving options for fulminant *Clostridium difficile* colitis (FCDC). *FMT* Fecal microbiota therapy, *TAC* Total abdominal colectomy

Operative Interventions

Loop Ileostomy and Colonic Lavage

In 2011, Neal et al. proposed a new surgical approach for FCDC which consisted of the creation of a loop ileostomy, intraoperative colonic lavage with warmed polyethylene glycol via the ileostomy, and postoperative antegrade instillation of vancomycin flushes into the diseased colon via the ileostomy (Fig. 10.2) [12]. In their single institution, single surgeon series, the authors compared 42 patients who underwent loop ileostomy and colonic lavage for FCDC with 42 historical patients who had undergone a TAC. Indications for operative management included a diagnosis of CDI either by endoscopy, laboratory assay, or evidence of colitis on imaging with any sign of clinical worsening (which included signs of peritonitis, worsening abdominal distention, sepsis, new-onset ventilator requirement, new or increasing vasopressor requirement, altered mental status, unexplained change in clinical status, non-improving leukocytosis, or bandemia despite appropriate antibiotic therapy). The primary endpoint was resolution of clinical signs associated with CDI and normalization of peripheral leukocyte count. Both the historical TAC and experimental groups were comparably critically ill as evidenced by similarities in their APACHE-II scores, white blood cell counts, intensive care unit admission, preoperative intubation, and need for vasopressors and pharmacologic immunosuppression. The authors found that all patients achieved resolution of disease. Moreover, they reported a significant reduction in the 30-day mortality in the loop ileostomy group compared to the historical control group who underwent a TAC (19% vs. 50%, respectively; $p = 0.006$). In addition to the survival benefit, the authors demonstrated an increase in ileostomy reversal rates (reported at 79% at 6 months), which is considerably higher than the reported 20% rate of gastrointestinal restoration rates following TAC [7]. The authors were also able to perform the lavage laparoscopically in the majority of patients (83%). In their series, one patient required immediate conversion to TAC due to persistent abdominal compartment syndrome (ACS) that was not improved with the lavage, and one patient developed

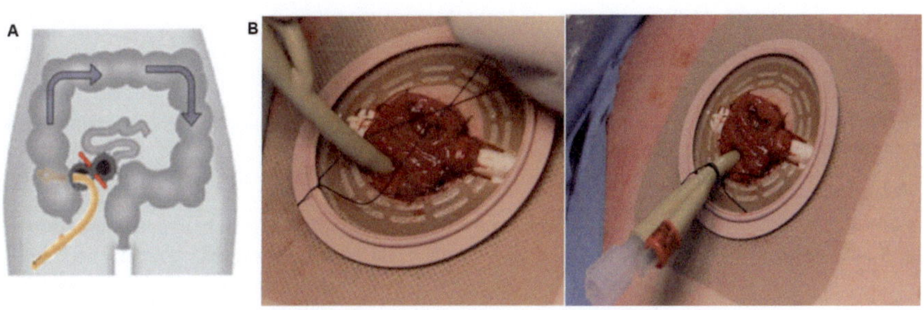

Fig. 10.2 (**a**) Schematic illustration of loop ileostomy with lavage technique. (**b**) Securing the Foley catheter. The Foley can be secured to the ileostomy appliance as shown here. Alternatively, it can be secured to the rod, or a tie around the catheter can be left long and held in place by the stoma bag. With permission from [11]. Copyright 2011 Wolters Kluwer

ACS 12 h after the lavage and required conversion to TAC. In their series of 42 patients, only one patient had recurrent vasopressor requirement 12 days after surgery and required conversion to a TAC. Thus, in a minority of patients who undergo a lavage, a second surgery may be necessary. The authors' hypotheses for the success of the lavage were that a diverting loop ileostomy poses minimal surgical stress for the critically ill patient and that since the fecal stream is diverted and the colonic lumen deprived of nutrition, mechanical lavage and local vancomycin delivery would result in successful removal of the bacteria and toxin. Many have speculated that the reason for success of this procedure is earlier time to surgical intervention. As earlier time to operation in patients with FCDC has been associated with faster recovery and better outcomes, surgeons might be more likely to intervene using this minimally invasive procedure at the first signs of severe or complicated disease, rather than delaying to the point where a TAC is the last resort (Table 10.1) [11]. Since the first description of this novel procedure, small retrospective series have been published comparing loop ileostomy and colonic lavage to TAC [13, 14]. In a single institution retrospective review of patients with surgical management of CDI, Fashandi et al. reviewed ten patients with loop ileostomy and colonic lavage compared to 13 patients with TAC. The 30-day mortality was similar in both groups (30 vs. 23%, $p = 0.1$) [13]. Similarly, there was no difference in the CDI recurrence rate (57 vs. 30%, $p = 0.35$). A recent multi-institutional retrospective chart review for patients with FCDC identified 21 patients who underwent loop ileostomy and colonic lavage and compared them to 77 patients who had a TAC [14]. The overall mortality rate was similar in both groups (23.8 vs. 33.8%, $p = 0.44$). Although likely underpowered, these reports demonstrate at least the equivalence of loop ileostomy and colonic lavage as a surgical option in patients with FCDC. A prospective national Canadian registry is currently recruiting patients to investigate this further and will hopefully better define the patient population who will best benefit from this procedure (https://clinicaltrials.gov/ct2/show/NCT02347280?term=Loop+ileostomy+c+difficile&rank=1). This registry will also collect information on strain of *C. difficile* to establish whether patients infected with some strains will be more likely to fail this minimally invasive operative management or suffer higher recurrence rates. Moreover, the registry will also allow for evaluation of the patient's quality of life and documentation of long-term outcomes.

Table 10.1 Summary table comparing total abdominal colectomy vs. loop ileostomy and colonic lavage for fulminant *Clostridium difficile* colitis

Procedure	Pros	Cons
Loop ileostomy and colonic lavage	• Minimally invasive option • Apparent survival benefit • Higher gastrointestinal restoration rates	• Limited available data to support use especially regarding recurrence rates • May fail and some patients would require reoperation
Total abdominal colectomy	• Definitive management, rare recurrence	• High morbidity and mortality • Low gastrointestinal restoration rates

Technical Details and Tips on Creation of Loop Ileostomy

The first step is exploratory laparotomy or diagnostic laparoscopy to confirm the diagnosis and ensure that there is no colonic necrosis or perforation. A laparoscopic approach is preferable if the patient is a good candidate and if the surgeon is comfortable with the procedure; otherwise it can be undertaken using an open approach. The second step involves the creation of a loop ileostomy. The loop ileostomy is ideally created 20 cm from the ileocecal valve so that an 18Fr Foley catheter, inserted into the distal limb of the ileostomy, can be positioned in the cecum. The Foley should be secured to the ileostomy at the end of the procedure using a 0-silk suture (Fig. 10.2b). Lavage of the colon is then performed with 8 L of polyethylene glycol (PEG) solution warmed to 37 °C. The colonic lavage is performed with the use of the Foley catheter connected to a bag with the PEG solution using urological connection tubing, similar to the one used in cystoscopy. A rectal tube or management device should be inserted into the rectum and attached to a large drainage bag until the lavage is complete. The PEG solution is administered in increments, liter by liter, ensuring that effluent drainage is collected in the rectal tube. If the procedure is performed laparoscopically, pneumoperitoneum can be maintained at 7–10 mmHg during lavage. Laparoscopic bowel graspers may be used to aid in pushing the fluid along the colon. If performed by a laparotomy, the abdomen is kept open, and the surgeon can manually aid the movement of the fluid through the colon. If trouble is encountered getting fluid through the colon, the patient may be moved into the Trendelenburg/reverse Trendelenburg positions as well as left side up/down and right side up/down to move the fluid along the colon. Alternatively, though rarely required, the hepatic and/or splenic flexures may be mobilized. Due to fluid sequestration in the diseased and atonic colon, an ACS may occur during or after the operation. Although the authors do not recommend routinely monitoring for ACS, the surgeon should be aware of this possibility. The surgeon may choose to leave a drain in the paracolic gutters to drain excessive ascites and potentially reduce the risk of an ACS. Postoperatively, vancomycin flushes (500 mg in 500 mL of Lactated Ringers) are delivered to the diseased colon through the Foley catheter that was left in the efferent limb of the ileostomy. The first vancomycin flush is given after completion of the PEG flushes, and administration should be continued every 8 h for 10 days or until the patient is clinically well.

Turnbull "Blowhole" Procedure

Although novel to the management of CDI, diverting loop ileostomy for fulminant colitis was advocated for decades ago. In 1971, Turnbull et al. described colonic decompression by a skin level colostomy and a loop ileostomy for toxic megacolon in patients with inflammatory bowel disease. This was proposed as a less invasive surgery to be performed in critically ill patients in order to decrease the morbidity and mortality associated with a total colectomy in the emergent setting [15]. In this publication, the authors described a diverting loop ileostomy and a transverse colostomy (Fig. 10.2). In the event that the sigmoid remained significantly dilated, a sigmoid colostomy was also created. Although this procedure has been used by surgeons for cases of FCDC, there has been little published literature to support its use, and no data is available to show how it compares with loop ileostomy and lavage as described by Neal et al. [16]. The authors believe this procedure could be an alternative in severely ill patients in whom intestinal lavage may lead to colonic perforation. Again, the rationale for the procedure would be diversion of the fecal stream and deprivation of the colonic mucosa of nutrition without the stress of a radical operation that is posed by TAC in a critically ill patient.

Non-Operative Interventions

Nasojejunal Lavage

As aforementioned, early intervention is key to improving the morbidity and mortality associated with operative management of FCDC. Drawing from this key aspect and from the success of the colonic lavage as proposed by Neal et al., some surgeons described the use of nasojejunal PEG administration as an alternative to surgical intervention. Although no study has yet assessed the efficacy or feasibility of this method of gastrointestinal lavage, it is a plausible alternative for patients who are not surgical candidates or who refuse surgery. It has not yet been established which patients would best benefit from this intervention. Nevertheless, the authors foresee this procedure as an option for the management of early severe disease, although it will have a limited role in replacing loop ileostomy and colonic lavage or TAC. A feasibility randomized trial of nasojejunal intestinal lavage for the treatment of *C. difficile* is underway and will hopefully shed more light on this procedure as a potential early alternative to surgical intervention (https://clinicaltrials.gov/ct2/show/NCT02466698).

Fecal Microbiota Therapy

Fecal microbiota therapy (FMT) has been described and recommended for cases of recurrent CDI. In recent years, there has been an increased interest regarding its role in severe or fulminant disease. Although sparse, some data suggest that FMT is a safe and potentially successful option in cases of severe and fulminant disease [17, 18]. Fischer et al. reported on the safety and efficacy of FMT delivered via colonoscopy after colonic lavage with bowel preparation solution in combination with continued vancomycin treatment in all of ten patients with severe CDI and 17 of 19 patients with severe/complicated CDI [17]. In this study, the authors used the severity score suggested by the American College of Gastroenterology in 2013, where severe CDI was defined as low serum albumin (<3 g/dL) with either leukocytosis (≥15,000 cells/mm^3) or abdominal pain and severe/complicated CDI was defined by any of the following: intensive care admission, hypotension, fever (≥38.5 °C), significant abdominal distension, ileus, mental status change, leukocytosis

(≥35,000 cells/mm^3) or leukopenia (<2000 cells/mm^3), lactate levels >2. Two millimoles per litre or evidence of end-organ failure [19]. Similar to nasojejunal lavage, perhaps these early interventions can prevent surgery for select patients and decrease the overall mortality associated with FCDC. Future research will better delineate the role of FMT in FCDC.

Conclusion

FCDC remains associated with high morbidity and mortality rates. Colon-preserving options have emerged as attractive alternatives. These options include minimally invasive surgical alternatives such as loop ileostomy with colonic lavage or non-operative interventions such as nasojejunal lavage or FMT. These strategies may optimize survival, minimize complications, and improve gastrointestinal restoration/preservation rates. Furthermore, these minimally invasive options may facilitate early management for FCDC. The patient and disease selection criteria have yet to be determined for each management option. However, it appears that despite these newer alternatives, some patients will still require a TAC. The commonality between the colon-preserving surgical procedures described is their less invasive nature causing minimal trauma to the critically ill patient and the potential for early surgical intervention, a key component of improved outcomes in surgery for FCDC. There remains a paucity of evidence for these new techniques, but the results of ongoing prospective trials will hopefully better delineate their specific roles in the management of FCDC (Fig. 10.3).

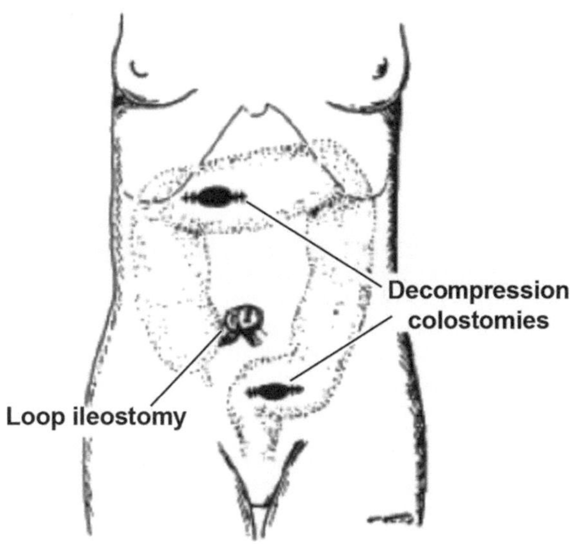

Fig. 10.3 Diverting loop ileostomy and decompression colostomies. With permission © Elsevier 1971 (https://clinicaltrials.gov/ct2/show/NCT02347280?term=Loop+ileostomy+c+difficile&rank=1)

References

1. Pepin J, Vo TT, Boutros M, Marcotte E, Dial S, Dube S, et al. Risk factors for mortality following emergency colectomy for fulminant Clostridium difficile infection. Dis Colon Rectum. 2009;52(3):400–5.
2. Sailhamer EA, Carson K, Chang Y, Zacharias N, Spaniolas K, Tabbara M, et al. Fulminant Clostridium difficile colitis: patterns of care and predictors of mortality. Arch Surg. 2009;144(5):433–9. discussion 9–40
3. Lamontagne F, Labbe AC, Haeck O, Lesur O, Lalancette M, Patino C, et al. Impact of emergency colectomy on survival of patients with fulminant Clostridium Difficile colitis during an epidemic caused by a hypervirulent strain. Ann Surg. 2007;245(2):267–72.
4. Dallal RM, Harbrecht BG, Boujoukas AJ, Sirio CA, Farkas LM, Lee KK, et al. Fulminant Clostridium difficile: an underappreciated and increasing cause of death and complications. Ann Surg. 2002;235(3):363–72.
5. Stewart DB, Hollenbeak CS, Wilson MZ. Is colectomy for fulminant Clostridium difficile colitis life saving? A systematic review. Color Dis. 2013;15(7):798–804.
6. Dallas KB, Condren A, Divino CM. Life after colectomy for fulminant Clostridium Difficile colitis: a 7-year follow up study. Am J Surg. 2014;207(4):533–9.
7. Miller AT, Tabrizian P, Greenstein AJ, Dikman A, Byrn J, Divino C. Long-term follow-up of patients with fulminant Clostridium difficile colitis. J Gastrointest Surg. 2009;13(5):956–9.
8. Ali SO, Welch JP, Dring RJ. Early surgical intervention for fulminant pseudomembranous colitis. Am Surg. 2008;74(1):20–6.
9. Markelov A, Livert D, Kohli H. Predictors of fatal outcome after colectomy for fulminant Clostridium difficile colitis: a 10-year experience. Am Surg. 2011;77(8):977–80.
10. Stokes AL, Bible A, Hollenbeak CS, Stewart DB Sr. Clostridium Difficile infection is associated with lower inpatient mortality when managed by GI surgeons. Dis Colon Rectum. 2016;59(9):855–61.
11. Hall JF, Berger D. Outcome of colectomy for Clostridium difficile colitis: a plea for early surgical management. Am J Surg. 2008;196(3):384–8.
12. Neal MD, Alverdy JC, Hall DE, Simmons RL, Zuckerbraun BS. Diverting loop ileostomy and colonic lavage: an alternative to total abdominal colectomy for the treatment of severe, complicated Clostridium difficile associated disease. Ann Surg. 2011;254(3):423–7. discussion 7–9
13. Fashandi AZ, Martin AN, Wang PT, Hedrick TL, Friel CM, Smith PW, et al. An institutional comparison of total abdominal colectomy and diverting loop ileostomy and colonic lavage in the treatment of severe, complicated Clostridium Difficile infections. Am J Surg. 2017;213(3):507–11.
14. Ferrada P, Callcut R, Zielinski MD, Bruns B, Yeh DD, Zakrison TL, et al. Loop ileostomy versus total colectomy as surgical treatment for Clostridium difficile-associated disease: an eastern Association for the Surgery of trauma multicenter trial. J Trauma Acute Care Surg. 2017;83(1):36–40.
15. Turnbull RB Jr, Hawk WA, Weakley FL. Surgical treatment of toxic megacolon. Ileostomy and colostomy to prepare patients for colectomy. Am J Surg. 1971;122(3):325–31.
16. Kerstens J, Diebels I, de Gheldere C, Vanclooster P. Blowhole colostomy for Clostridium difficile-associated toxic megacolon. Case Rep Surg. 2016;2016:5909248.
17. Fischer M, Sipe BW, Rogers NA, Cook GK, Robb BW, Vuppalanchi R, et al. Faecal microbiota transplantation plus selected use of vancomycin for severe-complicated Clostridium difficile infection: description of a protocol with high success rate. Aliment Pharmacol Ther. 2015;42(4):470–6.
18. Aroniadis OC, Brandt LJ, Greenberg A, Borody T, Kelly CR, Mellow M, et al. Long-term follow-up study of fecal microbiota transplantation for severe and/or complicated Clostridium difficile infection: a multicenter experience. J Clin Gastroenterol. 2016;50(5):398–402.
19. Surawicz CM, Brandt LJ, Binion DG, Ananthakrishnan AN, Curry SR, Gilligan PH, et al. Guidelines for diagnosis, treatment, and prevention of Clostridium Difficile infections. Am J Gastroenterol. 2013;108(4):478–98. quiz 99

Perforated Diverticulitis: Laparoscopic Lavage and Drainage

11

Morris E. Franklin Jr. and Miguel A. Hernández

Introduction

Whereas most people with diverticular disease remain asymptomatic, approximately 15% develop symptoms, and of these 15% develop significant complications, such as perforation [1]. Although the prevalence of perforated diverticulitis complicated by generalized peritonitis is low, its importance lies in the significant postoperative mortality, ranging from 4% to 26% regardless of selected surgical strategy [2].

Perforation with generalized peritonitis is one of the most common life-threatening emergencies requiring surgical intervention for diverticular disease of the colon [3].

The first report of surgical treatment for complicated diverticulitis was by Mayo in 1907 [4]. The classic three-stage operation includes an initial diverting colostomy and drainage followed by resection of the involved colon and, finally, a colostomy closure as the third stage. This nonresectional surgery strategy was reaffirmed and advocated by the experience at Mayo Clinic, which presented the results in 1924 [5].

During the next two decades, indications for emergency surgery evolved to include complicated diverticulitis, such as perforation, obstruction, and fistula formation. A preliminary transverse colostomy was advised in all cases in which resection was contemplated, and resection was delayed by three to six months [6, 7]. The rationale for this strategy was that primary resection is too difficult in the acute stage of the disease, often causing iatrogenic complications and hence mortality. After the fecal stream was diverted with a transverse colostomy created at the first stage, drainage of the abdomen and pelvic cavity was performed to diminish sigmoid inflammation. After several months, a second stage resection of the involved bowel could be performed to treat and prevent relapse of the disease.

M.E. Franklin Jr., (✉) • M.A. Hernández
Minimally Invasive Surgery, Texas Endosurgery Institute, San Antonio, TX, USA
e-mail: fellow@texasendosurgery.com; fellow@texasendosurgery.com

C.M. Schlachta, P. Sylla (eds.), *Current Common Dilemmas in Colorectal Surgery*,
https://doi.org/10.1007/978-3-319-70117-2_11

Since the 1960s, combinations of antibiotics have been used to treat Gram-negative and anaerobic bacteria. Combination antibacterial therapy has resulted in improved survival in septic patients [8]. Unfortunately, the mortality rate in patients with complicated diverticular disease remains high.

Until today the optimal treatment for perforated diverticulitis has been a matter of debate. During the last decades, the "gold standard" has changed several times.

The American Society of Colon and Rectal Surgeons Standards Committee and the Society for Surgery of Alimentary Tract have suggested sigmoid colon resection with end colostomy or Hartmann's procedure (HP) as the treatment of choice for patients with acute complicated diverticular disease. However, there has been increasing evidence demonstrating that HP is associated with high postoperative morbidity and mortality rates and a low colostomy closure rate (<40%).

Recently the concept of laparoscopic lavage and drainage (LLD) has been extended to manage non-trauma patients with critical conditions ranging from severe sepsis to hemorrhage [9]. With better understanding of the pathogenesis of perforated diverticulitis, we and other surgeons in the United States and Europe developed laparoscopic approach of peritoneal lavage and drainage to treat severe diverticulitis with generalized peritonitis. Because this nonresectional minimally invasive surgical strategy has been associated with a reduction in morbidity and mortality, it might be a promising alternative to the standard resection [10, 11].

We published a paper in 2012 titled damage control strategy for the management of perforated diverticulitis with generalized peritonitis: laparoscopic lavage and drainage vs. Hartmann's procedure. We included 47 patients in the group of LLD and 41 patients in the group of laparoscopic Hartmann's procedure (LHP). The aim of the study was to investigate a safer and more effective laparoscopic method for managing acute perforated diverticular disease with generalized peritonitis. The Hinchey staging for the LLD group was as follows: 5 patients with Hinchey II, 36 patients with Hinchey III, and 6 patients with Hinchey IV. In the other arm in the LHP group, we had 3 patients with Hinchey II, 31 patients with Hinchey III, and 7 patients with Hinchey IV. We found that in the group of LHP, the operative time and hospital stay were longer than in the LLD group. The morbidity and mortality were higher for the LHP group. One patient in the LLD was converted to an open Hartmann's procedure due to technical difficulty with multiple intestinal perforations. Additionally, 3 (6.4%) patients were reoperated for worsening symptoms during postoperative course: two underwent to open Hartmann's and one underwent to re-lavage. We concluded that LHP and LLD could be performed safely and effectively for managing severe diverticulitis with generalized peritonitis [12].

Cirocchi et al. in their systematic review of "Laparoscopic Peritoneal Lavage: A Definitive Treatment for Diverticular Peritonitis or a Bridge to Elective Laparoscopic Sigmoidectomy" performed a search in PubMed for case series and comparative studies published between January 1992 and February 2014 describing peritoneal lavage in patients with perforated diverticular disease. They found a total of 19 articles consisting in 10 cohorts, 8 case series, and 1 RCT. In total these studies analyzed 871 patients. In 11 studies the success rate of laparoscopic peritoneal lavage, defined as patients alive without surgical treatment for a recurrent episode of diverticulitis, was 24.3%. In patients with Hinchey stage III the incidence of laparotomy conversion was 1%, whereas in patients with stage IV, the incidence was 45%. Readmission rate after the first hospitalization for recurrence was 6%, and 69% of these patients required redo surgery. A two-stage procedure was performed in 18.3% of the patients. They concluded that laparoscopic peritoneal lavage should be considered an effective and safe option for the treatment of patients with sigmoid diverticulitis with Hinchey stage III and that it can also be considered as a "bridge" surgical step combined with a delayed and elective laparoscopic sigmoidectomy in order to avoid a Hartmann's procedure [13].

Angenete et al. published a RCT named "DILALA," which compared laparoscopic lavage with colon resection and stoma in a randomized multicenter control trial (9 surgical departments in Sweden and Denmark from February 2010 to February 2014). Clinical data was collected up to 12 weeks postoperatively. Eighty-three patients met the inclusion criteria but 4 patients were excluded in each group, leaving 39 patients in the laparoscopic lavage group and 36 in the Hartmann's procedure group. Morbidity and mortality did not differ between the groups. Laparoscopic lavage resulted in a shorter operative time, a shorter time in the recovery unit, and a shorter hospital stay. In conclusion they found that laparoscopic lavage as a treatment for patients with perforated diverticulitis Hinchey III was feasible and safe in the short term, although they suggested that widespread implementation of the technique should await long-term results from the ongoing randomized trials [14].

On the other hand, Galbraith et al. recently published a meta-analysis regarding laparoscopic lavage in the management of perforated diverticulitis. In this scientific paper, they included three randomized controlled trials (RCTs) with a total of 372 patients comparing laparoscopic lavage against colon resection for perforated diverticulitis. They showed that despite decreased rate of stoma formation within 90 days and equivalent mortality rates as compared with colon resection, laparoscopic lavage for Hinchey III diverticulitis fails to completely control the source of infection, with an increased rate of reoperations, and the need for subsequent percutaneous drainage [15].

Vennix et al. in their study of laparoscopy lavage or sigmoidectomy for perforated diverticulitis with purulent peritonitis: a multicenter parallel group, randomized, open label trial. This multicenter trial was conducted in 34 teaching hospitals and 8 academic hospitals from Belgium, Italy, and the Netherlands (Ladies trial), divided into two groups: LOLA comparing laparoscopic peritoneal lavage vs. sigmoidectomy and DIVA comparing Hartmann's procedure with sigmoidectomy plus primary anastomosis. LOLA study included 90 patients between July 1, 2010, and February 22, 2013. 47 were assigned to laparoscopic lavage and 43 to sigmoidectomy. Two patients were excluded for protocol violations. One patient in the group of peritoneal lavage was lost in the follow-up of 12 months. This study was terminated early for safety reasons for the patients of the lavage group because of the high short-term morbidity and reintervention rate. By 12 months of follow-up, no difference between the groups was reported regarding morbidity and mortality. Five patients died either postoperatively or during the follow-up in the lavage and sigmoidectomy group. The mean operative time in the lavage group was 60 min compared with 120 min in the sigmoidectomy group. The authors concluded that laparoscopic lavage is not superior to sigmoidectomy for the treatment of purulent perforated diverticulitis in terms to major morbidity and mortality at 12 months [16].

Recent guidelines recommend an individualized approach to recurrent uncomplicated diverticulitis disease, showing that non-operative treatment is safe for patients [17–19]. Thus, elective surgical intervention for diverticulitis may be reserved for complicated presentation. A laparoscopic approach may be used for both acute and chronic complicated diverticulitis in appropriately selected patients, as described in the American and European guidelines. However, a safe approach to minimally invasive surgery requires surgical expertise, recognition of when conditions deteriorate and/or are not suited for laparoscopy, as well as knowledge of a variety of technical maneuvers that elucidate difficult anatomy and facilitate resection. Primary anastomosis with or without diversion can be performed safely, and ileostomy reversal is significantly less morbid than Hartmann's reversal. Success in laparoscopy can be achieved with the use of adjunct techniques and technologies, including ureteral stents, hand ports, and hybrid approaches. When completed successfully, a laparoscopic approach has been shown to decrease the incidence of ileus, length of hospital stay, postoperative pain, surgical site infection rates, and incidence of incisional hernia compared to an open approach [20].

Surgical Technique for Laparoscopic Lavage and Drainage

The patient is placed in the Lloyd Davies position, with the hips and knees slightly flexed at 15° to facilitate intraoperative colonoscopy as needed. The patient's arms are tucked at the sides, and the shoulders are securely taped to the operating table to allow for the placement of the patient in steep Trendelenburg or right and left tilting position. Following proper preparation and draping of the abdomen and legs, the surgeon and the scope operator stand to the patient's right side while the assistant stands to the left side.

Pneumoperitoneum is established by inserting a Veress needle in the right flank of the abdomen, and the abdominal cavity is insufflated to a pressure of 14 mmHg. In addition, alternate sites, such as the right or left upper quadrant, may be selected in patients who have a history of prior lower abdominal surgery. Once adequate pneumoperitoneum has been achieved, a 5 mm trocar is placed and a 5 mm laparoscope (either 0° or 30°) is inserted into the cavity to survey the abdominal cavity. Following evaluation and placement of least one additional trocar, all adhesions to the anterior abdominal wall are taken down meticulously in a stepwise fashion. All attempts should be made to avoid excessive bleeding. Under laparoscopic visualization, the remaining working trocars are positioned in strategic locations along the abdominal wall. LLD proceeds sequentially by culturing and aspirating free purulent fluid in the peritoneal cavity, identifying and bluntly dissecting the diseased sigmoid colon, unroofing all purulent cavities, and washing out with copious amount of saline and iodine solution.

When sites of perforation have been found, they need to be closed with Lembert suture using slowly absorbable suture material, such as Vicryl in an interrupted fashion and further buttressed by a Graham patch with a portion of the appendiceal epiploic. Two 10 French Jackson-Pratt drains are routinely placed in the pelvis and near sites of repaired perforations. (Figs. 11.1, 11.2, 11.3, and 11.4)

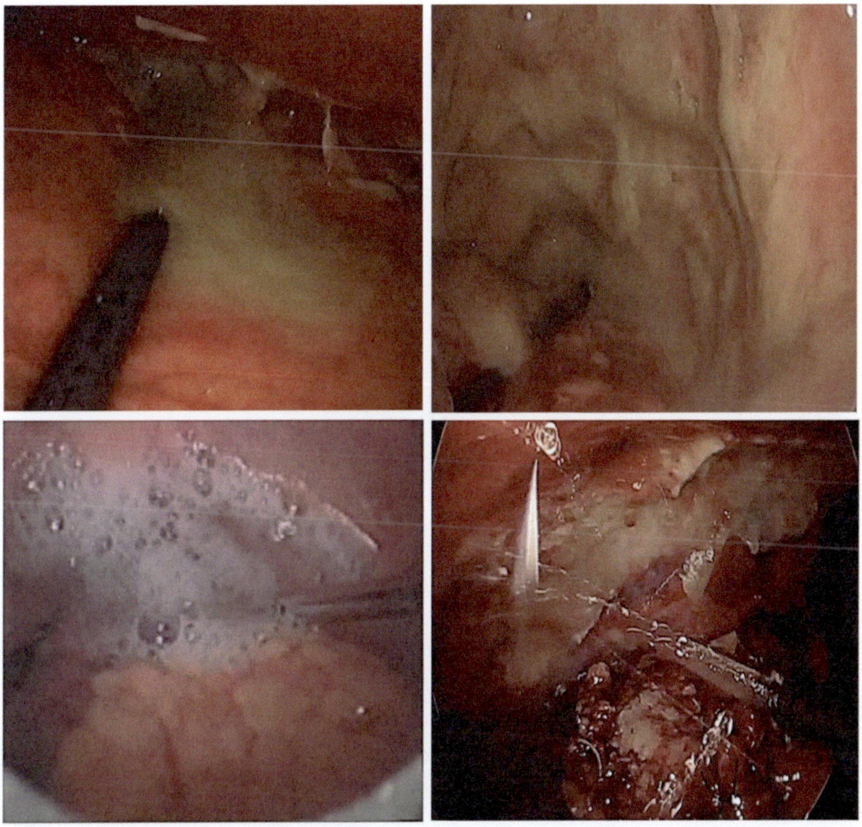

Fig. 11.1 Abdominal cavity drainage and lavage

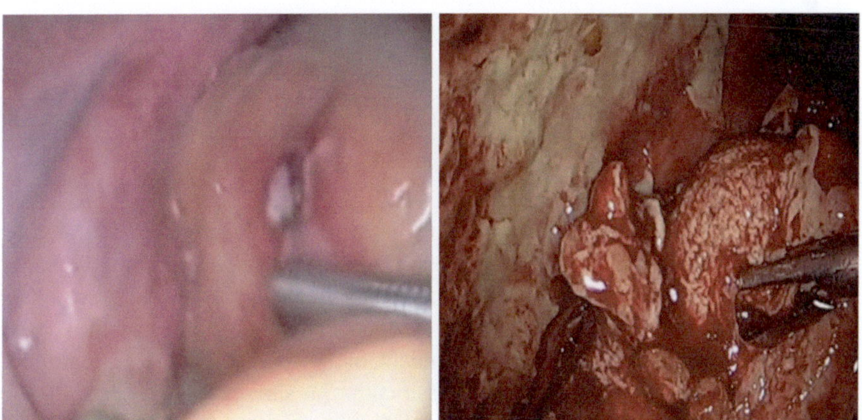

Fig. 11.2 Perforation site identification

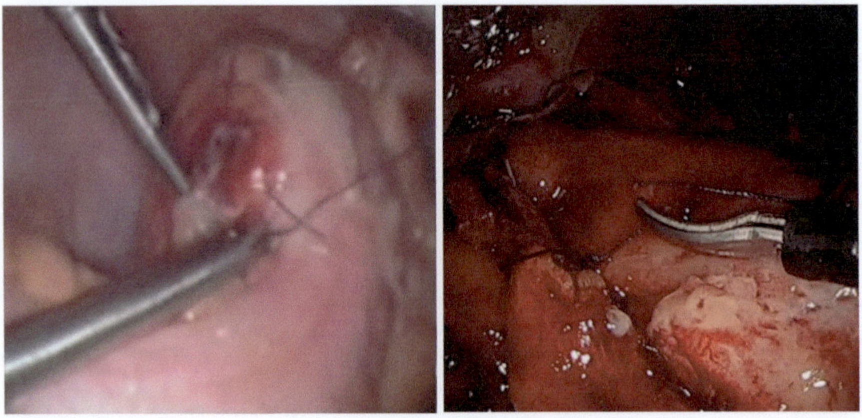

Fig. 11.3 Perforation closure with Graham's patch procedure

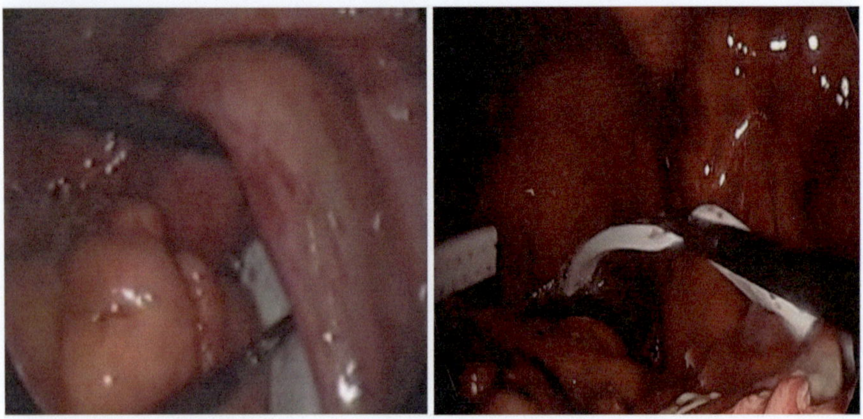

Fig. 11.4 Drains placement

Conclusions

There currently are a wide range of therapeutic options for treating complicated diverticular disease, ranging from non-operative approaches including percutaneous drainage procedures to diagnostic and therapeutic laparoscopic interventions and open surgical resections with or without fecal diversion. While selection of the appropriate intervention is largely dependent of the patient's general condition, hemodynamic stability, and Hinchey classification, it should also be based on the surgeon's skill, experience, and availability of an experienced surgical team to support more advanced laparoscopic interventions.

Despite the initial enthusiasm regarding the use of LLD as a less invasive and morbid alternative to HP, more recent studies have challenged its presumed superiority relative to other surgical approaches. Nevertheless in our experience at Texas Endosurgery Institute, in carefully selected patients, LLD has proven to be a safe alternative, decreasing morbidity and mortality, avoiding stoma formation, and improving patient's health immediately. The overall costs are decreased, and the diseased colon segment can be laparoscopically resected in a non-emergent fashion. Surgical therapy tailored to the patient appears appropriate.

References

1. Parks TG. Natural history of diverticular disease of colon. Clin Gastroenterol. 1975;4:53–69.
2. Morris CR, Harvey IM, Stebbings WS, Hart AR. Incidence of perforated diverticulitis and risk factors for death in a UK population. Br J Surg. 2008;95:876–81.
3. Vermeulen J, Gosselink MP, Hop WCJ, Lange JF, Coene PPLO, Van de Harst E, Weidema WF, Mannaerts GHH. Hospital mortality after emergency surgery for perforated diverticulitis. Ned Tijdschr Geneeskd. 2009;153:1209–14.
4. Mayo WJ, Wilson LB, Griffin HZ. Acquired diverticulitis of the large intestine. Surg Gynecol Obstet. 1907;5:8–15.
5. Judd ES, Pollack LW. Diverticulitis of the colon. Ann Surg. 1924;80:425–38.
6. Lockhart Mummery JP. Late results of diverticulitis. Lancet. 1938;2:1401–4.
7. Smithwick RH. Experiences with the surgical management of diverticulitis of the sigmoid. Ann Surg. 1942;115:969–83.
8. Jacobson MA, Young LS. New developments in the treatment of gram-negative bacteremia. West J Med. 1986;144:185–94.
9. Stawicki SP, Brooks A, Bilski T, Scaff D, Gupta R, Schwab CW. The concept of damage control: extending the paradigm to emergency general surgery. Injury. 2008;39(1):93–101.
10. Miller PR, Chang MC, Hoth JJ, Holmes JH, Meredith JW. Colonic resection in the setting of damage control laparotomy: is delayed anastomosis safe? Am Surg. 2007;73(6):606–9.
11. Bretagnol F, Pautrat K, Mor C, Benchellal Z, Huten N, De Calan L. Emergency laparoscopic management of perforated sigmoid diverticulitis: a promising alternative to more radical procedures. J Am Coll Surg. 2008;2006:654–7.
12. Liang S, Russek K, Franklin ME Jr. Damage control strategy for management of perforated diverticulitis with generalized peritonitis: laparoscopic lavage and drainage vs. laparoscopic Hartmann's procedure. Surg Endosc. 2012;26:2835–42.
13. Cirocchi R, Trastulli S, Vettoretto N, Milani D, Cavaliere D, Renzi C, Adamenko O, Desiderio J, Burattini MF, Parisi A, Arezzo A, Fingerhut A. Laparoscopic peritoneal lavage: a definitive treatment for diverticular peritonitis or a "bridge" to elective laparoscopic sigmoidectomy? A systematic review. Medicine. 2015;94(1):e334.
14. Angenete E, Thornell A, Burcharth J, Pommergaard H-C, Skullman S, Bisgaard T, Jess P, Läckberg Z, Matthiessen P, Heath J, Rosenberg J, Haglind E. Laparoscopic lavage is feasible and safe for the treatment of perforated diverticulitis with purulent peritonitis the first results from the randomized controlled trial DILALA. Ann Surg. 2016;263(1):117.
15. Galbraith N, Carter JV, Netz U, Yang D, Fry DE, McCafferty M, Galandiuk S. Laparoscopic lavage in the management of perforated diverticulitis: a contemporary meta-analysis. J Gastrointest Surg. 2017;21:1491.
16. Vennix S, Musters GD, Mulder IM, Swank HA, Consten EC, Belgers EH, van Geloven AA, Gerhards MF, Govaert MJ, van Grevenstein WM, Hoofwijk AG, Kruyt PM, Nienhuijs SW, Boermeester MA, Vermeulen J, van Dieren S, Lange JF, Bemelman WA. Laparoscopic peritoneal lavage or sigmoidectomy for perforated diverticulitis with purulent peritonitis: a multicenter, parallel-group, randomized, open-label trail. Lancet. 2015;386:1289–77.

17. Agresta F, et al. Laparoscopic approach to acute abdomen from the Consensus Development Conference of the Società Italiana di Chirurgia Endoscopica e nuove tecnologie (SICE), Associazione Chirurghi Ospedalieri Italiani (ACOI), Società Italiana di Chirurgia (SIC), Società Italiana di Chirurgia d'Urgenza e del Trauma (SICUT), Società Italiana di Chirurgia nell'Ospedalità Privata (SICOP), and the European Association for Endoscopic Surgery (EAES). Surg Endosc. 2012;26(8):2134–64.
18. Chabok A, Pahlman L, Hjern F, Haapaniemi S, Smedh K, AVOD Study Group. Randomized clinical trial of antibiotics in acute uncomplicated diverticulitis. Br J Surg. 2012;99:532–9.
19. Feingold D, Steele SR, Lee S, Kaiser A, Boushey R, Buie WD, Rafferty JF. Practice parameters for the treatment of sigmoid diverticulitis. Dis Colon Rectum. 2014;57(3):284–94.
20. Mahmoud NN, Riddle EW. Minimally invasive surgery for complicated diverticulitis. J Gastrointest Surg. 2017;21:731–8.

Perforated Diverticulitis: What Are the Options for Resection?

12

François Letarte and Carl J. Brown

Introduction

Diverticulosis typically involves the sigmoid colon and occurs in 50% of people aged over 50 years and up to 80% in those aged over 80 [1]. The vast majority of patients with colonic diverticulosis are asymptomatic, whereas 10–25% will develop at least a single episode of diverticulitis [2–4]. In these patients, 10–33% will eventually need surgical intervention [2, 5, 6] and only 1% of patients with diverticulosis will require surgery [7]. Of all admitted patients with a diagnosis of acute diverticulitis, 10–20% will require surgical treatment [8]. Urgent indications for surgery in patients with diverticulitis include obstruction, hemorrhage, failure of medical management, and free perforation. In this chapter, we will only consider options and issues related to the last two.

In essence, all presentations of diverticulitis are secondary to perforation of diverticula. However, most are microperforations that are walled off by adjacent organs or omentum. Free perforation necessitating urgent surgery is uncommon and is the indication to undergo emergent surgery in less than 25% of patients with acute complicated diverticulitis [7]. Rodkey and Welch [8] reviewed the indications for surgery in a series of 688 patients with acute diverticulitis: perforation with local peritonitis or pelvic abscess in 32.3%, generalized peritonitis in 14.6%, pain in 13.4%, obstruction in 10.9%, pericolic abscess in 10.9%, fistula in 9.7%, and bleeding in 8.2%. Free perforation following diverticulitis is especially common and lethal in immunosuppressed patients [9, 10].

F. Letarte • C.J. Brown (✉)
Department of Surgery, St. Paul's Hospital, University of British Columbia, Vancouver, BC, Canada
e-mail: fletarte@gmail.com; cbrown@providencehealth.bc.ca

C.M. Schlachta, P. Sylla (eds.), *Current Common Dilemmas in Colorectal Surgery*,
https://doi.org/10.1007/978-3-319-70117-2_12

Classification

Hughes was the first to present a practical clinical classification of diverticulitis based on the operative findings [11]. He divided patients according to the severity of their peritoneal contamination. Hinchey refined this classification into the widely adopted four-stage classification of presentations of diverticulitis [12]. In this classification, most patients treated by surgery for acute perforation are stage III or IV, representing generalized purulent and fecal peritonitis, respectively (Table 12.1). More recently, Killingback proposed a more complicated classification that differentiates abscess, perforation, and peritonitis into subclassifications [10].

Most cases of perforated diverticulitis will be walled off by adjacent structures preventing free perforation and generalized peritonitis (Hinchey I/II) and resolve with antibiotics and bowel rest. Rarely, purulent peritonitis may arise following a progressive leak from a diverticulum or presumed rupture of a previously contained perforation. In rare cases, patients initially presenting with early-stage diverticulitis will develop free perforation and generalized fecal peritonitis. This scenario is associated with a very high mortality rate [13–16].

The Hinchey classification system is used to determine both treatment and prognosis. Haglund et al. [5] confirmed the impact of free perforation on outcomes; in their series, patients experienced 33% surgical mortality in the presence of free perforation compared to a 3% mortality rate when only acute inflammation was present. Other reports have also shown that both localized peritonitis and abscess are associated with lower mortality when compared to diffuse fecal or purulent peritonitis [12, 17, 18].

Table 12.1 Clinical classification of complicated diverticulitis based on operative findings

Classification	Stage	Description
Hughes [11]	Stage I	Local peritonitis
	Stage II	Local pericolic or pelvic abscess
	Stage III	General peritonitis due to ruptured pericolic or pelvic abscess
	Stage IV	General peritonitis due to free perforation of the colon
Hinchey [12]	Stage I	Pericolic abscess or phlegmon
	Stage II	Pelvic, intraabdominal, or retroperitoneal abscess
	Stage III	Generalized purulent peritonitis
	Stage IV	Generalized fecal peritonitis
Killingback [10]	Stage I	Abscess
	a	Peridiverticular
	b	Mesenteric
	c	Pericolic (pelvic)
	Stage II	Perforation
	a	Free
	b	Concealed
	Stage III	Gangrenous sigmoiditis
	Stage IV	Peritonitis
	a	Serous, purulent or fecal
	b	Local, pelvic or generalized

Indications for Surgery

As previously described, we consider two scenarios that require surgery for perforated diverticulitis. The first indication includes patients who present with generalized peritonitis due to free perforation. Typically, these patients present with diffuse peritonitis, tachycardia, hypotension, and free air on x-ray and/or CT scan. The decision to operate is not usually difficult. The second indication includes patients who fail to respond to non-operative management. Most will be patients with a phlegmon or abscess with persistent fevers, leukocytosis, tachycardia, pain and tenderness on examination despite intravenous antibiotics, bowel rest, and fluid resuscitation. It is important to note that most patients with evidence of "perforation" on CT imaging may present with localized peritonitis and non-operative management can safely be attempted. Free air will often result from the initial microperforation that is quickly contained by the adjacent structures, preventing free perforation and generalized peritonitis in most cases.

Surgical Management of Perforated Diverticulitis

The main objective of surgical resection for perforated diverticulitis is to eliminate the source of ongoing sepsis as quickly and safely as possible. Laparoscopic lavage has been proposed as an alternative to resection, and this option is discussed in detail in a different chapter.

Limitations of the Available Evidence

The current literature on the management of perforated diverticulitis consists mostly of case series and retrospective reports increasing the risk for bias. Another concern is the lack of consistent classification of diverticular disease that can lead to comparison of patients with different severity of disease. Most studies do not specify precisely the extent of peritonitis (i.e., localized vs. purulent vs. feculent peritonitis). The authors also compare series from different eras where there are numerous confounding factors influencing patient outcomes (e.g., antibiotic use, improvements in perioperative care). Hence, their conclusions and recommendations should be interpreted with caution.

Historic Management

In the early-mid twentieth century, the recommendation for patients presenting with perforated diverticulitis was a three-stage procedure: an initial transverse loop colostomy and drainage, followed 3 to 6 months later by a subsequent resection, and finally, closure of the loop colostomy [19, 20]. This procedure has largely been abandoned in favor of either the Hartmann's procedure or resection with primary anastomosis with or without proximal diversion. In 1984, Krukowski and Matheson reviewed the world literature on emergency surgery for diverticular disease complicated by generalized peritonitis [14]. They demonstrated a clear advantage in terms of mortality and morbidity after resection of the diseased segment rather than performing an operation where the colon was retained. Their review included 1282 patients from 57 publications. The mortality rates in operations where the colon was resected ranged 6.1–12.2%. When the diseased segment was diverted but not resected, mortality was 25.7–28.1%. The authors recommended that segmental resection should be performed. While the three-stage procedure has been abandoned, there continues to be debate on which surgical procedure to choose when facing perforated diverticulitis. We will review the controversies and highlight the circumstances when each may be applied.

Technical Considerations

The extent of resection is determined intraoperatively based on the quality of the tissues and should include the entire thickened contracted segment, including the inflammatory process. Proximal and distal margins should be healthy colon and rectum. The most important factor to prevent recurrence of diverticulitis is to extend the distal margin of resection to the proximal rectum to create a colorectal anastomosis.

Thaler et al. examined the impact of surgery-related variables on recurrence rate after sigmoid resection for diverticulitis [21]. The level of the anastomosis was the only predictor of recurrence; patients with colosigmoid anastomosis had a recurrence rate fourfold higher than patients with colorectal anastomosis (2.8% vs. 12.5%, $p = 0.033$). Similarly, Benn et al. in a series of 501 patients reported a diverticulitis recurrence rate that was doubled in patients whom the distal margin used in the anastomosis was the sigmoid colon rather than the rectum (6.7% vs. 12.5%) [22]. In both series, the segment harboring diverticulitis was in the sigmoid colon.

In cases where the diseased colonic segment is proximal to a healthy sigmoid, it is likely safe to proceed with a colo-colonic anastomosis as long as the entire thickened segment is removed. While there are no comparative studies supporting this approach, it is clear that removing all colonic diverticula en bloc is not advisable in patients with diverticulitis. While it is not necessary to remove all diverticula-bearing colon, efforts should be made to avoid including diverticula in the anastomosis to decrease the risk of leak.

It is not clear whether effort should be made to preserve the inferior mesenteric artery and its branches. The rationale behind preserving this artery is that it may improve blood supply to the distal aspect of the anastomosis and, hence, reduce the risk of anastomotic leakage. A retrospective review of 130 patients with diverticulitis who underwent elective resection, where the primary outcome was to evaluate the impact of inferior mesenteric artery (IMA) or superior rectal artery (SRA) preservation with respect to anastomotic leak rates, showed that preservation of the major vascular pedicle was not associated with improved outcomes [23]. However, a randomized controlled study looking at 86 patients undergoing sigmoidectomy for complicated diverticular disease observed a lower clinical leak rate when preserving the SRA (2% vs. 7%, $p = 0.03$) [24]. Of note, the authors used liberal definitions of leak that may not represent actual or clinically significant anastomotic leaks and may have influenced the results.

While the evidence is marginal, it appears that preservation of the IMA may be beneficial. However, the diagnosis of diverticulitis is often in doubt at the time of emergency surgery, as there is a possibility of undiagnosed cancer. Bacon et al. [25] found an underlying carcinoma in 7.7% of 351 patients undergoing elective resection for diverticulitis. In cases of emergent colectomy for presumed diverticulitis, two series report 20–25% rates of unexpected underlying carcinoma [26, 27]. While our experience more closely reflects cancer incidence similar to those reported by Bacon et al., we believe that patients having emergency surgery where endoscopic exclusion of a malignancy is not possible should undergo an oncologic resection including high ligation of the IMA.

Hartmann's Vs. Primary Anastomosis

Hartmann's procedure, consisting of sigmoid resection, terminal colostomy, and closure of the rectal stump, is the easiest, fastest, and safest operation to clear the sepsis-inducing segment of the colon and avoid the risk of anastomotic leak. The disadvantages of interval colostomy include rectal stump leak, stoma complications, and long hospital stay. Most importantly, intestinal reconstruction can be quite challenging and is associated with a significant risk of complications, with observed morbidity of up to 40% [28]. Data from large administrative database studies show that more than a third of patients never undergo Hartmann reversal and that the number increases up to 70% when patients are aged over 77 years [29, 30]. These factors make a primary colorectal anastomosis an enticing alternative.

The available comparative data are mostly observational studies suggesting primary anastomosis (PRA), and Hartmann's procedure (HP) is associated with similar outcomes in terms of morbidity and mortality. However, these studies are marred by considerable selection bias, where younger, healthier patients tend to be managed with a restorative approach. Abbas et al. reviewed this literature comparing the safety and feasibility of PRA compared to HP for patients with acute complicated diverticulitis [31]. Eighteen studies including 884 patients were included in the review, none of which were randomized controlled trials. When compared to HP, PRA was associated with lower mortality rate (9% vs. 19%) and similar postoperative morbidity rates (29% vs. 33.4%). He found an anastomotic leak rate of 5.5% in the PRA patients compared to 8% in the HP patients. Constantinides et al. conducted a prospective study to assess adverse events following PRA versus HP for complicated diverticular disease [32]. Over a 12-month period across 42 centers in Great Britain, data were collected for 248 patients who underwent PRA and 167 patients who underwent HP. After adjusting for risk factors for selection of patients for a non-restorative procedure, HP was found to be associated with similar 30-day mortality (OR 1.76, $p = 0.223$), increased surgical complications (OR 1.90, $p = 0.025$), and increased overall medical complications (OR 2.08, $p = 0.026$) when compared to PRA. Constantinides also published a second systematic review comparing PRA and HP [33]. It included 963 patients (57% PRA and 43% HP) from 15 studies. Overall mortality was significantly reduced with PRA (4.9% vs. 15.1%; OR 0.41). Subgroup analyses were performed, and PRA was associated with decreased mortality when trials were matched for emergency operations (6.4% vs. 15.6%; OR 0.44). However, when trials were matched for severity of peritonitis of Hinchey III or IV, there was no significant difference in mortality (14.1% vs. 14.4%, OR = 0.85) (see Table 12.2). Salem et al. also conducted a systematic review on the topic. Their paper included 1051 patients undergoing HP and 569 patients undergoing PRA. Mortality rates were, respectively, 19.6% for HP and 9.9% for PRA. However, no subgroup analyses were performed. A study by Aydin, one of the largest single institution retrospective reviews, aimed to assess the likelihood of Hartmann versus primary anastomosis in patients with perforated diverticulitis. They described a diverticulitis disease propensity score which showed that the strongest predictors of Hartmann's procedure were urgent or emergent cases, BMI over 30, Manheim peritonitis index of 10 and over, immunosuppression, and Hinchey grade III or IV [36]. These factors have also been recognized in other studies as predictors of end-colostomy formation, including a prospective study showing an association between higher Manheim peritonitis index and likelihood of end colostomy [34, 35, 37]. A more recent systematic review and meta-analysis addressing the treatment of Hinchey III and IV diverticulitis found comparable mortality between patients undergoing primary anastomosis versus Hartmann's procedure [38]. Marked heterogeneity and potential for selection bias once again limit the interpretation of the results as well as the possibility to draw any conclusion.

A single small randomized trial has tried to address the issue of selection bias [39]. Oberkofler et al. randomized 64 patients with Hinchey III and IV diverticulitis to HP or PRA. The study was discontinued early as an interim safety analysis showed HP to be associated with significantly more serious complications when compared to ileostomy reversal. The majority of patients included were Hinchey stage III diverticulitis. There was no significant difference in terms of mortality and morbidity between the two groups, but stoma reversal was significantly higher in the primary anastomosis group. PRA was also associated with shorter hospital stay and lower in-hospital costs.

The Dutch Diverticular Disease (3D) Collaborative Study group started the Ladies trial in 2010 in an effort to answer two important questions. The first, comparing laparoscopic lavage with sigmoidectomy for purulent perforated diverticulitis, was stopped early by the data safety monitoring committee and is discussed in another chapter. In the DIVA arm (perforated DIVerticulitis: sigmoid resection with or without Anastomosis), patients randomized to resection were then randomized to either HP or PRA [40]. The results of this trial are still pending, but this will provide more clarity for surgeons.

Since no strong evidence is available to allow for general guidelines, surgeons must weigh the benefits of primary anastomosis versus the risks linked to anastomotic failure and longer operating times. In clinical practice, the decision to perform primary anastomosis should be individualized to each patient, and surgeons should ask themselves if the patient could withstand and survive an anastomotic leak. Presence of any one of the parameters including hemodynamic instability, acidosis, acute organ failure, and any significant comorbidity such as diabetes, malnutrition, chronic end-stage organ failure, or immunosuppression should prompt the

Table 12.2 Mortality comparing PRA vs. HP

Outcome Mortality comperison in diverticular disease

Study or sub category	PRA n/N	Hartmann's Procedure n/N	OR (random) 95% CI	Weight %	OR (random) 95% CI	Year
02 Mortality - diverticular disease						
Drumm [24]	2/3	1/5		2.85	8.00 [0.31, 206.37]	1984
Gregg [26]	0/35	2/25		3.15	0.13 [0.01, 2.88]	1984
Underwood [34]	0/6	1/15		2.72	0.74 [0.03, 20.81]	1984
Kourtesis [28]	1/23	0/10		2.80	1.40 [0.05, 37.33]	1988
Alenis [21]	1/34	4/26		5.50	0.17 [0.02, 1.59]	1989
Hold [27]	4/99	9/76		14.25	0.31 [0.09, 1.06]	1990
Peoples [30]	2/11	8/43		8.69	0.97 [0.18, 5.40]	1990
Medina [29]	0/3	1/3		2.37	0.24 [0.01, 8.62]	1991
Sarin [33]	2/19	0/8		3.03	2.43 [0.10, 56.39]	1991
Saccomani [32]	1/26	3/7		4.61	0.05 [0.00, 0.65]	1993
Wedel [35]	2/183	7/31		9.41	0.04 [0.01, 0.19]	1997
Goozsen [25]	5/32	6/28		12.88	0.68 [0.18, 2.53]	2001
Schiling [36]	1/13	4/42		5.38	0.79 [0.08, 7.78]	2001
Blair [22]	3/33	13/64		12.61	0.39 [0.10, 1.49]	2002
Regenet [31]	3/27	4/33		9.75	0.91 [0.18, 4.45]	2003
Subtotal (95% CI)	547	416		100.00	0.41 [0.22, 0.77]	
Total events: 27 (PRA), 63 (Hartman's procedure)						
Test for heterogeneity: Chi² = 20.10, df = 14 (P = 0.13), I^2 = 30.4%						
Test for overall effect: Z = 2.77 (P = 0.006)						
03 Mortality - diverticular disease and emergency operations only						
Hold [27]	4/99	9/76		23.95	0.31 [0.09, 1.06]	1990
Saccomani [32]	1/26	3/7		7.75	0.05 [0.00, 0.65]	1993
Goozsen [25]	5/32	6/28		21.66	0.69 [0.18, 2.53]	2001
Schiling [36]	1/13	4/42		9.05	0.79 [0.08, 7.78]	2001
Blair [22]	3/33	13/64		21.20	0.39 [0.10, 1.49]	2002
Regenet [31]	3/27	4/33		16.39	0.91 [0.18, 4.45]	2003
Subtotal (95% CI)	230	250		100.00	0.44 [0.24, 0.83]	
Total events: 17 (PRA), 39 (Hartman's procedure)						
Test for heterogeneity: Chi² = 4.53, df = 5 (P = 0.48), I^2 = 0%						
Test for overall effect: Z = 2.55 (P = 0.01)						
05 Mortality - diverticular disease and Hinchey >2						
Drumm [24]	2/3	1/5		8.58	8.00 [0.31, 206.37]	1984
Medina [29]	0/3	1/3		7.12	0.24 [0.01, 8.62]	1991
Goozsen [25]	5/32	6/28		38.77	0.68 [0.18, 2.53]	2001
Schiling [36]	1/13	4/42		16.20	0.79 [0.08, 7.78]	2001
Regenet [31]	3/27	4/33		29.33	0.91 [0.18, 4.45]	2003
Subtotal (95% CI)	78	111		100.00	0.85 [0.36, 2.01]	
Total events: 11 (PRA), 16 (Hartman's procedure)						
Test for heterogeneity: Chi² = 2.43, df = 4 (P = 0.66), I^2 = 0%						
Test for overall effect: Z = 0.38 (P = 0.71)						
07 Mortality - diverticular disease and abscess/peritonitis						
Drumm [24]	2/3	1/5		3.30	8.00 [0.31, 206.37]	1984
Underwood [34]	0/6	1/15		3.15	0.74 [0.03, 20.81]	1984
Alanis [21]	1/34	4/26		6.37	0.17 [0.02, 1.59]	1989
Hold [27]	4/99	9/76		16.49	0.31 [0.09, 1.06]	1990
Peoples [30]	2/11	8/43		10.05	0.97 [0.18, 5.40]	1990
Medina [29]	0/3	1/3		2.74	0.24 [0.01, 8.62]	1991
Wedel [35]	2/183	7/31		10.89	0.04 [0.01, 0.19]	1997
Goozsen [25]	5/32	6/28		14.91	0.68 [0.18, 2.53]	2001
Schiling [36]	1/13	4/42		6.23	0.79 [0.08, 7.78]	2001
Blair [22]	3/33	13/64		14.59	0.39 [0.10, 1.49]	2002
Regenet [31]	3/27	4/33		11.28	0.91 [0.18, 4.45]	2003
Subtotal (95% CI)	444	366		100.00	0.43 [0.21, 0.85]	
Total events: 23 (PRA), 58 (Hartman's procedure)						
Test for heterogeneity: Chi² = 15.26, df = 10 (P = 0.12), I^2 = 34.5%						
Test for overall effect: Z = 2.41 (P = 0.02)						

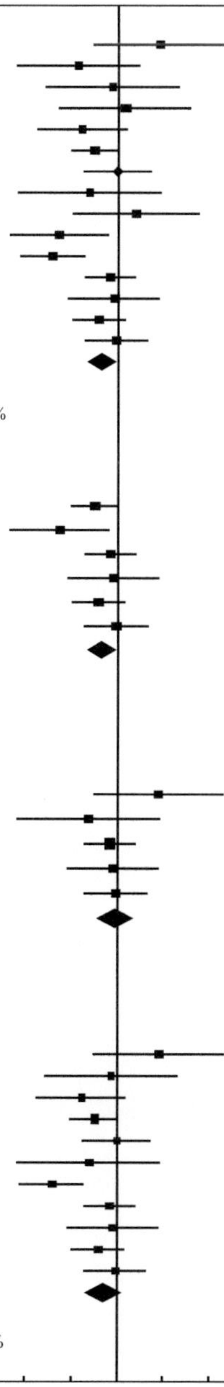

Modified from Constantinides et al. systematic review [33]

operating surgeon to strongly consider end colostomy. Diffuse peritonitis, either purulent or feculent, is often considered as a strong contraindication for primary anastomosis. However, it is our opinion that select young patients, hemodynamically stable with healthy tissues and without any significant comorbidities, could undergo safely primary anastomosis even in the presence of diffuse peritonitis. Diverting loop ileostomy should be strongly considered in any of the cases.

Damage Control Surgery for Perforated Diverticulitis

Initially described for patients with major abdominal injuries, indications for damage control surgery (DCS) have expanded to include patients with severe peritonitis and instability [41–43]. DCS for perforated diverticulitis has been reported as an alternative treatment strategy by several authors [7, 44–49]. DCS for perforated diverticulitis involves a three-stage approach: stage I, an abbreviated initial operative procedure with temporary abdominal closure; stage II, continued resuscitation and management of physiologic and acid–base derangements; and stage III, definitive treatment and closure. This alternative approach allows for rapid source control and patient resuscitation in the intensive care, postponing the decision on the definitive surgical resolution to a semi-elective setting in a hemodynamically stable patient. In a series by Kafka-Ritsch et al. [46], they achieved a low mortality rate (9.8%), and most patients were discharged with their colon reconstructed (77% overall, 50% for fecal peritonitis). All of this despite a median Manheim peritonitis index of 26 and a high rate of severe comorbidities (Table 12.3). This alternative concept should be taken into consideration before choosing to perform a Hartmann's procedure in patients presenting with extensive peritonitis from perforated diverticulitis.

Table 12.3 Outcomes of damage control surgery for complicated diverticulitis

Study	Outcomes	Primary definitive surgery	Damage control surgery
Sohn et al. [42]	*N*	18	19
	Postoperative complication rate	39%	32%
	Mortality	11%	10.5%
	Primary anastomosis	22.2%	78.9%
Kafka-Ritsch et al. [46]	*N*	Not applicable	51
	Postoperative complication rate		Not available
	Mortality		9.8%
	Primary anastomosis		76%
Finlay et al. [43]	*N*	Not applicable	14
	Postoperative complication rate		Not available
	Mortality		7.1%
	Primary anastomosis		85.7%

The Role of Laparoscopic Colectomy for Perforated Diverticulitis

Laparoscopic surgery is now considered the procedure of choice for elective management of diverticular disease. Many randomized controlled trials have demonstrated that laparoscopic colectomy by experienced surgeons is safe and results in better short-term outcomes, including less postoperative pain, shorter length of hospital stay, lower ileus rates, reduced complication rates, and improved quality of life when compared to open surgery [50–56]. The American Society of Colon and Rectal Surgeons (ASCRS) recommends that "when expertise is available, the laparoscopic approach to elective colectomy for diverticulitis is preferred. Grade of Recommendation: Strong recommendation based on high-quality evidence, 1A" [57]. Those benefits have led some to investigate the role of laparoscopic colectomy for perforated diverticulitis in the acute setting. There are concerns regarding the safety of this approach when dealing with an acutely inflamed surgical field resulting in friable mesentery, obliterated surgical planes, distended small bowel, and distorted anatomy. Another concern is the hypothetical risk of increased bacteremia and hypercapnia secondary to the pneumoperitoneum [58]. Increasing experience with abdominal sepsis does not support this theory [59]. In 2006, the European Association of Endoscopic Surgeons (EAES) published their guidelines and suggested that acute diverticulitis should not be treated laparoscopically, except for the use of laparoscopic lavage in some selected cases. The ASCRS practice parameters for sigmoid diverticulitis do not comment on the use of laparoscopy for emergent colonic resection.

The current literature on the use of laparoscopic colectomy for perforated diverticulitis is composed of mainly single-center retrospective case series which demonstrate it to be safe, with similar benefits found in the elective setting [60–79]. A systematic review assessed the safety of laparoscopic sigmoidectomy for perforated diverticulitis with generalized peritonitis. This included 4 case series and one cohort study for a total of 104 patients of which 20 had PRA. Their results suggest that laparoscopic sigmoidectomy in selected patients with Hinchey III and IV diverticulitis has an acceptable conversion rate, a low reintervention rate, a low morbidity rate, and a low mortality rate. Laparoscopic sigmoidectomy for perforated diverticulitis was also shown to be superior to open surgery in a propensity-matched cohort. Laparoscopic surgery was associated with better postoperative morbidity rates, shorter hospital stay, lower cost, and similar mortality rates [80].

In experienced hands and in well-selected patients, laparoscopic colectomy for perforated diverticulitis appears to be safe and feasible and might be associated with short-term benefit when compared to open surgery.

Perforated Diverticulitis in Immunosuppressed Patients

The number of patients with diverticulitis and concomitant immunosuppression (e.g., transplant, steroid dependency, chronic renal failure, etc.) is rising [81–84]. Diverticulitis complicated with free perforation is a major concern in this population since they have impaired ability to mount a response to severe sepsis. This combination can mask the clinical symptoms of perforation, leading to delayed diagnosis and increased morbidity and mortality [85–88]. Most experts recommend proceeding with HP in this population as the risk of anastomotic failure is high. Most studies of outcomes in immunosuppressed patients with perforated diverticulitis have demonstrated worse postoperative morbidity and mortality when compared to the general population [38, 89, 90]. The current standard of care in immunocompromised patients presenting with perforated diverticulitis is resection with colostomy; PRA should be avoided [83, 91].

Conclusion

Diffuse peritonitis from diverticulitis with free perforation is one the most severe acute conditions that surgeons have to manage. The primary objective is to control the sepsis by removing the diseased segment of the colon. Once this is accomplished, the surgeon is left with the choice of either proceeding with an end colostomy or creating a primary anastomosis. The available evidence to support this decision has significant limits, and hence, the decision should be individualized for each patient based on the clinical scenario.

References

1. Weizman AV, Nguyen GC. Diverticular disease: epidemiology and management. Can J Gastroenterol. 2011;25:385–9.
2. Parks TG. Natural history of diverticular disease of the colon. Clin Gastroenterol. 1975;4:53–69.
3. Connell AM. Pathogenesis of diverticular disease of the colon. Adv Intern Med. 1977;22:377–95.
4. Hackford AW, Veidenheimer MC. Diverticular disease of the colon. Current concepts and management. Surg Clin North Am. 1985;65:347–63.
5. Haglund U, Hellberg R, Johnsen C, et al. Complicated diverticular disease of the sigmoid colon. An analysis of short- and long-term outcome in 392 patients. Ann Chir Gynaecol. 1979;68:41–6.
6. Thorn M, Graf W, Stefansson T, Pahlman L. Clinical and functional results after elective colonic resection in 75 consecutive patients with diverticular disease. Am J Surg. 2002;183:7–11.
7. Vermeulen J, Lange JF. Treatment of perforated diverticulitis with generalized peritonitis: past, present, and future. World J Surg. 2010;34:587–93.
8. Hughes ES, Cuthbertson AM, Carden AB. The surgical management of acute diverticulitis. Med J Aust. 1963;50(1):780–2.
9. Hinchey EJ, Schaal PG, Richards GK. Treatment of perforated diverticular disease of the colon. Adv Surg. 1978;12:85–109.
10. Killingback M. Management of perforative diverticulitis. Surg Clin North Am. 1983;63:97–115.
11. Hughes ESR, Cuthbertson AM, Carden ABG. The surgical management of acute diverticulitis. Med J Aust. 1963;1:780–2.
12. Hinchey EJ, Schaal PGH, Richards GK. Treatment of perforated disease of the colon. Adv Surg. 1978;12:86–109.
13. Nagorney DM, Adson MA, Pemberton JH. Sigmoid diverticulitis with perforation-and generalized peritonitis. Dis Colon Rectum. 1985;28:71.

14. Krukowski ZH, Matheson NA. Emergency surgery for diverticular disease complicated by generalized and fecal peritonitis: a review. Br J Surg. 1984;71:921–7.
15. Hollender LF, Meyer CH, Alexiou D, et al. Therapeutic principles in emergency colonic surgery. Int Surg. 1981;66:307–10.
16. Miller DW, Wichern WA. Perforated diverticulitis. Appraisal of primary versus delayed resection. Am J Surg. 1971;121:536–40.
17. Cullen KW, Ferguson JC. Diverticular disease as a surgical emergency. Br J Clin Pract. 1984;38:20–4.
18. Killingback M. Diverticulitis of the colon. In: Fazio VW, editor. Current therapy in colon and Rectal surgery. Toronto: BC Decker; 1990. p. 222–31.
19. Smithwick RH. Experiences with the surgical management of diverticulitis of the sigmoid. Ann Surg. 1942;115:969–85.
20. Lockhart-Mummery JP. Late results of diverticulitis. Lancet. 1938;2:1401–4.
21. Thaler K, Baig MK, Berho M, et al. Determinants of recurrence after sigmoid resection for uncomplicated diverticulitis. Dis Colon Rectum. 2003;46:385–8.
22. Benn PL, Wolff BG, Ilstrup DM. Levels of anastomosis and recurrent colonic diverticulitis. Am J Surg. 1986;151:269–71.
23. Lehmann RK, Brounts LR, Johnson EK, Rizzo JA, Steele SR. Does sacrifice of the inferior mesenteric artery or superior rectal artery affect anastomotic leak following sigmoidectomy for diverticulitis? Am J Surg. 2011;201:623–7.
24. Tocchi A, Mazzoni G, Fornasari V, Miccini M, Daddi G, Tagliacozzo S. Preservation of the inferior mesenteric artery in colorectal resection for complicated diverticular disease. Am J Surg. 2001;182:162–7.
25. Bacon HE, Tse GN, Herabat T. Co-existing carcinoma with peridiverticulitis of the colon. Dis Colon Rectum. 1973;16:500–3.
26. Krukowski ZH, Koruth NM, Matheson NA. Evolving practice in acute diverticulitis. Br J Surg. 1985;72:684–6.
27. Smallwood JA. Diverticular disease: emergency surgical problems. Hosp Updat. 1982;8:1554–61.
28. Keck JO, Collopy BT, Ryan PJ, et al. Reversal of Hartmann's procedure: effect of timing and technique on ease and safety. Dis Colon Rectum. 1994;37:243–8.
29. Macias AM, Haukoos JS, Dixon MR, Sorial E, Arnell TD, Stamos MJ, et al. Diverticulitis: truly minimally invasive management. Am Surg. 2004;70(10):932–5.
30. Maggard MA, Zingmoud D, O'Connell JB, Ko CY. What proportion of patients with an ostomy for diverticulitis get reversed? Am Surg. 2004;70:928–32.
31. Abbas S. Resection and primary anastomosis in acute complicated diverticulitis, a systematic review of the literature. Int J Color Dis. 2007;22:351–7.
32. Constantinides VA, Tekkis PP, Senapati A. Prospective multicentre evaluation of adverse outcomes following treatment for complicated diverticular disease. Br J Surg. 2006;93:1503–13.
33. Constantinides VA, Tekkis PP, Athanasiou T, et al. Primary resection with anastomosis vs. Hartmann's procedure in nonelective surgery for acute colonic diverticulitis: a systematic review. Dis Colon Rectum. 2006;49:966–81.
34. Aydin HN, Tekkis PP, Remzi FH, Constantinides V, Fazio VW. Evaluation of the risk of a nonrestorative resection for the treatment of diverticular disease: the Cleveland Clinic diverticular disease propensity score. Dis Colon Rectum. 2006;49:629–39.
35. Constantinides VA, Heriot A, Remzi F, et al. Operative strategies for diverticular peritonitis: a decision analysis between primary resection and anastomosis versus Hartmann procedures. Ann Surg. 2007;245:94–103.
36. Salem L, Flum DR. Primary anastomosis or Hartmann's procedure for patients with diverticular peritonitis? A systematic review. Dis Colon Rectum. 2004;47:1953–64.
37. Richter S, Lindemann W, Kollmar O, Pistorius GA, Maurer CA, Schilling MK. One-stage sigmoid colon resection for perforated sigmoid diverticulitis (Hinchey stages III and IV). World J Surg. 2006;30:1027–32.

38. Cirocchi R, trastulli S, Desiderio J, Listorti C, Boselli C, Parisi A, Noya G, Liu L. Treatment of Hinchey stage III-IV diverticulitis: a systematic review and meta-analysis. Int J Color Dis. 2013;28:447–57.
39. Oberkofler CE, Rickenbacher A, Raptis DA, et al. A multicenter randomized clinical trial of primary anastomosis or Hartmann's procedure for perforated left colonic diverticulitis with purulent or fecal peritonitis. Ann Surg. 2012;256:819–27.
40. Vennix S, Musters GD, Mulder IM, et al. Laparoscopic peritoneal lavage or sigmoidectomy for perforated diverticulitis with purulent peritonitis: a multicentre, parallel-group, randomised, open-label trial. Lancet. 2015;386(10000):1269–77.
41. Rotondo MF, Schwab CW, McGonigal MD, et al. 'Damage control': an approach for improved survival in exsanguinating penetrating abdominal injury. J Trauma. 1993;35:375–82.
42. Sohn M, Agha A, Heitland W, Gundling F, Steiner P, Iesalnieks I. Damage control strategy for the treatment of perforated diverticulitis with generalized peritonitis. Tech Coloproctol. 2016;20:577–83.
43. Finlay IG, Edwards TJ, Lambert AW. Damage control laparotomy. Br J Surg. 2004;91:83–5.
44. Kwon E, Browder T, Fildes J. Surgical management of fulminant diverticulitis. Curr Surg Rep. 2013;2:40.
45. Moore FA, Coimbra R, Davis JW, et al. Mandatory exploration is not necessary for patients with acute diverticulitis and free intraperitoneal air. J Trauma Acute Care Surg. 2013;74:1376–7.
46. Kafka-Ritsch R, Birkfellner F, Perathoner A, et al. Damage control surgery with abdominal vacuum and delayed bowel reconstruction in patients with perforated diverticulitis Hinchey III/IV. J Gastrointest Surg. 2012;16:1915–22.
47. Liang S, Russek K, Franklin ME Jr. Damage control strategy for the management of perforated diverticulitis with generalized peritonitis: laparoscopic lavage and drainage vs. laparoscopic Hartmann's procedure. Surg Endosc. 2012;26:2835–42.
48. Moore FA, Moore EE, Burlew CC, et al. Western Trauma Association critical decisions in trauma: management of complicated diverticulitis. J Trauma Acute Care Surg. 2012;73:1365–71.
49. Perathoner A, Klaus A, Mühlmann G, et al. Damage control with abdominal vacuum therapy (VAC) to manage perforated diverticulitis with advanced generalized peritonitis—a proof of concept. Int J Color Dis. 2010;25:767–74.
50. Klarenbeek BR, Veenhof AA, Bergamaschi R, et al. Laparoscopic sigmoid resection for diverticulitis decreases major morbidity rates: a randomized control trial. Ann Surg. 2009;249:39–44.
51. Gervaz P, Inan I, Perneger T, Schiffer E, Morel P. A prospective, randomized, single-blind comparison of laparoscopic versus open sigmoid colectomy for diverticulitis. Ann Surg. 2010;252:3–8.
52. Schwenk W, Haase O, Neudecker JJ, Müller JM. Short-term benefits for laparoscopic colorectal resection. Cochrane Database Syst Rev. 2005;(3):CD003145.
53. Masoomi H, Buchberg B, Nguyen B, Tung V, Stamos MJ, Mills S. Outcomes of laparoscopic versus open colectomy in elective surgery for diverticulitis. World J Surg. 2011;35:2143–8.
54. Scheidbach H, Schneider C, Rose J, et al. Laparoscopic approach to treatment of sigmoid diverticulitis: changes in the spectrum of indications and results of a prospective, multicenter study on 1,545 patients. Dis Colon Rectum. 2004;47:1883–8.
55. Bartus CM, Lipof T, Sarwar CM, et al. Colovesical fistula: not a contraindication to elective laparoscopic colectomy. Dis Colon Rectum. 2005;48:233–6.
56. Jones OM, Stevenson AR, Clark D, Stitz RW, Lumley JW. Laparoscopic resection for diverticular disease: follow-up of 500 consecutive patients. Ann Surg. 2008;248:1092–7.
57. Feingold D, Steele SR, Lee S, et al. Practice parameters for the treatment of sigmoid diverticulitis. Dis Colon Rectum. 2014;57:2284–94.
58. Pearl JP, Marks JM, Hardacre JM, Ponsky JL, Delaney CP, Rosen MJ. Laparoscopic treatment of complex small bowel obstruction: is it safe? Surg Innov. 2008;15:110–3.
59. Sartelli M, Viale P, Catena F, Ansaloni L, Moore E, et al. 2013 WSES guidelines for management of intra-abdominal infections. World J Emerg Surg. 2013;8:3.

60. Catani M, De Milito R, Romagnoli F, Romeo V, Modini C. Laparoscopic colorectal surgery in urgent and emergent settings. Surg Laparosc Endosc Percutan Tech. 2011;21:340–3.
61. Champagne B, Stulberg JJ, Fan Z, Delaney CP. The feasibility of laparoscopic colectomy in urgent and emergent settings. Surg Endosc. 2009;23:1791–6.
62. Fine AP. Laparoscopic surgery for inflammatory complications of acute sigmoid diverticulitis. JSLS. 2001;5:233–5.
63. Koh FH, Tan KK, Tsang CB, Koh DC. Laparoscopic versus an open colectomy in an emergency setting: a case-controlled study. Ann Coloproctol. 2013;29:12–6.
64. Uematsu D, Akiyama G, Magishi A, Sano T, Niitsu H, Narita M, Komatsu H. Laparoscopic Hartmann's procedure for fecal peritonitis resulting from perforation of the left-sided colon in elderly and severely ill patients. Tech Coloproctol. 2012;16:243–6.
65. Kwon JW, Kim BS, Park HC, HK O, Shin R, Ryoo SB, Park KJ, Lee BH. Surgical treatment of complicated right colonic diverticulitis: laparoscopic versus open surgery. Surg Endosc. 2012;26:2926–30.
66. Li JC, Ng SS, Lee JF, Yiu RY, Hon SS, Leung WW, Leung KL. Emergency laparoscopic-assisted versus open right hemicolectomy for complicated cecal diverticulitis: a comparative study. J Laparoendosc Adv Surg Tech A. 2009;19:479–83.
67. Binda GA, Karas JR, Serventi A, Sokmen S, Amato A, Hydo L, Bergamaschi R, Study Group on Diverticulitis. Primary anastomosis vs nonrestorative resection for perforated diverticulitis with peritonitis: a prematurely terminated randomized controlled trial. Color Dis. 2012;14:1403–10.
68. Morks AN, Klarenbeek BR, Flikweert ER, van der Peet DL, Karsten TM, Eddes EH, Cuesta MA, de Graaf PW. Current surgical treatment of diverticular disease in the Netherlands. World J Gastroenterol. 2010;16:1742–6.
69. Tadlock MD, Karamanos E, Skiada D, Inaba K, Talving P, Senagore A, Demetriades D. Emergency surgery for acute diverticulitis: which operation? A national surgical quality improvement program study. J Trauma Acute Care Surg. 2013;74:1385–91. Quiz1610.
70. Franklin ME Jr, Dorman JP, Jacobs M, Plasencia G. Is laparoscopic surgery applicable to complicated colonic diverticular disease? Surg Endosc. 1997;11:1021–5.
71. Lam HD, Tinton N, Cambier E, Navez B. Laparoscopic treatment in acute complicated diverticulitis: a review of 11 cases. Acta Chir Belg. 2009;109:56–60.
72. Mbadiwe T, Obirieze AC, Cornwell EE 3rd, Turner P, Fullum TM. Surgical management of complicated diverticulitis: a comparison of the laparoscopic and open approaches. J Am Coll Surg. 2013;216:782–8. Discussion 788–90.
73. Zdichavsky M, Granderath FA, Blumenstock G, Kramer M, Kuper MA, Konigsrainer A. Acute laparoscopic intervention for diverticular disease (AIDD): a feasible approach. Langenbeck's Arch Surg. 2010;395:41–8.
74. Zdichavsky M, Kratt T, Stuker D, Meile T, Feilitzsch MV, Wichmann D, Konigsrainer A. Acute and elective laparoscopic resection for complicated sigmoid diverticulitis: clinical and histological outcome. J Gastrointest Surg. 2013;17:1966–71.
75. Strik MW, Comman A, Staab M, Benecke C. Perforated diverticulitis of the sigmoid colon. indication for laparoscopic resection and primary anastomosis [German]. Coloproctology 2008:30.
76. El Zarrok Elgazwi K, Baca I, Grzybowski L, Jaacks A. Laparoscopic sigmoidectomy for diverticulitis: a prospective study. JSLS. 2010;14:469–75.
77. Kockerling F, Schneider C, Reymond MA, Scheidbach H, Scheuerlein H, Konradt J, Bruch HP, Zornig C, Kohler L, Barlehner E, Kuthe A, Szinicz G, Richter HA, Hohenberger W. Laparoscopic resection of sigmoid diverticulitis. Results of a multicenter study. Laparoscopic Colorectal Surgery Study Group. Surg Endosc. 1999;13:567–71.
78. Letarte F, Hallet J, Drolet S, Charles Gregoire R, Bouchard A, Gagne JP, Thibault C, Bouchard P. Laparoscopic emergency surgery for diverticular disease that failed medical treatment: a valuable option? Results of a retrospective comparative cohort study. Dis Colon Rectum. 2013;56:1395–402.

79. Rea JD, Herzig DO, Diggs BS, Cone MM, KC L. Use and outcomes of emergent laparoscopic resection for acute diverticulitis. Am J Surg. 2012;203:639–43.
80. Vennix S, Boersema GS, Buskens CJ, et al. Emergency laparoscopic sigmoidectomy for perforated diverticulitis with generalised peritonitis: a systematic review. Dig Surg. 2016;33:1–7.
81. Biondo S, Borao JL, Kreisler E, et al. Recurrence and virulence of colonic diverticulitis in immunocompromised patients. Am J Surg. 2012;204:1729.
82. Dalla Valle R, Capocasale E, Mazzoni MP, et al. Acute diverticulitis with colon perforation in renal transplantation. Transplant Proc. 2005;37:2507–10.
83. Hesterberg R, Muller F, Schmidt WU, Moslein G, Lammers B. Sigmoid diverticulitis in immunosuppressive drug therapy. Chirurg. 1994;65:873–6.
84. Perkins JD, Shield CF 3rd, Chang FC, Farha GJ. Acute diverticulitis. Comparison of treatment in immunocompromised and nonimmunocompromised patients. Am J Surg. 1984;148:745–8.
85. Pourfarziani V, Mousavi-Nayeeni SM, Ghaheri H, et al. The outcome of diverticulosis in kidney recipients with polycystic kidney disease. Transplant Proc. 2007;39:1054–6.
86. Qasabian RA, Meagher AP, Lee R, Dore GJ, Keogh A. Severe diverticulitis after heart, lung, and heart-lung transplantation. J Heart Lung Transplant. 2004;23:845–9.
87. Sachar DB. Diverticulitis in immunosuppressed patients. J Clin Gastroenterol. 2008;42:1154–5.
88. Tyau ES, Prystowsky JB, Joehl RJ, Nahrwold DL. Acute diverticulitis. A complicated problem in the immunocompromised patient. Arch Surg. 1991;126:855–8. Discussion 858–59.
89. Hwang SS, Cannom RR, Abbas MA, Etzioni D. Diverticulitis in transplant patients and patients on chronic corticosteroid therapy: a systematic review. Dis Colon Rectum. 2010;53:1699–707.
90. Zingg U, Pasternak I, Dietrich M, Seifert B, Oertli D, Metzger U. Primary anastomosis vs Hartmann's procedure in patients undergoing emergency left colectomy for perforated diverticulitis. Color Dis. 2010;12:54–60.
91. Golda T, Kreisler E, Mercader C, Frago R, Trenti L, biondo S. Emergency surgery for perforated diverticulitis in the immunosuppressed patient. Color Dis. 2014;16:723–31.

Perforated Diverticulitis: When Is Interval Resection Really Indicated?

13

Abe Fingerhut, Luigi Boni, Viktor Justin, and Selman Uranues

Abbreviations

ACPGBI	Association of Coloproctology of Great Britain and Ireland
ASCRS	American Society of Colon and Rectal Surgeons
ASN	Association of Surgeons of the Netherlands
DSS	Danish Surgical Society
EAES	European Association for Endoscopic Surgery
WSES	World Society for Emergency Surgery

Introduction

The dilemma of whether to perform interval colectomy after perforated diverticular disease has long been a subject of discussion, but has given rise to a surge of current interest today, parallel to the increasing use of laparoscopy to treat colonic diverticular disease.

A. Fingerhut (✉) • S. Uranues
Department of Surgery, University Hospital of Graz, Graz, Austria
e-mail: abefingerhut@aol.com; selman.uranues@aon.at

L. Boni
Department of General and Emergency IRCCS-Ca' Granda-Policlinico Hospital, University of Milan, Milan, Italy
e-mail: luigi.boni@unimi.it

V. Justin
Department of Surgery, Section for Surgical Research, Medical University of Graz, Graz, Austria
e-mail: viktor.justin@gmail.com

C.M. Schlachta, P. Sylla (eds.), *Current Common Dilemmas in Colorectal Surgery*, https://doi.org/10.1007/978-3-319-70117-2_13

Perforated diverticulitis can be *microscopic*, also called covered perforations, which usually give rise to phlegmon or localized abscesses, amenable under specific circumstances to percutaneous drainage by interventional radiology, or *macroscopic*, free perforations, which typically give rise to purulent or feculent peritonitis, which customarily requires surgical resolution.

The scope of therapy for perforated diverticular disease ranges from antibiotics, percutaneous drainage, or simple surgical drainage with or without suturing, usually for microscopic perforations, to resection with an end-colostomy or primary anastomosis, usually for macroscopic perforations. All types of surgical interventions can be performed laparoscopically. The indication for interval resection after perforated diverticular disease depends on the type of perforation (microscopic or macroscopic) and the management initially proposed for the perforation: after microscopic perforations, usually after resolution by percutaneous drainage, or after macroscopic perforations, when initial resection was not performed. Additional resection for diseased proximal colon once a colectomy has been performed for source control is rarely indicated.

Interval Colectomy

Elective interval colectomy has traditionally been recommended for patients (a) under 50 years of age at initial presentation and who are immunocompromised, after one acute episode of diverticulitis [1], (b) who have experienced two or more episodes of uncomplicated bouts of diverticulitis [1–3], or (c) who have had complicated diverticular disease (abscess, perforation, fistula), not treated by emergency colectomy.

Age

Young age has recently been challenged as an absolute indication for elective colectomy; effectively diverticular disease has not been proven irrevocably to be more virulent in this population, albeit that the increased life span of patients after the initial bout might increase the chance over time that another event occurs [4–6]. The practice of elective surgical resection based on age alone has gradually disappeared and is no longer recommended routinely [6, 7].

Immune Compromise

Immunocompromised patients including transplant patients, patients on chronic corticosteroid therapy, and patients with chronic renal failure or collagen-vascular disease, constitute a unique subgroup in which medical management is more likely to fail [7, 8] and/or has a greater risk of recurrent, complicated diverticulitis requiring emergency surgery [9]; they may be candidates for interval colectomy earlier in the course of diverticular disease. Elective colectomy in anticipation of organ transplantation remains controversial [7].

Recurrent Episodes

Interval resection after a certain, predetermined number of acute flares of diverticulitis has been a dogma among colorectal and general surgeons for decades [10, 11]. The rationale was that the probability of recurrence was such that elective "prophylactic" colectomy would be preferable to another episode of acute inflammation of diverticular disease, eventually complicated by an adverse event such as an abscess or perforation with ensuing peritonitis, and/or the need for a stoma. However, this dogma was mainly based on studies performed more than 50 years ago. There is increasing evidence to challenge the hypothesis that patients with recurrent disease are at increased risk of subsequent adverse events [10, 12, 13], and some reports have observed that the index presentation may be the most severe [4, 13, 14]. The optimal or cutoff number of recurrences before interval colectomy should be entertained may be more cost-effective when applied after four episodes [15].

Ritz et al. suggested that an episode of severe diverticulitis may result in a buttressing effect around the affected portion of the colon, thereby protecting it from subsequent attacks [13]. The most recent (2014) ASCRS practice parameters have now indicated that the number of attacks of uncomplicated diverticulitis is not a necessary factor in defining the need for surgery [7], similar to what was already recommended in 2006 [6].

Perforated Diverticulitis

Microperforation

For microperforations, leading to abscess formation, retrospective observational, mostly uncontrolled studies continue to indicate that interval resection should be proposed to patients because of the risk of recurrence after successful non-operative management of a diverticular abscess (antibiotics or percutaneous drainage). In these studies, recurrence was noted in 112 of 185 (60.5%) [16] and in 5 of 12 (41.2%) of patients with pelvic abscesses [17]. Ambrosetti et al. [17] followed 73 patients (45 with a mesocolic abscess and 28 with a pelvic abscess) for a median of 43 months. Just over half of patients with mesocolic abscess required interval surgery, compared to 71% of those with pelvic abscess. The authors concluded that it would be possible not to perform interval colectomy for patients with success percutaneous drainage, but recommended interval colectomy for patients with pelvic abscess [17].

The recent ASCRS guidelines recommended elective interval surgery following successful medical treatment of mesocolic abscesses ≥5 cm or pelvic abscesses with or without percutaneous drainage, because of high recurrence rates (40%), but acknowledged that this is based on retrospective data and that non-operative management was also possible [6]. The ACPGBI and the WSES guidelines recommend elective surgical treatment only for pelvic abscesses because of their poor long-term prognosis and that successfully treated mesocolic abscesses do not routinely require surgery [18].

Lastly, a recent analysis of more than 2,00,000 patients with diverticulitis in the USA, Rose et al. [19] reported an increased risk for recurrence after medically treated episodes ranging from 16.2% after the first to 30% after the second, with a cumulative incidence of 75% after three medically managed attacks. Furthermore, they described a higher risk for adverse outcomes among patients with complicated disease at the first episode. As the mortality rate after interval elective colectomy following the first complicated episode was 0.3% as compared to a 4.6% mortality rate after surgical intervention during a second episode, these authors strongly proposed to consider surgical management in patients who present with a complicated disease or are older than 50 years [19]. However, limitations of this study included the sole inclusion of inpatient records, the lack of further imaging, and procedural details of surgical approaches.

Notwithstanding the recommendations for interval colectomy as indicated above, in a population-based retrospective cohort study using administrative discharge data conducted in Ontario, Canada, the outcomes of 14,124 patients with a prior episode of diverticulitis managed non-operatively and who were eligible for elective colectomy from 2002 to 2012, were analyzed [20]. There was a statistically significant drop in the proportion of patients who underwent elective colectomy following an episode of diverticulitis treated non-operatively. After a median follow-up of 3.9 years (maximum, 10; interquartile range, 1.7–6.4), 1342 (9.5%) patients underwent elective colectomy, 76% within 1 year of discharge (median, 160 days; interquartile range, 88–346). The proportion of patients undergoing elective colectomy within 1 year of discharge declined from 9.6% of patients in 2002 to 3.9% by 2011 ($p < 0.001$), especially in patients <50 years of age (from 17% to 5%) and those with complicated disease (from 28% to 8%) (all $p < 0.001$). After adjusting for changes in patient characteristics, the odds of elective surgery decreased by 0.93 per annum (adjusted OR; 95% CI, 0.90–0.95).

In conclusion, there is no high level evidence for routine elective surgery after nonsurgical treatment of abscesses. Mesocolic abscesses ≥5 cm or pelvic abscesses might have a higher recurrence rate and could justify surgery, but the level of evidence is not strong [17, 20].

Macroperforation

Concerning macroscopic or overt perforations, the conundrum remains wide open. Whereas several studies have looked at the actual occurrence of recurrence after acute bouts of diverticular disease [14, 15], very few have studied the natural history specifically after macroscopic perforation whether treated by resection or not. As most recent guidelines recommend source control, that is, resection for overt perforations, the question of secondary or interval resection was rarely raised. However, today, more and more patients are treated with drainage alone, whether because they are deemed unfit for major surgery or since the provoking publications of O'Sullivan [21] and then Myers [22] initiated the current trend of managing perforated diverticular disease by laparoscopic lavage and drainage only. This has led to the conundrum of whether prior perforation is a marker of disease severity such that colectomy should be performed after simple initial lavage and drainage. However, the literature on this specific question is sparse. Two randomized controlled trials have compared one-stage to two-stage treatment (initial suturing, drainage, colostomy) of perforated diverticular disease [23, 24], with conflicting results, the former favoring secondary resection, the latter favoring initial primary resection. However, both of these studies included patients undergoing laparotomy, and interval colectomy (two-stage) procedure was performed for all patients surviving the initial operation, as part of the protocol. There is a lack of data and consensus on the natural history of unresected diverticulitis [25].

In the study by Myers et al., only two patients (out of 88 with Hinchey III) were reported to require readmission and be treated for recurrent diverticulitis: both resolved with antibiotics alone and did not require surgery [22]. Of note, median follow-up for the 88 patients was 36 (range 12–84) months. Myers et al. concluded that subsequent elective resection was probably unnecessary [22]. Conversely, other tenors of laparoscopic lavage only in the acute phase recommend elective interval resection of the diseased portion of the bowel [26, 27]. The main argument in favor of this strategy is that laparoscopy is less aggressive and that both operations can be performed laparoscopically without the need for a stoma [27].

In a recent systematic review [28], the research committee of the European Society of Coloproctology indicated that all societies but the ASCRS have approved the option of laparoscopic lavage as a safe approach for selected patients with purulent perforated diverticulitis (Hinchey III), but no clear recommendations were made regarding lavage as a bridge to elective resection or as a final treatment option [6].

Looking at the outcomes from recent randomized trials, indications for further surgery after simple laparoscopic lavage were not always provided. In the LOLA trial [29], 47 patients underwent laparoscopic lavage without resection and were followed for 12 months. At one-year follow-up, recurrent diverticulitis was observed in 9 patients of 46 (20%) in the laparoscopic lavage group compared to 1 patient of 42 in the resection group (2%) ($p = 0.0315$). Of the patients in the lavage group, surgery was necessary for 13. Seven patients underwent elective laparoscopic sigmoidectomy, of whom two had to be converted to laparotomy; the fourth presented with a colovesical fistula 8 months later. Two patients who had acute reoperation after laparoscopic lavage needed additional surgical re-intervention, including treatment of a hematoma after Hartmann's reversal.

In the DILALA study, although the main endpoint was reoperations within 12 months, the first paper reported only the short-term follow-up results after 12 weeks, and therefore, no information was available concerning interval colectomy [30]. Similarly, no long-term recommendations were made in the SCANDIV study [31].

In the systematic review of the literature by Afshar and Kurer, 51% of patients who had initial lavage and drainage only underwent elective resection with primary anastomosis with the majority being completed laparoscopically [32]. However, these numbers were from observational studies only and cannot be used to recommend interval colectomy nor to estimate the true prevalence of interval colectomies being performed after initial laparoscopic lavage and drainage.

Cuomo et al. performed an excellent review of the literature to back their recommendations in a 2014 Italian Consensus paper [33]: the conclusions and recommendations were similar to the ASCRS as concerns the management of abscess, fistula, and stenosis [6], but there were no specific recommendations for interval colectomy after management of perforated diverticular disease by simple lavage [33].

Diverticular Fistula and Stenosis

The ASN [34], the DSS [35], and the EAES [1] guidelines (revised by Agresta et al. [36]) recommend routine sigmoid resection for diverticulitis complicated by fistula or stenosis. The DSS guideline recommends individualized treatment in high-risk patients: patients with a high surgical risk may benefit from colostomy without resection of the diseased segment [34]. In conclusion, diverticular disease complicated by stenosis or fistula is an indication for elective surgery, although more conservative options are possible for high-risk patients, but the level of evidence is low [37].

Risk of Cancer

The risk of perforation secondary to colonic cancer mimicking complicated diverticular disease and similitude of CT findings seen in patients with diverticulitis and colon cancer have given rise to the indication of colonoscopy after the initial episode. This have received a strong recommendation (1C) from the Clinical Practice Guideline Committee of the ASCRS in 2014 (according to the Grading of Recommendations, Assessment, Development, and Evaluation (GRADE) system), even though this is based on low-quality evidence [6].

In a report from Sallinen et al., of 633 patients with CT-diagnosed acute diverticulitis, 536 were treated conservatively, 394 of whom subsequently underwent colonoscopy [38]. Seventeen patients (2.7%) with an initial diagnosis of acute diverticulitis were found to have a colon carcinoma, 16 of whom (94%) had an abscess. Similar results (2.8% colorectal cancer rate) have been reported by Lau et al. [39], who observed a fourfold increased risk for malignancy in the presence of local perforation, a more than sixfold increased risk in patients with an abscess, as well as an 18-fold increase in case of fistulization, after adjusting for sex and age. Both groups of authors concluded that routine colonoscopy was not necessary after CT-proven uncomplicated diverticulitis but should be performed in patients with a diagnosis of diverticular abscess.

In their meta-analysis including 1970 patients across 11 studies, Sharma et al. [40] reported an overall carcinoma rate of 1.6% (95% confidence interval [CI], 0.9–2.8%). Of note, while uncomplicated diverticulitis was associated with a proportional estimated risk of 0.7% (CI, 0.3–1.4%) for colon cancer, malignancy was observed in 7.6% of complicated cases (proportion estimate of risk 10.8%; CI, 5.2–21.0%).

In the LOLA study, four patients in the lavage-only group had open surgery for colorectal cancer, of whom three were diagnosed during follow-up colonoscopy [29]. In the SCANDIV study, 12 of 199 patients enrolled actually had perforated sigmoid carcinoma at the origin of what was thought to be perforated diverticular disease, and 8 were found on the resection specimen [31]. However, 4 out of 74 patients randomized to lavage alone had a missed sigmoid carcinoma requiring secondary resection [31]. This is one of the arguments in favor of routine postoperative colonoscopy and interval resection [31].

Conclusion

In conclusion and in accordance with Fozard et al. [41], the majority of the evidence in support of elective interval resection in diverticular disease is of poor quality. The decision to perform interval colectomy therefore cannot be determined with any high level of evidence. The decision regarding whether or not to offer interval resection should be made on an individual basis, and the surgeon should involve the radiologists and pathologists in this decision, in addition to the patients themselves. In support of interval colectomy is the fact that elective surgery may be associated with improved quality of life [6, 42] and reduced episodes of abdominal pain, hospital admission, and readmission [6, 43]. Moreover, elective resection has an advantage over emergency resection in that it (should) remove all diseased segments [6].

References

1. Kohler L, Sauerland S, Neugebauer E. Diagnosis and treatment of diverticular disease: results of a consensus development conference. Surg Endosc. 1999;13:430–6.
2. Stollman NH, Raskin JB. Diagnosis and management of diverticular disease of the colon in adults. Ad Hoc Practice Parameters Committee of the American College of Gastroenterology. Am J Gastroenterol. 1999;94:3110–21.
3. Wong WD, Wexner SD, Lowry A, Vernava A, Burnstein M, Denstman F, Fazio V, Kerner B, Moore R, Olivier G, Peters W, Ross T, Senagore P, Simmang C. Practice parameters for the treatment of sigmoid diverticulitis. The Standards Task Force. The American Society of Colon and Rectal Surgeons. Dis Colon Rectum. 2000;43:289–97.
4. Janes S, Meagher A, Frizelle FA. Elective surgery after acute diverticulitis. Br J Surg. 2005; 92:133–42.
5. Murphy SF, Waters PS, Waldron RM, Bennani F, Ryan RS, Khan W, Khan IZ, Barry K. Predictive factors for colonic resection in patients less than 49 years with symptomatic diverticular disease. Am J Surg. 2016;212(1):47–52.

6. Feingold D, Steele SR, Lee S, Kaiser A, Boushey R, Buie WD, Rafferty JF. Practice parameters for the treatment of sigmoid diverticulitis. Dis Colon Rectum. 2014;57:284–94.
7. Rafferty J, Shellito P, Hyman NH, Buie WD, The Standards Committee of The American Society of Colon and Rectal Surgeons. Practice parameters for sigmoid diverticulitis. Dis Colon Rectum. 2006;49:939–44.
8. Hwang SS, Cannom RR, Abbas MA, Etzioni D. Diverticulitis in transplant patients and patients on chronic corticosteroid therapy: a systematic review. Dis Colon Rectum. 2010;53:1699–707.
9. Klarenbeek BR, Samuels M, van der Wal MA, van der Peet DL, Meijerink WJ, Cuesta MA. Indications for elective sigmoid resection in diverticular disease. Ann Surg. 2010;251:670–4.
10. Chapman J, Davies M, Wolff B, et al. Complicated diverticulitis: is it time to rethink the rules? Ann Surg. 2005;242:576–81.
11. Shaikh S, Krukowski ZH. Outcome of a conservative policy for managing acute sigmoid diverticulitis. Br J Surg. 2007;94:876–9.
12. Binda GA, Arezzo A, Serventi A, Italian Study Group on Complicated Diverticulosis (GISDIC), et al. Multicentre observational study of the natural history of left-sided acute diverticulitis. Br J Surg. 2012;99:276–85.
13. Ritz JP, Lehmann KS, Frericks B, Stroux A, Buhr HJ, Holmer C. Outcome of patients with acute sigmoid diverticulitis: multivariate analysis of risk factors for free perforation. Surgery. 2011;149:606–13.
14. Salem L, Veenstra DL, Sullivan SD, Flum DR. The timing of elective colectomy in diverticulitis: a decision analysis. J Am Coll Surg. 2004;199:904–12.
15. Salem TA, Molloy RG, O'Dwyer PJ. Prospective, five-year follow-up study of patients with symptomatic uncomplicated diverticular disease. Dis Colon Rectum. 2007;50:1460–4.
16. Kaiser AM, Jiang JK, Lake JP, et al. The management of complicated diverticulitis and the role of computed tomography. Am J Gastroenterol. 2005;100:910–7.
17. Ambrosetti P, Chautems R, Soravia C, Peiris-Waser N, Terrier F. Long-term outcome of mesocolic and pelvic diverticular abscesses of the left colon: a prospective study of 73 cases. Dis Colon Rectum. 2005;48:787–91.
18. Tursi A, Papa A, Danese S. Review article: the pathophysiology and medical management of diverticulosis and diverticular disease of the colon. Aliment Pharmacol Ther. 2015;42:664–84.
19. Rose J, Parina RP, Faiz O, Chang DC, Talamini MA. Long-term outcomes after initial presentation of diverticulitis. Ann Surg. 2015;262(6):1046–53.
20. Li D, Baxter NN, McLeod RS, Moineddin R, Nathens AB. The decline of elective colectomy following diverticulitis: a population-based analysis. Dis Colon Rectum. 2016;59:332–9.
21. O'Sullivan GC, Murphy D, O'Brien MG, Ireland A. Laparoscopic management of generalized peritonitis due to perforated colonic diverticula. Am J Surg. 1996;171:432–4.
22. Myers E, Hurley M, O'Sullivan GC, Kavanagh D, Wilson I, Winter DC. Laparoscopic peritoneal lavage for generalized peritonitis due to perforated diverticulitis. Br J Surg. 2008;95:97–101.
23. Kronborg O. Treatment of perforated sigmoid diverticulitis: a prospective randomized trial. Br J Surg. 1993;80:505–7.
24. Zeitoun G, Laurent A, Rouffet F, Hay JM, Fingerhut A, Paquet JC, Peillon C. Multicentre randomized clinical trial of primary vs. secondary sigmoid resection in generalized peritonitis complicating sigmoid diverticulitis. Br J Surg. 2000;87:1366–74.
25. Devaraj B, Liu W, Tatum J, Cologne K, Kaiser AM. Medically treated diverticular abscess associated with high risk of recurrence and disease complications. Dis Colon Rectum. 2016;59:208–15.
26. Faranda C, Barrat C, Catheline JM, Champault GG. Two-stage laparoscopic management of generalised peritonitis due to perforated sigmoid diverticula: eighteen cases. Surg Laparosc Endosc Percutan Tech. 2000;10(3):135–8.
27. Taylor CJ, Layani L, Ghusin MA, White SI. Perforated diverticulitis managed by laparoscopic lavage. ANZ J Surg. 2006;76:962–5.
28. Vennix S, Morton DG, Hahnloser D, Lange JF, Bemelman WA, Research Committee of the European Society of Coloproctocology. Systematic review of evidence and consensus on diverticulitis: an analysis of national and international guidelines. Color Dis. 2014;16:866–78.

29. Vennix S, Musters GD, Mulder IM, Swank HA, Consten EC, Belgers EH, van Geloven AA, Gerhards MF, Govaert MJ, van Grevenstein WM, Hoofwijk AG, Kruyt PM, Nienhuijs SW, Boermeester MA, Vermeulen J, van Dieren S, Lange JF, Bemelman WA, Ladies Trial Collaborators. Laparoscopic peritoneal lavage or sigmoidectomy for perforated diverticulitis with purulent peritonitis: a multicentre, parallel-group, randomised, open-label trial. Lancet. 2015;386:1269–77.
30. Angenete E, Thornell A, Burcharth J, Pommergaard H-C, Skullman S, Bisgaard T, Jess P, Lackberg Z, Matthiessen P, Heath J, Rosenberg J, Haglind E. Laparoscopic lavage is feasible and safe for the treatment of perforated diverticulitis with purulent peritonitis. The first results from the randomized controlled trial DILALA. Ann Surg. 2016;263:117–22.
31. Schultz JK, Yaqub S, Wallon C, Blecic L, Forsmo HM, Folkesson J, Buchwald P, Korner H, Dahl FA, Oresland T, SCANDIV Study Group. Laparoscopic lavage vs primary resection for acute perforated diverticulitis the SCANDIV randomized clinical trial. JAMA. 2015;314(13):1364–75.
32. Afshar S, Kurer MA. Laparoscopic peritoneal lavage for perforated sigmoid diverticulitis. Color Dis. 2011;14:135–42.
33. Cuomo R, Barbara G, Pace F, Annese V, Bassotti G, Binda GA, Casetti T, Colecchia A, Festi D, Fiocca R, Laghi A, Maconi G, Nascimbeni R, Scarpignato C, Villanacci V, Annibale B. Italian consensus conference for colonic diverticulosis and diverticular disease. United European Gastroenterol J. 2014;2(5):413–42.
34. Andersen JC, Bundgaard L, Elbrond H, et al. Danish national guidelines for treatment of diverticular disease. Dan Med J. 2012;59:C4453.
35. Andeweg CS, Mulder IM, Felt-Bersma RJ, et al. Guidelines of diagnostics and treatment of acute left-sided colonic diverticulitis. Dig Surg. 2013;30:278–92.
36. Agresta F, Ansaloni L, Baiocchi GL, et al. Laparoscopic approach to acute abdomen from the Consensus Development Conference of the Societa Italiana di Chirurgia Endoscopica e nuove tecnologie (SICE), Associazione Chirurghi Ospedalieri Italiani (ACOI), Societa Italiana di Chirurgia (SIC), Societa Italiana di Chirurgia d'Urgenza e del Trauma (SICUT), Societa Italiana di Chirurgia nell'Ospedalita Priv ata (SICOP), and the European Association for Endoscopic Surgery (EAES). Surg Endosc. 2012;26:2134–64.
37. Solkar MH, Forshaw MJ, Sankararajah D, Stewart M, Parker MC. Colovesical fistula–is a surgical approach always justified? Color Dis. 2005;7:467–71.
38. Sallinen V, Mentula P, Leppaniemi A. Risk of colon cancer after computed tomography-diagnosed acute diverticulitis: is routine colonoscopy necessary? Surg Endosc. 2014;28:961–6.
39. Lau KC, Spilsbury K, Farooque Y, Kariyawasam SB, Owen RG, Wallace Afshar S, Kurer MA. Laparoscopic peritoneal lavage for perforated sigmoid diverticulitis. Color Dis. 2011;14: 135–42.
40. Sharma PV, Eglinton T, Hider P, Frizelle F. Systematic review and meta-analysis of the role of routine colonic evaluation after radiologically confirmed acute diverticulitis. Ann Surg. 2014; 259(2):263–72.
41. Fozard JB, Armitage NC, Schofield JB, Jones OM. ACPGBI position statement on elective resection for diverticulitis. Color Dis. 2011;13(Suppl 3):1–11.
42. van de Wall BJ, Draaisma WA, van Iersel JJ, Consten EC, Wiezer MJ, Broeders IA. Elective resection for ongoing diverticular disease significantly improves quality of life. Dig Surg. 2013; 30:190–7.
43. Mäkelä JT, Kiviniemi HO, Laitinen ST. Elective surgery for recurrent diverticulitis. Hepato-Gastroenterology. 2007;54:1412–6.

Part IV

Optimizing Surgical Management of Pelvic Floor Disorders

14 Utility of Pelvic Floor Testing for Clinical Assessment of Pelvic Floor Disorders?

Julia Saraidaridis and Liliana Bordeianou

Introduction

Pelvic floor disorders as they relate to the colorectal surgeon focus primarily on fecal incontinence and functional constipation. Both disorders incorporate the use of pelvic floor testing differently and therefore will be described separately. First the types of diagnostic tests used in the assessment of the pelvic floor will be explained followed by a discussion of how the workup of fecal incontinence and functional constipation incorporates these diagnostic maneuvers.

Pelvic Floor Testing

Anal Manometry

A small, thin, flexible catheter attached to a pressure transducer is introduced into the patient's rectum. Resting and squeeze (straining) pressures are calculated at each centimeter starting 6 cm from the anal verge. Maximal resting pressure is obtained at the area of highest pressure with the patient at rest (ranging from 40–80 mmHg). Maximum squeeze pressure is defined as the difference between the baseline pressure and the highest pressure that is recorded at any level during an episode of straining. Anal manometry also assesses the rectoanal inhibitory reflex (RAIR) wherein the internal sphincter relaxes with distension of the rectum. Finally, anal manometry

J. Saraidaridis (✉)
Division of Colon and Rectal Surgery, Lahey Clinic, Burlington, MA 01805, USA
e-mail: julia.t.saraidaridis@lahey.org

L. Bordeianou
Department of General Surgery, Massachusetts General Hospital, Boston, MA 02114, USA
e-mail: LBORDEIANOU@mgh.harvard.edu

C.M. Schlachta, P. Sylla (eds.), *Current Common Dilemmas in Colorectal Surgery*,
https://doi.org/10.1007/978-3-319-70117-2_14

allows quantification of rectal sensation and rectal compliance. A rectal balloon is slowly filled and the volume required to give the sensation of rectal distension, the urge to defecate, and intolerable distension are recorded [1, 2]. Normal volunteers usually describe a sensation of rectal distension at around 40 mL of air.

Balloon Expulsion Testing

This test is performed by inserting a balloon attached to a catheter into the rectum and then filling the balloon with 50–60 mL of air or water. The patient is then asked to defecate the balloon within 5 min. Most healthy patients can evacuate the balloon within 1 min [3].

Electromyography (EMG)

This test is performed by inserting a small EMG sponge with imbedded electrodes into the anal sphincter. Measurements of electrical activity are obtained with the patient at rest, squeeze, and push. Normally the sphincter complex relaxes during attempted evacuation, therefore the presence of contraction of the sphincter during attempted defecation is defined as abnormal.

Anal Endosonography

This test is performed using a 2D ultrasound scanner with a rotating endoprobe allowing for a 360° view of the anal canal. The probe is inserted 6 cm into the rectal cavity and then slowly removed obtaining cross-sectional images of the puborectalis, the external anal sphincter, and the internal anal sphincter. Defects in the external anal sphincter are visualized as hypoechogenic areas. Anal endosonography also allows assessment of sphincter muscle thickness and integrity.

Defecography

This test allows for a real time, dynamic evaluation of the act of defecation. All potential cavities or areas of prolapse are opacified with contrast to assist with visualization of the anatomy. The test begins 2 h prior to the actual examination with the patient drinking a liquid barium or gastrograffin slurry to opacify the small bowel. Opacification of the small bowel and colon is confirmed by performing a scout abdominal radiograph after 1 h. Once contrast is confirmed in the colon, approximately 10 ccs of barium paste is placed in the vagina (if the patient is female) and approximately 250–400 mL of thick barium paste (stool consistency) is inserted into the rectum. The patient is then placed onto a radiolucent upright commode. Fluoroscopic images are then obtained in video format while the patient is asked to rest, strain, and evacuate. Measurements are made of the anorectal angle and perineal descent. Normal patients demonstrate relaxation of the puborectal sling and a widening of the anorectal angle from 90° at rest to 135° with defecation [4]. Defecography is also helpful in identifying anatomic barriers to defecation including rectocele, sigmoidocele, enterocele, and internal rectal prolapse.

Pudendal Nerve Terminal Motor Latency

This test is performed by placing a disposable electrode onto the physician's finger which is then inserted into the anus and towards the ischial spines bilaterally. An electrical impulse is then delivered to the pudendal nerve and the time it takes for the external anal sphincter to respond is noted. Normal response is within 2.0+/−0.2 ms. A bilaterally prolonged motor latency is associated with a decreased maximum mean resting pressure and an increased fecal incontinence score [5].

Normal Physiology

While seemingly simple, the act of defecation requires a complex interplay of factors. The internal anal sphincter is a continuation of the smooth muscle layers of the rectum. This muscle thickens as it reaches the anal verge and undergoes continuous, tonic contraction that helps maintain continence. When rectal distension is encountered, the internal anal sphincter relaxes slightly in response to allow sampling of the rectal contents by the sensory nerves of the transition zone—this reflex is called the rectoanal inhibitory reflex (RAIR). This sampling allows discrimination of the nature of rectal contents. The internal anal sphincter provides approximately 80% of the resting anal pressure to provide continence with the external anal sphincter providing the rest. The external anal sphincter surrounds the internal sphincter and the puborectalis slings posteriorly around the sphincters. The puborectalis and external anal sphincter are under voluntary control and have somatic innervation (the external anal sphincter via the pudendal nerve and the puborectalis via pelvic branches of S3 and S4). When normal defecation occurs, a patient must relax both the external anal sphincter and the puborectalis muscle to allow the anorectal canal to straighten and the opening of the rectum. To prevent fecal incontinence, there is a spinal reflex that causes the external anal sphincter to contract during sudden increases in intra-abdominal pressure to aid in maintaining continence. While fecal incontinence and functional constipation can be due to a multitude of different factors, pelvic floor testing can be of significant utility in determining the etiology and subsequent management strategy of these disorders.

Fecal Incontinence

Fecal incontinence is characterized by the involuntary loss of solid or liquid feces for at least 1 month in a person over 4 years of age who had previously achieved fecal continence [6]. The prevalence of the disease is variable, but in an assessment of the Nurses' Health Study population was proposed to be around 4% in women 62–87 years [7]. The maintenance of fecal continence is a complex interplay of a number of factors including mental status, type of stool, colonic transit time, sphincter function, and anorectal sensation. Therefore fecal incontinence can have a number of different etiologies including decreased mental status, sphincter injury (obstetric or post-surgical), anatomic pathophysiology (rectocele, rectal prolapse, internal intussusception), pudendal nerve malfunction, overall neuropathy, decreased capacitance, and poorly controlled diarrhea.

Evaluation of fecal incontinence begins with obtaining a thorough history from the patient. The severity, onset, duration, and type of symptoms must be assessed. Validated surveys such as the Fecal Incontinence Severity Index are useful in this regard [8]. The patient must be questioned regarding the risk factors for incontinence including obstetric history, previous anorectal surgery, and other medical conditions such as diabetes mellitus, inflammatory bowel disease, neurologic disorders, and systemic sclerosis. After a thorough history, a physical exam including anoscopy is performed. Patients with concerns for loose stools or inflammatory processes should also undergo flexible sigmoidoscopy or colonoscopy if the situation merits. Physical exam includes an assessment of the external perineum for evidence of fistula, hemorrhoids, or rectal prolapse. The digital rectal exam should assess the patient's resting and squeeze sphincter tones. Once the history and physical exam has been performed, the clinician should have a good working theory as to the etiology of the fecal incontinence.

After the initial evaluation of fecal incontinence, regardless of potential cause, the first line treatment is medical therapy. There is no actual medication for FI but symptomatic control can be achieved by supplementing the diet with a bulking agent (such as methylcellulose). For those patients whose primary issue seems to be poorly controlled diarrhea, loperamide should be recommended (after infectious etiologies ruled out) [9]. And, finally, for those with overflow incontinence, laxatives and disimpaction to promote regular, soft, daily bowel movements are helpful. After assessment of the improvement after these lifestyle changes, our group recommends physical therapy and biofeedback (pelvic floor rehabilitation) to recoordinate pelvic floor and sphincter muscles. Biofeedback is thought to be helpful in 50–70% of patients with fecal incontinence [10, 11]. Most patients find the combination of medical symptomatic control and biofeedback to be of significant utility.

However, if fecal incontinence is not significantly improved by these initial measures, we then move on to pelvic floor testing to further elucidate potential treatable areas of fecal incontinence. For fecal incontinence there are three studies of significant utility: anal endosonography, anal manometry, and defecography. Our group usually starts with anal endosonography to assess for sphincter integrity. This test is thought to have a sensitivity of 68–100% and a specificity of 83% for identifying a sphincter defect (either of the internal or external anal sphincter) [12–14]. Anal endosonography is useful even if there is no clinical evidence of sphincter injury: in one study examining postpartum patients without clinically obvious tear, 28% had an anal injury that could be identified by anal endosonography. These patients subsequently had an odds ratio of 8.8 towards developing fecal incontinence in 3 months in comparison to their compatriots without occult injury [13]. Anal endosonography, like other ultrasonographic diagnostic tests, is operator dependent, however, in one study, intra-observer agreement was substantial (kappa 0.63) and inter-observer agreement was moderate (kappa 0.42). The true benefit of this test is that a sphincter defect demonstrated in ultrasound can be a surgically amenable etiology of fecal incontinence.

Regardless of anal endosonography results, patients should undergo anal manometry to delineate the function of the pelvic floor. The information gleaned from anal manometry is not specific or diagnostic for fecal incontinence but allows clinicians to better understand the etiology of present fecal incontinence and to better troubleshoot therapeutic benefit. Patients with fecal incontinence have significantly lower maximum resting pressure, maximal squeeze pressure, and decreased rectal capacitance than those who are continent, but there is significant overlap between subjects. Actual values of maximum resting pressure <40 mmHg, a maximal squeeze pressure <60 mmHg, and a rectal capacitance <200 mLs in women are thought to be seen primarily with incontinence [15, 16]. As stated, the results of anal manometry are heterogeneous between those with FI and those without, and there have been studies that demonstrate no correlation between the severity of FI and anal manometry [17]. Despite these misgivings, the information from anal manometry is helpful to the clinician. For patients with decreased MRP or MSP with sphincter defect, operative repair would be recommended. For those with decreased MRP and MSP without sphincter defect, biofeedback or sacral nerve stimulation would be recommended. For those with decreased capacitance, efforts towards frequent, scheduled stooling would be emphasized. Overall, anal manometry while not specifically diagnostic of fecal incontinence provides useful information for potential intervention in the disorder.

For patients in whom anal endosonography and anal manometry have been utilized and still there is clinical uncertainty, defecography is of benefit. While labor and resource intensive (radiolucent commode), defecography provides excellent information to the clinician. A decrease in the anorectal angle has been seen to be predictive of FI score [18]. More importantly, defecography can point to internal prolapse and rectocele which can both be repaired surgically.

In the past, PNTML has been hailed as one of the pillars of pelvic floor testing for fecal incontinence. More recently, however, it has been acknowledged to be of little utility. Pudendal neuropathy is present in up to 70% of patients with FI making this test's ability to differentiate the disease minimal. Some studies have shown that patients with prolonged PNTML would not benefit from sphincteroplasty [19], but this has been contested in other studies. Overall, PNTML provides little additional information to a clinician, and therefore we recommend that it not be part of the armamentarium for evaluating fecal incontinence.

Functional Constipation

Constipation is one of the most common gastrointestinal complaints and the etiologies of the complaint are variable. It is estimated to affect approximately 15% of the population [20]. For diagnosis of functional constipation a patient must fulfill the Rome III criteria including symptoms for 12 weeks in the last 6 months including: straining during at least 25% of defecations, lumpy or hard stools in 25% of defecations, sensation of incomplete evacuation for at least 25% of defecations, sensation of anorectal blockage for at least 25% of defecations, manual maneuvers to facilitate at least 25% of defecations, fewer than three defecations per week, loose stools rarely present without laxatives, and insufficient criteria for IBS [21]. Given these diagnostic criteria, it is important to start with a full history and physical with careful attention to other medical disorders that can cause constipation (diabetes, hypothyroidism) and medications (opioids) that exacerbate it. Clinicians should consider having their patients perform a 2-week diary tracking their bowel habits. Physical exam should rule out hemorrhoids, fissure, rectal mass, or rectal prolapse. Digital rectal exam should be performed feeling for tenderness, mass, stricture, and stool. The patient should be asked to strain looking for prolapse or rectocele. Based on symptomatology and physical exam, constipation can further be broken down into IBS constipation predominant, colonic transit disorder, and defecatory disorders. Obstructive defecation syndrome accounts for 50% of constipation cases. Colorectal surgeons are primarily interested in identifying dyssynergia and obstructive defecation.

Unless patients have worrisome symptoms including age >50, nocturnal diarrhea, bloody stools, family hx of colon cancer, the patient can be started empirically on fiber supplementation. However, if routine medical therapy fails, the patient should undergo pelvic floor evaluation. There are two types of constipation that can be treated by colorectal surgeons that require pelvic floor testing to elucidate: dyssynergia and obstructive defecation. Failure of coordination of the pelvic floor and rectoanal muscles can result in dyssynergia and this should be evaluated by pelvic floor testing. Additionally there are certain anatomic pathologies (internal rectal prolapse, for example) that prevent evacuation via obstruction that can only be discovered via pelvic floor testing.

Our group recommends four tests to evaluate the patient with suspected obstructive defecation: the balloon expulsion test, anal manometry, EMG, and defecography. The first pelvic floor test to evaluate the patient with suspected defecatory disorder is the balloon expulsion test, which is a quick and inexpensive way of ruling patients in for further evaluation. Most patients without defecatory disorders are able to expel the balloon in 1 min [22]. Patients unable to expel the balloon within 5 min are considered to have obstructive defecation although the test does discriminate between dyssynergia and anatomic obstruction.

Following the balloon expulsion test, we move onto anorectal manometry which allows an assessment of the coordination of movements involved in defecation. Three types of dysfunction of anal pressure have been identified on anal manometry: type 1 adequate pushing force with paradoxical increase in sphincter pressure, type 2 inadequate pushing force, type 3 adequate pushing force with incomplete sphincter relaxation [3]. All three of these types of dysfunction are consistent with dyssynergia and require biofeedback for amelioration. Anal manometry can also demonstrate an absence of a rectoanal inhibitory reflex which is consistent with a diagnosis of Hirschsprung's disease. Finally, patients with impaired rectal sensation and increased rectal capacitance (megarectum) are also identified via anal manometry. Overall, the test is useful in allowing understanding in the etiology of some types of functional constipation and can guide future attempts at biofeedback.

EMG can also assist in the diagnosis of dyssynergia due to a non-relaxing puborectalis or external anal sphincter. EMG tracings demonstrating contraction during attempted evacuation demonstrate non-relaxation and are consistent with dyssynergia. Patients with EMG findings of either contraction of puborectalis or external anal sphincter benefit from biofeedback therapy in ameliorating their constipation.

Finally, patients with suspected defecatory disorder that is not fully delineated by the three previous diagnostic maneuvers should undergo defecography. Defecography allows real-time evaluation of defecation, which can be the only way a clinician can identify the presence of internal intussusception, enteroceles, sigmoidoceles, and rectoceles.

After pelvic floor testing, clinicians are able to identify patients as having obstructive defecatory syndrome or dyssynergia. These patients benefit from biofeedback as it teaches patients to relax the anus and puborectalis during defecation. Additionally only pelvic floor testing can identify certain anatomic obstructions that can be repaired surgically. Overall, pelvic floor testing is an integral aspect of the workup of functional constipation.

Conclusion

Fecal incontinence and functional constipation are multifactorial conditions that require a nuanced workup by the clinician. The intelligent use of pelvic floor testing for these conditions can assist in identifying surgically correctable etiologies of these two disorders.

References

1. Kim JH. How to interpret conventional anorectal manometry. J Neurogastroenterol Motil. 2010;16(4):437–9.
2. Lam TJ, Mulder CJ, Felt-Bersma RJ. Critical reappraisal of anorectal function tests in patients with faecal incontinence who have failed conservative treatment. Int J Color Dis. 2012;27(7):931–7.
3. Rao SS. Constipation: evaluation and treatment of colonic and anorectal motility disorders. Gastroenterol Clin N Am. 2007;36(3):687–711, x.
4. Karasick S, Karasick D, Karasick SR. Functional disorders of the anus and rectum: findings on defecography. AJR Am J Roentgenol. 1993;160(4):777–82.
5. Ricciardi R, et al. The utility of pudendal nerve terminal motor latencies in idiopathic incontinence. Dis Colon Rectum. 2006;49(6):852–7.
6. Paquette IM, et al. The American Society of Colon and Rectal Surgeons' clinical practice guideline for the treatment of fecal incontinence. Dis Colon Rectum. 2015;58(7):623–36.
7. Matthews CA, et al. Risk factors for urinary, fecal, or dual incontinence in the Nurses' Health Study. Obstet Gynecol. 2013;122(3):539–45.
8. Rockwood TH, et al. Patient and surgeon ranking of the severity of symptoms associated with fecal incontinence: the fecal incontinence severity index. Dis Colon Rectum. 1999;42(12):1525–32.
9. Omar MI, Alexander CE. Drug treatment for faecal incontinence in adults. Cochrane Database Syst Rev. 2013;6:CD002116.
10. Keck JO, et al. Biofeedback training is useful in fecal incontinence but disappointing in constipation. Dis Colon Rectum. 1994;37(12):1271–6.
11. Pager CK, et al. Long-term outcomes of pelvic floor exercise and biofeedback treatment for patients with fecal incontinence. Dis Colon Rectum. 2002;45(8):997–1003.
12. Meyenberger C, et al. Anal sphincter defects in fecal incontinence: correlation between endosonography and surgery. Endoscopy. 1996;28(2):217–24.
13. Faltin DL, et al. Diagnosis of anal sphincter tears by postpartum endosonography to predict fecal incontinence. Obstet Gynecol. 2000;95(5):643–7.
14. Sultan AH, et al. Anal endosonography for identifying external sphincter defects confirmed histologically. Br J Surg. 1994;81(3):463–5.
15. Felt-Bersma RJ, Klinkenberg-Knol EC, Meuwissen SG. Anorectal function investigations in incontinent and continent patients. Differences and discriminatory value. Dis Colon Rectum. 1990;33(6):479–85. discussion 485–6.
16. Lam TJ, Kuik DJ, Felt-Bersma RJ. Anorectal function evaluation and predictive factors for faecal incontinence in 600 patients. Color Dis. 2012;14(2):214–23.
17. Zutshi M, et al. Anal physiology testing in fecal incontinence: is it of any value? Int J Color Dis. 2010;25(2):277–82.
18. Piloni V, et al. Measurement of the anorectal angle by defecography for the diagnosis of fecal incontinence. Int J Color Dis. 1999;14(2):131–5.
19. Birnbaum EH, et al. Pudendal nerve terminal motor latency influences surgical outcome in treatment of rectal prolapse. Dis Colon Rectum. 1996;39(11):1215–21.
20. Suares NC, Ford AC. Prevalence of, and risk factors for, chronic idiopathic constipation in the community: systematic review and meta-analysis. Am J Gastroenterol. 2011;106(9):1582–91. quiz 1581, 1592.
21. Drossman DA. The functional gastrointestinal disorders and the Rome III process. Gastroenterology. 2006;130(5):1377–90.
22. Rao SS, et al. Manometric tests of anorectal function in healthy adults. Am J Gastroenterol. 1999;94(3):773–83.

Rectal Prolapse in the Healthy Patient: Is Perineal Approach Ever Indicated?

15

Skandan Shanmugan and Joshua I.S. Bleier

Introduction

Perineal proctosigmoidectomy was first described in 1882 by Auffret [1] in France and later popularized by Miles [2] in 1930 at the famed St. Marks institution in London. This approach quickly became the preferred surgical remedy for rectal prolapse in the early twentieth century, but very few of Miles' successors were able to duplicate his early success [3, 4]. This discrepancy led to a marked increase in the recurrence rates in the early reports, and the procedure was less utilized. Resurgence in the technique occurred almost two decades later when William Altemeier at the University of Cincinnati theorized that the high recurrence rates seen in early perineal proctosigmoidectomies was due to the lack of rectal mobilization in the setting of a widened pelvic hiatus [5]. He therefore pioneered a technique of circumferential rectal dissection and resection of excess rectum and sigmoid along with a levatorplasty to narrow the pelvic defect. The Altemeier procedure, the eponym now most commonly attached to the perineal approach, quickly returned perineal proctosigmoidectomy to prominence only to be short lived, as over 100 surgical procedures for repair of full-thickness prolapse have since been described. Due to this heterogeneity in techniques, the Altemeier procedure has been relegated, albeit unfairly, to elderly or other high-risk patients who are not candidates for transabdominal repair [6]. This chapter will show that perineal proctosigmoidectomy has excellent results and decreased morbidity even in a wider spectrum of patients, including the young and healthy [7, 8].

Perineal Procto-(recto)-sigmoidectomy

The principal components of perineal proctosigmoidectomy are illustrated in Fig. 15.1. Prior to surgery, full-thickness rectal prolapse should clearly have been visualized and demonstrated to the surgeon in the clinic or with photo documentation.

S. Shanmugan • J.I.S. Bleier (✉)
Department of Surgery, PENN Presbyterian Medical Center, Philadelphia, PA, USA
e-mail: skandan.shanmugan@uphs.upenn.edu; joshua.bleier@uphs.upenn.edu

C.M. Schlachta, P. Sylla (eds.), *Current Common Dilemmas in Colorectal Surgery*,
https://doi.org/10.1007/978-3-319-70117-2_15

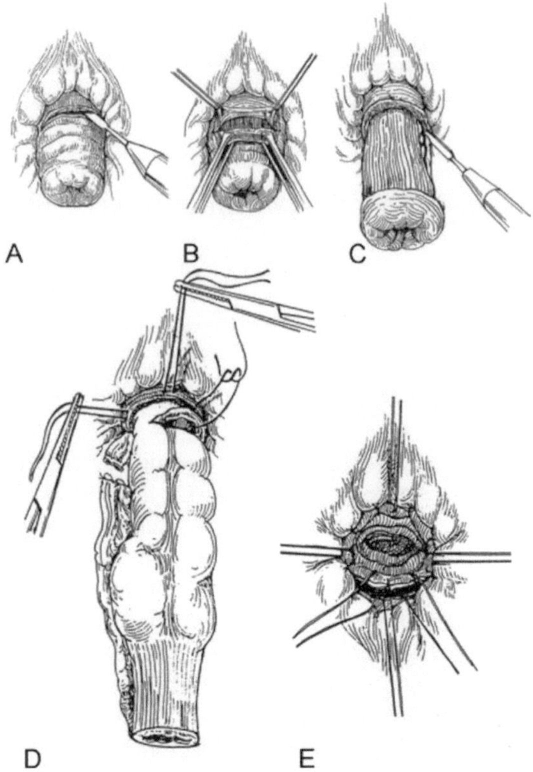

Fig. 15.1 Perineal rectosigmoidectomy. (**a**, **b**) Incision of rectal wall. (**c**) Division of vessel adjacent to bowel wall. (**d**) The prolapsed segment is amputated. Stay sutures previously placed in distal edge of outer cylinder are placed in cut edge of inner cylinder. (**e**) Anastomosis of distal aspect of remaining colon to the short rectal stump. [From Beck and Whitlow. Copyright 2003 by Taylor & Francis Group LLC (B). Reproduced with permission of Taylor & Francis Group (B) in the format Textbook via Copyright Clearance Center]

Consideration should be given to a preoperative barium enema to delineate a "road map" of the degree of redundancy, which can help the surgeon get a sense of how much bowel can be removed. Preoperative colonoscopy should have been accomplished in the immediate preoperative period or in the recent past. It is our preference that all patients receive mechanical bowel preparation with oral antibiotics. Patient positioning can vary based on surgeon preference but is usually done in a high lithotomy position. This will facilitate an emergent laparotomy if warranted, in rare but fatal complications of intra-abdominal bleeding, inadequate reach or anastomotic dehiscence, both of which may require an abdominal approach for further mobilization. However, the prone jackknife position offers better visualization and working space for the surgeon and assistants [9].

Anesthetic options include general endotracheal anesthesia or spinal anesthesia with local anesthetics. The procedure begins by prolapsing an adequate amount of rectum with Babcock or Allis clamps such that the distal rectum and dentate line are everted and easily visualized [10]. The use of a Lone Star® retractor (CooperSurgical, Trumbull, CT) or everting perianal sutures can also significantly improve exposure. A circumferential full-thickness incision is then made 1–2 cm above the dentate line. Some authors inject the rectal wall with an epinephrine solution to promote hemostasis prior to incision, but this is not absolutely necessary and can sometimes distort tissue planes. The circumferential incision is then deepened with electrocautery until the rectal wall has been divided. The redundant rectum and sigmoid colon are then sequentially withdrawn cephalad while progressively dividing and ligating the surrounding mesorectum and ligamentous attachments.

Newer generation bipolar devices such as a LigaSure™ (Covidien-Medtronic, Minneapolis, MN) or Harmonic® (Ethicon US, LLC) may facilitate the division of mesorectum and mesentery while being cautious to ensure complete hemostasis since some of these vascular pedicles may retract into the abdominal cavity once divided. The most difficult plane will most likely appear anteriorly at the level of the peritoneal reflection and the redundant hernia sac. This layer must be divided to enter the intra-abdominal cavity. The proximal dissection continues until there is no further redundancy remaining in the rectum and/or sigmoid colon. Applying differential traction first, on the pedicle and then the bowel itself helps elucidate whether additional bowel redundancy exists. The colon is then amputated at this level and held in place with one coloanal stitch. A levatorplasty is then undertaken either anteriorly or posteriorly by suturing the levator muscles together so as to allow 1–1½ fingers alongside the rectum. A circumferential handsewn coloanal anastomosis is then completed, usually in a single layer either in an interrupted or running fashion. Sequential division of the colon wall with serial sutures placed full thickness through distal rectal mucosa and proximal sphincter serves to complete the first layer of anastomosis as the bowel is being divided, so that by the time a circumferential division is complete, the anastomosis is grossly intact, with minimal risk of inadvertent retraction and loss of the bowel into the abdominal cavity. A completion rigid proctoscopy should be performed afterward to ensure a patent lumen without any signs of ischemia, obvious redundancy, or other pathologies.

Following the procedure, patients are placed in an enhanced recovery after surgery (ERAS) pathway that promotes early feeding, multimodal analgesia, and ambulation. The mortality rate from this procedure is nil, and morbidity is low and mostly stems from pre-existing medical conditions [11]. Ironically, this procedure results in the most distal of anastomoses, and one placed deliberately on tension, two of the primary hallmarks of a high-risk anastomosis—factors which would traditionally mandate proximal diversion, yet anastomotic dehiscence and pelvic sepsis are exceedingly rare but can occur and require a high index of suspicion and urgent intervention. Most study endpoints revolve around the rate of recurrence which can range from a cumulative rate of 40% in earlier studies prior to 1980 compared to a cumulative recurrence rate of 0–20% in later studies with a follow-up ranging from 6 months to 5 years [12]. In the past decade, excellent outcomes have been reported in many series prompting a reevaluation and resurgence of the perineal approach in the younger, healthy patient.

Glasgow et al. evaluated 103 consecutive patients undergoing perineal proctosigmoidectomy independent of age or other comorbidities. [7] The recurrence rate at 36 months was 8.5% with a significant improvement in fecal incontinence and constipation. Kim et al. evaluated 38 consecutive patients undergoing transperineal rectosigmoidectomy with excellent postoperative quality of life scores and functional results [13]. Their recurrence rate at 5 months was 2.6% (1/39). Finally, in perhaps the most conclusive testament to the Altemeier procedure, Cirocco et al. reviewed 103 consecutive patients [14]. Twelve of these patients presented with recurrent rectal prolapse following various abdominal procedures. The mean time for the operation was 97.7 min with a mean 7.2 cm of rectum resected. There was no mortality, minimal morbidity (14%), and no recurrence with mean follow-up of 43 months (range, 3 months to 10 years). These results are so convincing that these authors prefer the perineal approach as the initial operation regardless of age.

How then can we account for the conventional dogma that perineal proctosigmoidectomy has a perceived higher recurrence rate than most transabdominal approaches? Perhaps this can best be explained for the immense amount of heterogeneity among the literature and the fact that various perineal techniques are being incorporated into the category of perineal approaches. For instance, the Delorme procedure, which has become favored in Europe, is a substantially different technique than the Altemeier.

Delorme Procedure

The Delorme procedure entails mucosal stripping and not a full-thickness excision. A circumferential incision within the submucosal plane is made 1 cm proximal to the dentate line, and mucosal stripping is performed to the most proximal portion of prolapsed bowel and the stripped mucosa is then excised. After the circumferential mucosal sleeve resection, the muscularis layer is imbricated with serial vertical sutures (Fig. 15.2). Finally, an anastomosis is performed between the mucosal edges as is done with a handsewn coloanal anastomosis. Similar to the Altemeier procedure, hospital stay after Delorme is short, and complication rates are lower than abdominal approaches. Nevertheless, urinary retention, fecal impaction, infection, and bleeding have been reported in 4–12% [15–17]. Stricture and suture line dehiscence has also been reported.

Overall Delorme recurrence rates are higher than the Altemeier procedure likely because the peritoneal cavity is not entered and mucosal resection is limited. Nevertheless, incontinence rates and constipation are improved. Watts and Thompson in 2000 reviewed 101 patients and reported 27% recurrence rate, but 25% of patients displayed improvement in continence, and 13% showed improvement in constipation [17]. Additionally, Tobin and Scott reviewed 43 patients noting a 26% recurrence rate and 50% of patients noting improvement in continence [15]. Overall recurrence rates in literature range from 7% to 27%. Reported improvement rates in continence and constipation range from 25% to 70% and 13% to 100%, respectively. Recurrence rates are unequivocally higher than the abdominal approaches, and head-to-head comparisons have shown the Delorme procedure to also be inferior to the Altemeier in terms of recurrence. For instance, the only level I randomized control trial to evaluate the Altemeier versus Delorme procedures showed a recurrence rate of 23% (24/102) and 31% (31/99) favoring the former [18]. However, the Delorme may have a role in short-segment rectal prolapse or mucosal prolapse.

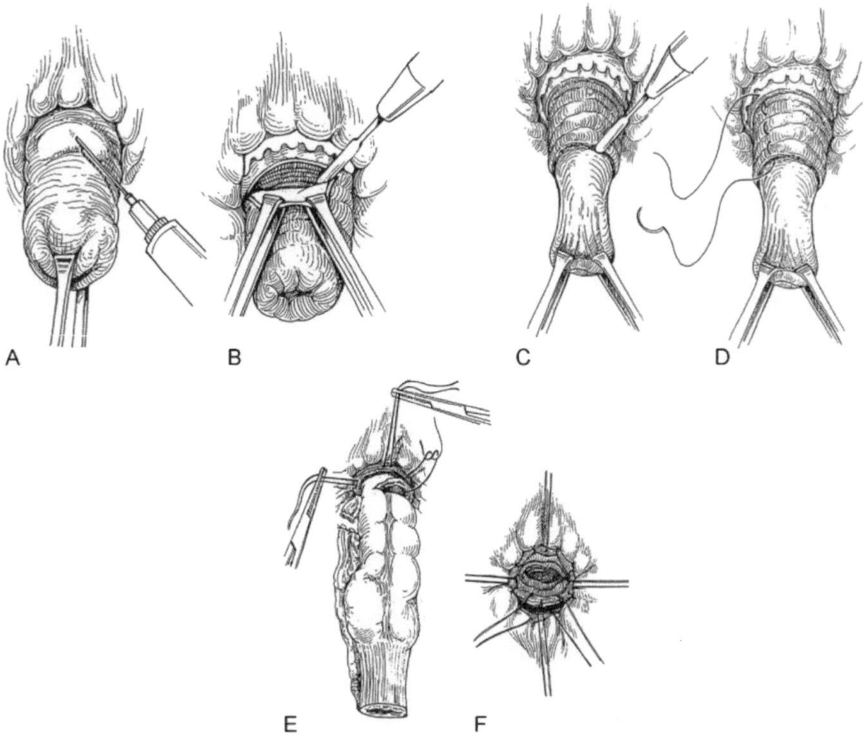

Fig. 15.2 Delorme's procedure. (**a**) Subcutaneous infiltration of dilute epinephrine solution. (**b**) Circumferential mucosal incision. (**c**) Dissection of mucosa off muscular layer. (**d**) Plicating stitch approximating cut edge of mucosa, muscular wall, and mucosa just proximal to dentate line. (**e**) Plicating stitch tied. (**f**) Completed anastomosis. [From Beck and Whitlow. Copyright 2003 by Taylor & Francis Group LLC (B). Reproduced with permission of Taylor & Francis Group (B) in the format Textbook via Copyright Clearance Center]

In addition to the Delorme procedure, some authors also include another technique where a semicircular stapling device is utilized. Ram et al. describe this perineal stapled prolapse resection with a recurrence rate of 29% in an alarmingly brief period of time [19]. Ironically all of these patients then underwent an Altemeier procedure as described earlier with improved results. Tschuor et al. echoed this conclusion and note that their 44% recurrence rate with a stapled perineal repair is higher than for the other perineal procedures [20]. Further alternations in technique include the fact that some surgeons perform perineal proctosigmoidectomy without a levatorplasty, which has been shown to have higher recurrence rate and a shorter time to recurrence than perineal rectosigmoidectomy with levatorplasty [21]. Therefore, technique matters and studies should be closely evaluated to elucidate which specific perineal procedure was utilized.

Historically, patients undergoing perineal proctosigmoidectomy are generally older with significantly more comorbidities than those who are considered for abdominal repair. Furthermore, recurrence rates have been reported to be as high as

16–30%. However, the studies of which these rates were inferred from are older, heterogeneous, and low quality (i.e., level IV) and involved small numbers of patients. In fact, a recent literature review showed that the cumulative rate of recurrence for studies up to 1971 was 37% (146 recurrences of 396 cases) and only 10% (126 recurrences of 1239 cases) for studies published after 1971 [13]. In fact, there have only been two randomized trials that compared abdominal repair to perineal proctosigmoidectomy. The earlier trial (1994) by Deen et al. [22] randomized ten patients to either a resection rectopexy vs. rectosigmoidectomy with only one recurrence in the perineal group. Senapati et al. [18] then compared 25 patients undergoing a perineal repair to 19 patients in the abdominal repair group, with recurrence rates measured at 20% (5/25) and 26% (5/19), respectively, at median 36 months follow-up. In a comprehensive Cochrane Review including 15 randomized controlled trials with 1007 participants, the authors concluded that "there was insufficient data to confidently comment on the difference in complications" and that they "did not see any obvious difference in recurrence between abdominal or perineal approaches [11].

Conclusion

A well-established dogma and older, heterogeneous literature seem to indicate that from the standpoint of recurrence, the perineal proctectomy offers an increased recurrence rate. However, recent, well-designed studies of perineal proctosigmoidectomy with levatorplasty do not uniformly bear this out. We do not mean to report that the perineal proctosigmoidectomy is superior to the various abdominal approaches, but it certainly should be included in same breadth of the surgical procedures for repair of rectal prolapse. If performed properly, the Altemeier procedure can achieve excellent results in any age group and should not only be relegated to older patients with significant comorbidities.

References

1. Auffret M. Un cas de procidence du gros intestin d'une longueur de 90 centimetres: operation par excision: double rangee de suture; mort. Prog Med. 1882;10:650–2.
2. Thompson HR. Discussion on prolapse of the rectum. Proc R Soc Med. 1949;41:1011.
3. Hughes ES. Discussion on prolapse of the rectum. Proc R Soc Med. 1949;41:1007–11.
4. Porter N. Collective results of operations for rectal prolapse. Proc R Soc Med. 1962;55:1087–91.
5. Altemeier WA, Hoxworth PI, Giuseffi J. Further experiences with the treatment of prolapse of the rectum. Surg Clin N Am. 1955;35:1437–47.
6. Varma M, Rafferty J, Buie D. Practice parameters for the management of rectal prolapse. Dis Colon Rectum. 2011;54:1339–46.
7. Glasgow SC, Birnbaum EH, Kodner IJ, Fleshman JW Jr, Dietz DW. Recurrence and quality of life following perineal proctectomy for rectal prolapse. J Gastrointest Surg. 2008;12:1446–51.
8. Goldberg SM, Mayoral JL. Rectal prolapse: perineal approach. In: Baker RJ, Fischer JE, editors. Mastery of surgery. 4th ed. Philadelphia: Lippincott Williams & Wilkins; 2001. p. 1626–32.

9. Showalter SL, Kelz RR, Mahmoud NN. Effect of technique on postoperative perineal wound infections in abdominoperineal resection. Am J Surg. 2013;206(1):80–5.
10. Steele SR, Hull TL, Read TE, Saclarides TJ, Senagore AJ, Whitlow CB, editors. The ASCRS textbook of colon and rectal surgery. Cham: Springer; 2007. p. 1077–89.
11. Tou S, Brown SR, Nelson RL. Surgery for complete (full-thickness) rectal prolapse in adults. Cochrane Database Syst Rev. 2015 Nov 24;(11):CD001758. doi: 10.1002/14651858.CD001758.pub3.
12. Barfield LR. Perineal approaches to rectal prolapse. Clin Colon Rectal Surg. 2017;30(1):12–5. https://doi.org/10.1055/s-0036-1593432.
13. M K, Reibetanz J, Boenicke L, Germer CT, Jayne D, Isbert C. Quality of life after transperineal rectosigmoidectomy. Br J Surg. 2010;97(2):269–72.
14. Cirocco W. The Altemeier procedure for rectal prolapse: an operation for all ages. Dis Colon Rectum. 2010;53:1618–23.
15. Tobin SA, Scott IHK. Delorme operation for rectal prolapse. Br J Surg. 1994;81:1681.
16. Pidala MJ. Rectal prolapse. In: Bailey HR, Billingham RP, Stamos MJ, Snyder MJ, editors. Colorectal surgery. Philadelphia: Elsevier Saunders; 2013. p. 475–87.
17. Watts AMI, Thompson MR. Evaluation of Delorme's procedure as a treatment for full-thickness rectal prolapse. Br J Surg. 2000;87(2):218–22.
18. Senapati A, Gray RG, Middleton LJ, Harding J, Hills RK, Armitage NCM, et al. PROSPER: a randomized comparison of surgical treatments for rectal prolapse. Color Dis. 2013;15(7):858–68.
19. Ram E, Krissi H, Zbar A, Atar E, Joubran S, Rath-Wolfson L. Perineal stapled prolapse resection (PSPR) in elderly patients for external rectal prolapse: early experience. Tech Coloproctol. 2014;18:1003. https://doi.org/10.1007/s10151-014-1137-9.
20. Tschuor C, Limani P, Nocito A, Dindo D, Clavien P-A, Hahnloser D. Perineal stapled prolapse resection for external rectal prolapse: is it worthwhile in the long-term? Tech Coloproctol. 2013;17:537–40.
21. Chun SW, Pikarsky AJ, You SY, Gervaz P, Efron J, Weiss E, Nogueras JJ, Wexner SD. Perineal rectosigmoidectomy for rectal prolapse: role of levatorplasty. Tech Coloproctol. 2004;8(1):3–8; discussion 8-9.
22. Deen KI, Grant E, Billingham C, Keighley MR. Abdominal resection rectopexy with pelvic floor repair versus perianal rectosigmoidectomy and pelvic floor repair for full-thickness rectal prolapse. Br J Surg. 1994;81(2):302–4.

Rectal Prolapse in the Health Patient: Which Abdominal Approach?

16

Peter Alexander Newman and Tony Dixon

Introduction

Surgery is the treatment for rectal prolapse, yet there is no such uniformly accepted operation. Part of this reason is that rectal prolapse is not a singular diagnosis due to a singular pathophysiological mechanism. It is part of a spectrum of disorders of the pelvic floor and it does not occur in isolation. The (dys)functionality of each compartment may be interpreted differently by patients, hence resulting in a wide spectrum of symptomatology. The published data from which we can make informed decisions is a myriad of low-level evidence at high risk of bias with a paucity of good quality randomised control trials. The PROSPER trial attempts to plug this gap and yet suffered difficulty in patient recruitment highlighting difficulties in clinical research within this field [1]. However, there have been dramatic changes in the approach to these patients with pioneering surgeons questioning traditionally held beliefs, for example, in the recognition of internal rectal prolapse as a separate pathological entity and the development of laparoscopic ventral mesh rectopexy (LVMR). Clearly there is a huge capacity for further research, and with the increasing uptake of minimally invasive modalities of treatment, most recently robotic surgery, this is a rapidly advancing and exciting area of colorectal surgery.

In order to answer the question posed 'which abdominal approach?' the disease entity, aetiology and underlying pathophysiology must be considered. With these in mind, the principles of different interventions can be considered critically, the approach which can be perineal (discussed earlier) or abdominal (open, laparoscopic or robotic), the degree of mobilisation and the method of fixation, which materials should be employed and whether or not resection should be considered.

P.A. Newman • T. Dixon (✉)
Department of Colorectal Surgery, North Bristol NHS Trust, Southmead Hospital Bristol, Bristol, UK
e-mail: peteralex.newman@nbt.nhs.uk; anthony.dixon@nbt.nhs.uk

C.M. Schlachta, P. Sylla (eds.), *Current Common Dilemmas in Colorectal Surgery*,
https://doi.org/10.1007/978-3-319-70117-2_16

The evidence base to inform decision making practices will continue to progress and must be viewed regularly and critically by any surgeon seeking to treat patients with rectal prolapse.

Definitions

Rectal prolapse (RP) represents a failure in the functional supportive mechanisms of the posterior pelvic compartment. External rectal prolapse (ERP) is a full-thickness protrusion or intussusception of all the layers of the rectum beyond the anal canal and classically is diagnosed by the presence of concentric rings of rectal mucosa on examination. Internal rectal prolapse (IRP) precedes ERP and is the progressive internal intussusception of rectal tissue; this is graded according to the most proximal or origin of the intussusception site and the most distal anatomical level into which it proceeds, recto-rectal high or low (grades 1 and 2, respectively) and recto-anal high or low (grades 3 and 4, respectively) and ERP (grade 5) [2].

Aetiology

When considering management for these patients, a clear understanding of the anatomy of the pelvic floor and the associated functional effects of pelvic floor prolapse is required in order to select optimal intervention. The aetiology is unclear, although prolapse is associated with conditions that increase intra-abdominal/intra-pelvic pressure (e.g. obesity) and reduction in the quantity (e.g. post hysterectomy) or quality (e.g. connective tissue disorder) of the supportive structures to withstand the pressure effects and behavioural factors (e.g. chronic straining). Postulated mechanisms include a disruption of the collagen-rich extracellular matrix of connective tissue that envelopes the pelvic viscera, supported by histological findings [3–5] and the change in intra-luminal force vectors during defaecation [6]. Anatomical features include a redundant sigmoid colon, the loss of a vertical position of the rectum and a deep pouch of Douglas [7]. Importantly, the underpinning pathophysiology is not limited to the posterior compartment and will also affect the middle and anterior compartments to a greater or lesser extent.

Symptoms

Patients with ERP may present with a bulge that may or may not reduce spontaneously. The symptoms for IRP may be less clear including a sensation of a lump or dragging sensation during defaecation. Often there are associated functional symptoms such as constipation, obstruction and faecal incontinence, and there may be a history of rectal bleeding, mucous discharge or pain. As ERP or IRP occurs in tandem with other pelvic organ prolapse (POP) disorders, there may be vaginal vault prolapse, dyspareunia and urinary incontinence [7]. RP is a debilitating condition which can severely impair quality of life (QoL).

Patient Assessment

A proctological, gynaecological and urological history should be obtained along with the use of validated symptom questionnaires to provide preoperative information and for follow-up purposes. All compartments require examination. Investigations should be tailored to the individual patient, endoscopic studies are useful in excluding other pathologies and imaging and physiology investigations may help surgical approach in patients with constipation or incontinence. Patients should, if possible, be discussed at a pelvic floor multidisciplinary team meeting in order to provide an individualised treatment care plan [8].

Surgical Options

The management of RP is surgical, either via an abdominal or perineal approach. This area of speciality has seen dramatic changes over the past decade with the popular uptake of minimal invasive technique utilising and the modifying of traditional open techniques. There is a myriad of published literature with over 300 operations described, yet there is a significant heterogeneity between studies and a paucity of good quality randomised controlled trials (RCTs) to draw conclusions, and as such no evidence-based guidelines exist [9]. This chapter will focus on abdominal approaches to the management of RP; perineal approaches will be considered here as a comparator to the abdominal approaches but are discussed in an earlier chapter.

Abdominal approaches can be considered in terms of access, open versus minimally invasive laparoscopic versus robotic techniques, mobilisation of the rectum, method of fixation and whether or not colonic resection is performed. Each broad category will be discussed. Surgical principles are to correct the underlying anatomical abnormality rather than just focusing on the pathological consequence, hence improving the symptoms and the functional effects these patients suffer.

Access

Perineal, open, laparoscopic and robotic access will be reviewed in general. Historically, an open operation is more effective than a perineal but with greater morbidity due to the patient undergoing a laparotomy [10], yet mortality rates between perineal procedures and open abdominal procedures are comparable at 0–5% and 0–7%, respectively [11]. Perineal procedures have a high recurrence rate, up to 16% with Altemeier's and 38% with Delorme's procedure [11]; this is part explained by selection bias towards older patients with poorer tissue quality and medical comorbidities and part explained by perineal procedures not addressing the underlying pathology but rather treating the external consequence. From a functional perspective, resecting colon via a local approach, i.e. rectosigmoidectomy, can unsurprisingly result in worsening faecal continence; however, constipation is usually less of a problem.

Table 16.1 shows data from observational studies for patients undergoing these different surgical procedures [11, 12].

The advantage of a trans-abdominal route is that it allows the surgeon to address the underlying pathology that results in rectal prolapse. The extent of mobilisation, fixation and whether or not resection is needed can all be finalised and performed trans-abdominally rather than locally. Indeed, decision making may change due to intraoperative findings, and there is an option for treating the middle or anterior pelvic compartment as well. There are two small RCTs that compare open with perineal surgery [1, 13], and a recently updated Cochrane review reports no significant difference between the groups in terms of recurrence, incontinence, morbidity or QoL as measured by the EQ-5D at 3 years post-surgery [14].

Table 16.2 shows data from randomised trials undergoing interventions for rectal prolapse [1, 13, 15–17].

In the laparoscopic era, a trans-abdominal approach to the pelvis using minimal invasive techniques has become increasingly popular. A comprehensive systematic review on ventral rectopexy for ERP and IRP, including 12 studies, demonstrated an improvement in continence and constipation in those undergoing laparoscopic ventral mesh rectopexy (LVMR) of 30–73% and 15–83%, respectively [12]. The advantages of this approach specific to treatment of RP are that it provides good visualisation and surgical access within the rigid confines of the pelvis and avoids placing the patient prone, the pneumoperitoneum can aid in dissection and associated POP can be treated simultaneously. More general advantages include lower post-operative morbidity and less pain.

Laparoscopy is safe in the elderly. In a case series, Wijffels et al. assessed the outcomes of patients over the age of 80 undergoing laparoscopic ventral mesh rectopexy (LVMR) and reported a recurrence rate of 3% at a median follow-up of 23 months with no mortality and only one major complication [18]. This has called into question the use of a perineal approach in this cohort.

An economic evaluation of laparoscopic versus open abdominal rectopexy demonstrated a significantly shorter hospital stay (mean 3.9 vs. 6.6 days, $P = 0.001$) and reduced overall cost by 11% [19]. Tou et al. identified two RCTs which compared open with laparoscopic surgery and identified fewer complications (30% vs. 73%), a shorter length of stay (mean 2.35 days less) and no recurrence (0% vs. 5%) in the laparoscopic group [14]; see Table 16.2. A contemporaneous RCT—the DeloRes trial (German Clinic Trial Number DRKS00000482)—seeks to compare Delorme's procedure with laparoscopic resection rectopexy with recurrence as the primary outcome measure [20], results of which will help inform surgeons.

The use of robotic systems to assist in performing rectopexy (RR) for rectal prolapse has also been reported [17, 21–23]. This is theoretically advantageous with improved ergonomics, allowing for a more controlled dissection with greater visualisation, but offset by no tactile feedback and high cost. There is no significant difference in complications between LVMR and RR, and the functional outcomes are in keeping with laparoscopic surgery [9].

The current use of open surgery should be limited to those who have been converted from minimally invasive techniques, for example, due to adhesions. Perineal

Table 16.1 Adapted data from observational studies for surgical treatment of rectal prolapse

		Procedure	Number of studies	Number of participants	Follow-up (months)	Recurrence (%)	Functional outcomes (% improvement)		Mortality (%)
							Incontinence	Constipation	
Perineal		Delorme's [11]	10	410	11–47	0–38	32–67	13–100	0–4
		Altemeier's [11]	12	579	12–228	0–16	−22–91	61	0–5
Abdominal	Open	Suture rectopexy [11]	5	206	47–144	0–9	−12–75	−31–83	0
		Posterior rectopexy [11]	14	753	12–84	0–6	3–75	−48–100	0–3
		Resection with suture rectopexy [11]	9	511	12–98	0–5	11–100	18–80	0–7
		Division of lateral ligaments [11]	8	307	n/a	n/a	−10–64	−48–18	n/a
		Preservation of lateral ligaments [11]	16	1010	n/a	n/a	−10–75	−17–89	n/a
		Ventral rectopexy with posterior mobilisation [12]	7	476	24–60	0–9	14–60	−14–29	n/a
	Laparoscopic	Suture rectopexy [11]	5	124	24–48	0–7	50–82	−11–76	0
		Posterior rectopexy [11]	5	119	8–30	0–4	10–92	−38–0	0
		Resection with suture rectopexy [11]	3	60	12–18	0	70–100	0–64	0
		Division of lateral ligaments [11]	4	112	n/a	n/a	50–100	14	n/a
		Preservation of lateral ligaments [11]	4	93	n/a	n/a	64–82	64–76	n/a
		Ventral rectopexy without posterior mobilisation [12]	5	217	3–61	0–15	30–73	15–83	n/a

n/a not applicable or data not available

Table 16.2 Adapted data from randomised trials for surgical treatment of rectal prolapse

Author	Comparison	Year	Number of patients	Indication	Follow-up months	Recurrence %	Functional outcomes: Incontinence	Functional outcomes: Constipation	QoL	Mortality
Senapati et al. [1][a]		2013	293[b]	ERP	Median 36		Vaizey	Bowel thermometer	EQ-5D	
	Abdominal vs. perineal		23 vs. 26			20 vs. 26 (NS)	4.6 vs. 5.0 (NS)	52 vs. 50 (NS)	0.73 vs. 0.86 (NS)	13 vs. 0 (NS)
	Suture rectopexy vs. resection		38 vs. 40			26 vs. 13 (NS)	4.8 vs. 4.5 (NS)	63 vs. 66 (NS)	0.7 vs. 0.82 (NS)	5 vs. 13 (NS)
	Altemeier's vs. delorme's		106 vs. 107			24 vs. 31 (NS)	7.6 vs. 7.4 (NS)	68 vs. 68 (NS)	0.72 vs. 0.68 (NS)	22 vs. 22 (NS)
Deen et al. [13]	Abdominal resection vs. Altemeier's	1994	10 vs. 10	ERP with FI	Median 17	0 vs. 10 (NS)	20% vs. 60% (NS)[c]	0%	n/a	0 vs. 0 (NS)
Boccasanta et al. [15]	Open Well's vs. laparoscopic Well's	1998	13 vs. 8	ERP with FI	Mean 29.5	8 vs. 0 (NS)	n/a	23% vs. 0%	n/a	n/a
Solomon et al. [16]	Open vs. laparoscopic lateral rectopexy	2002	19 vs. 20	ERP	Mean 24	5 vs. 0 (NS)	2 vs. 1.6 (NS)	n/a	n/a	n/a
Mäkelä-Kaikkonen et al. [17]	Laparoscopic vs. robotic ventral rectopexy	2016	14 vs. 16	ERP or IRP	3	0 vs. 0	n/a	n/a	n/a	n/a

[a]Essentially three RCTs in one study
[b]293 patients of which 47 were in two arms, hence 340 randomised comparisons
[c]Faecal soiling based on A–D grading system
NS nonstatistically significant, *n/a* not applicable or data not available, *ERP* external rectal prolapse, *IRP* internal rectal prolapse, *FI* faecal incontinence

procedures will continue to play a role for those who are deemed unfit for a general anaesthetic; but given the safety of modern anaesthetic [24] and the proven safety profile of laparoscopic approach in elderly patients along with the greater functional results, minimally invasive techniques will continue to be adopted and should become the mainstay of practice. Both the complex redo surgical patient and those with a failed perineal procedure can be managed laparoscopically in the appropriate tertiary setting with good outcomes [25, 26].

Mobilisation

The degree of mobilisation of the rectum is an important factor in determining functional results. Posterior rectopexy with complete circumferential mobilisation of the rectum (Wells) has a low recurrence rate [27] but an unacceptably high rate of constipation, with worsening in 20–30% of patients [28]. D'Hoore et al. (2004) noted that constipation rates were in the region of 50% after posterior rectopexy [29]. Anterior and posterior mobilisation (Orr-Loygue) has been shown to have a low recurrence rate but high levels of constipation although this is improved with limited lateral dissection [30]. Observational studies report that division of lateral ligaments can worsen constipation by up to 48%; this contrasts with ventral mesh rectopexy without posterior mobilisation improving constipation by up to 83% [12]. Two small RCTs comparing preservation vs. division of the lateral ligaments of the pelvic side wall report nonsignificantly higher rates of recurrence (33% vs. 0%) but lower rates of constipation (8% vs. 50%, OR 0.32); however, these were open procedures using different fixation methods [14]. Ventral mobilisation spares the lateral pelvic side wall ligaments hence preserving the intrinsic autonomic nerve supply to the rectum with reduced post-operative constipation and is the basis for the development of LVMR.

Fixation

Rectal fixation or rectopexy can be performed with sutures or mesh, the material can be synthetic or biological and location of fixation can vary. There is disagreement between trials which assess the need for rectopexy following rectal mobilisation; however, those showing no benefit from rectopexy are poor-quality studies with no level 1 evidence [31]. A large international non-inferiority RCT involving over 250 patients demonstrated the advantage of rectopexy over no rectopexy with recurrence rates of 1.5% vs. 8.6% ($P = 0.003$), respectively, at 5-year follow-up [32].

Sutured rectopexy involves dorsal mobilisation in order to tack the rectum to the sacrum. A 5-year recurrence was reported as 6%, but this increased to 20% at 10 years highlighting the importance of long-term follow-up for these patients [33]. Interestingly an analysis of a variety of abdominal operations for ERP did not show that the surgical technique employed had any effect on the rate of recurrence suggesting the significance of the scarring process [34]. There is a need for a RCT comparing sutured with mesh rectopexy.

Mesh can be biological or synthetic with a panel of experts recommending the use of titanium-coated lightweight polypropylene mesh [35]. Polyester mesh is a predictor for mesh-related complications, recurrence and further intervention and hence should not be used [36]. The results from 13 observational studies suggest that biological mesh is as effective as synthetic mesh, although they represented only 11.4% of the patient cohort with limited long-term follow-up [37]. Mesh-related complications have been shown to be amenable to laparoscopic correction with revisional surgery being equally effective for failed interventions or complications ensuing from xenografts [26].

LVMR combines the autonomic nerve sparring mobilisation with placement of mesh. In their study of 190 LVMRs followed up for a median of 73 months, Randall et al. reported 60-day mortality, recurrence and mesh-related complication at 1%, 3% and 3.7%, respectively, and also sustained improvement in QoL [25]. The Belgian and Dutch observational study reported a 10-year recurrence rate of 8.2% which is in line with the more classic types of mesh rectopexy [38]. The advantage of this procedure is that all compartments of the pelvic floor can be addressed. It has a proven safety profile and is effective in the treatment of ERP, IRP and solitary rectal ulcer syndrome (SRUS), and it gives the surgeons access to the middle and anterior compartment; hence, genital prolapse and cystoceles can be managed simultaneously [25, 39–41]. Indeed, during LVMR, a window can be made, and a sutured posterior rectopexy can be performed if needed. LVMR is technically demanding using laparoscopic instruments, and there is a protracted learning curve of over 100 cases prior to achieving predictable functional results [36].

Resection

Bowel resection as part of the surgical treatment was described by Frykman and Goldberg [42]. The principle of resection is logical given the finding of redundant sigmoid and the mechanical effect of performing an anastomosis. This is particularly true for patients who have pre-existing constipation. In the abdominal procedure arm of the PROPSER trial, patients were further randomised into sutured rectopexy with or without resection which found no significant difference in rates of recurrence [1]. Pooled analysis of three RCTs shows lower rates of post-operative constipation with bowel resection (0.14, 95% CI 0.04–0.44) and no difference in incontinence [14]. However, performing a resection is a major undertaking, will increase the risk of complications (although not significant in the three RCTs) and should not be performed if it can be avoided.

Conclusion

Evaluation of different techniques for the treatment of prolapse is difficult due to the poor quality of studies and the lack of a consistent definition of outcome parameters. There is a desperate need for adequately powered trials with defined primary outcome measures, long-term follow-up, which incorporates validated functional symptom questionnaires with formal QoL assessments and cost analysis, in order to evaluate the reliability of each repair technique.

There is a large variety of operations that can be employed to treat RP. In answer to the question posed—which abdominal approach?—simply put, this depends on the individual patient: age, health status, underlying pathology and functional disorders, as well as the available surgical service and expertise. As such, all patients should be discussed at a pelvic floor multidisciplinary team meeting and options considered with the patient in order to create an individualised treatment plan. This is especially the case with benign functional disorders with significant psychological sequelae. Minimally invasive surgery is safe even in the elderly and has a lower recurrence profile than perineal operations. Ventral mobilisation preserves the lateral nerves of the pelvis, and hence there are lower rates of post-operative constipation. With LVMR, the anterior wall of the posterior compartment and the posterior wall of the middle compartment are treated with the option of correcting the posterior wall of the posterior and anterior compartment and the anterior wall of the middle compartment. Pelvic floor surgery is ideally suited for robotic assistance given the fixed and confined space.

Current areas for further consideration include an up-to-date review of current practice of treatment of RP, a further cross-speciality collaboration with gynaecologists and urologists and the development of a national if not international database in order to provide live real-time feedback and comparisons to surgeons, especially given the difficulty, cost and 'time-decay' nature of RCTs.

References

1. Senapati A, Gray RG, Middleton LJ, Harding J, Hills RK, Armitage NCM, et al. PROSPER: a randomised comparison of surgical treatments for rectal prolapse. Color Dis. 2013;15(7):858–68.
2. Collinson R, Cunningham C, D'Costa H, Lindsey I. Rectal intussusception and unexplained faecal incontinence: findings of a proctographic study. Color Dis. 2009;11(1):77–83.
3. Soderberg MW, Falconer C, Bystrom B, Malmstrom A, Ekman G. Young women with genital prolapse have a low collagen concentration. Acta Obstet Gynecol Scand. 2004;83(12):1193–8.
4. Jackson S, Avery NC, Tarlton JF, Eckford SD, Abrams P, Bailey AJ. Changes in metabolism of collagen in genitourinary prolapse. Lancet. 1996;347(9016):1658–61.
5. Moalli PA, Shand SH, Zyczynski HM, Gordy SC, Men LA. Remodelling of vaginal connective tissue in patients with prolapse. Obstet Gynecol. 2005;106(5):593–63.
6. Dixon AR. Pathophysiological approach to obstruction defecation. In: Lindsey I, Nugent K, Dixon AR, editors. Pelvic floor disorders for the colorectal surgeon. Oxford: Oxford University Press; 2010. p. 57–68.

7. Bordeianou L, Hicks CW, Kaiser AM, Alavi K, Sudan R, Wise PE. Rectal prolapse: an overview of clinical features, diagnosis, and patient-specific management strategies. J Gastrointest Surg. 2014;18(5):1059–69.
8. The Pelvic Floor Society. 2014. QA and Standards. (Online). Available from http://thepelvicfloorsociety.co.uk/pages.php?t=QA-&-standards&s=QA-&-Governance&id=101. Accessed 10 June 2016.
9. Van Iersel JJ, Paulides TJ, Verheijen PM, Lumley JW, Broeders IA, Consten EC. Current status of laparoscopic and robotic ventral mesh rectopexy for external and internal rectal prolapse. World J Gastroenterol. 2016;22(21):4977–87.
10. Melton GB, Kwaan MR. Rectal prolapse. Surg Clin North Am. 2013;93(1):187–98.
11. Madiba TE, Baig MK, Wexner SD. Surgical management of rectal prolapse. Arch Surg. 2005;140(1):63–73.
12. Samaranayake CB, Luo C, Plank AW, Merrie AE, Plank LD, Bissett IP. Systematic review on ventral rectopexy for rectal prolapse and intussusception. Color Dis. 2010;12(6):504–12.
13. Deen KI, Grant E, Billingham C, Keighley MR. Abdominal resection rectopexy with pelvic floor repair versus perianal rectosigmoidectomy and pelvic floor repair for full-thickness rectal prolapse. Br J Surg. 1994;81(2):302–4.
14. Tou S, Brown SR, Nelson RL. Surgery for complete (full-thickness) rectal prolapse in adults. Cochrane Database Syst Rev. 2015;(11):CD001758. https://doi.org/10.1002/14651858.CD002758.pub3.
15. Boccasanta P, Rosati R, Venturi M, Montorsi M, Cioffi U, De Simone M, et al. Comparison of laparoscopic rectopexy with open technique in the treatment of complete rectal prolapse: clinical and functional results. Surg Laparosc Endosc. 1998;8(6):460–5.
16. Solomon MJ, Young CJ, Eyers AA, Roberts RA. Randomized clinical trial of laparoscopic versus open abdominal rectopexy for rectal prolapse. Br J Surg. 2002;89(1):35–9.
17. Mäkelä-Kaikkonen J, Rautio T, Klintrup K, Takala H, Vierimaa M, Ohtonen P, Mäkelä J. Robotic-assisted and laparoscopic ventral rectopexy in the treatment of rectal prolapse: a matched-pairs study of operative details and complications. Tech Coloproctol. 2014;18(2):151–5.
18. Wijffels N, Cunningham C, Dixon A, Greenslade G, Lindsey I. Laparoscopic ventral rectopexy for external rectal prolapse is safe and effective in the elderly. Does this make perineal procedures obsolete? Color Dis. 2011;13(5):561–6.
19. Salkeld G, Bagia M, Solomon M. Economic impact of laparoscopic versus open abdominal rectopexy. Br J Surg. 2004;91(9):1188–91.
20. Rothenhoefer S, Herrle F, Herold A, Joos A, Bussen D, Kieser M, Schiller P, Klose C, Seiler CM, Kienle P, Post S. DeloRes trial: study protocol for a randomized trial comparing two standardized surgical approaches in rectal prolapse – Delorme's procedure versus resection rectopexy. Trials. 2012;13(1):155.
21. Wong MT, Meurette G, Rigaud J, Regenet N, Lehur PA. Robotic versus laparoscopic rectopexy for complex rectocele: a prospective comparison of short-term outcomes. Dis Colon Rectum. 2011;54(3):342–6.
22. Mantoo S, Podevin J, Regenet N, Rigaud J, Lehur PA, Meurette G. Is robotic-assisted ventral mesh rectopexy superior to laparoscopic ventral mesh rectopexy in the management of obstructed defaecation? Color Dis. 2013;15(8):469–75.
23. de Hoog DE, Heemskerk J, Nieman FH, van Gemert WG, Baeten CG, Bouvy ND. Recurrence and functional results after open versus conventional laparoscopic versus robot-assisted laparoscopic rectopexy for rectal prolapse: a case-control study. Int J Color Dis. 2009;24(10):1201–6.
24. Lagasse RS. Anesthesia safety: model or myth? A review of the published literature and analysis of current original data. Anesthesiology. 2002;97(6):1609–17.
25. Randall J, Smyth E, McCarthy K, Dixon AR. Outcome of laparoscopic ventral mesh rectopexy for external rectal prolapse. Color Dis. 2014;16(11):914–9.
26. Badrek-Al Amoudi AH, Greenslade GL, Dixon AR. How to deal with complications after laparoscopic ventral mesh rectopexy: lessons learnt from a tertiary referral centre. Color Dis. 2013;15(6):707–12.

27. Dulucq JL, Wintringer P, Mahajna A. Clinical and functional outcome of laparoscopic posterior rectopexy (Wells) for full-thickness rectal prolapse. A prospective study. Surg Endosc. 2007;21(12):2226–30.
28. Himpens J, Cadière GB, Bruyns J, Vertruyen M. Laparoscopic rectopexy according to Wells. Surg Endosc. 1999;13(2):139–41.
29. D'Hoore A, Cadoni R, Penninckx F. Long-term outcome of laparoscopic ventral rectopexy for total rectal prolapse. Br J Surg. 2004;91(11):1500–5.
30. Portier G, Iovino F, Lazorthes F. Surgery for rectal prolapse: Orr-Loygue ventral rectopexy with limited dissection prevents postoperative-induced constipation without increasing recurrence. Dis Colon Rectum. 2006;49(8):1136–40.
31. Nelson R, Spitz J, Pearl RK, Abcarian H. What role does full rectal mobilisation play in the treatment of rectal prolapse? Tech Coloproctol. 2001;5(1):3–5.
32. Karas JR, Uranues S, Altomare DF, Sokmen S, Krivokapic Z, Hoch J, Bartha I, Bergamaschi R, Rectal Prolapse Recurrence Study Group. No rectopexy versus rectopexy following rectal mobilization for full-thickness rectal prolapse: a randomized controlled trial. Dis Colon Rectum. 2011;54(1):29–34.
33. Foppa C, Martinek L, Arnaud JP, Bergamaschi R. Ten-year follow up after laparoscopic suture rectopexy for full-thickness rectal prolapse. Color Dis. 2014;16(10):809–14.
34. Raftopoulos Y, Senagore AJ, Di Giuro G, Bergamaschi R, Rectal Prolapse Recurrence Study Group. Recurrence rates after abdominal surgery for complete rectal prolapse: a multicenter pooled analysis of 643 individual patient data. Dis Colon Rectum. 2005;48(6):1200–6.
35. Mercer-Jones MA, D'Hoore A, Dixon AR, Lehur P, Lindsey I, Mellgren A, Stevenson AR. Consensus on ventral rectopexy: report of a panel of experts. Color Dis. 2014;16(2):82–8.
36. Mackenzie H, Dixon AR. Proficiency gain curve and predictors of outcome for laparoscopic ventral mesh rectopexy. Surgery. 2014;156(1):158–67.
37. Smart NJ, Pathak S, Boorman P, Daniels IR. Synthetic or biological mesh use in laparoscopic ventral mesh rectopexy--a systematic review. Color Dis. 2013;15(6):650–4.
38. Consten EC, van Iersel JJ, Verheijen PM, Broeders IA, Wolthuis AM, D'Hoore A. Long-term outcome after laparoscopic ventral mesh rectopexy: an observational study of 919 consecutive patients. Ann Surg. 2015;262(5):742–7.
39. Collinson R, Wijffels N, Cunningham C, Lindsey I. Laparoscopic ventral rectopexy for internal rectal prolapse: short-term functional results. Color Dis. 2010;12(2):97–104.
40. Badrek-Amoudi AH, Roe T, Mabey K, Carter H, Mills A, Dixon AR. Laparoscopic ventral mesh rectopexy in the management of solitary rectal ulcer syndrome: a cause for optimism? Color Dis. 2013;15(5):575–81.
41. Slawik S, Soulsby R, Carter H, Payne H, Dixon AR. Laparoscopic ventral rectopexy, posterior colporrhaphy and vaginal sacrocolpopexy for the treatment of recto-genital prolapse and mechanical outlet obstruction. Color Dis. 2008;10(2):138–43.
42. Frykman HM, Goldberg SM. The surgical treatment of rectal procidentia. Surg Gynecol Obstet. 1969;129(6):1225–30.

Obstructed Defecation: When Is Surgery Indicated?

17

Maria Emilia Carvalho e Carvalho and Brooke H. Gurland

Introduction

The defecation process requires normal colonic motility, rectal sensation, expulsion force, and coordination of the pelvic floor muscles. Individuals with obstructed defecation syndrome (ODS) as defined by the Rome criteria may complain of one or more of the following: straining at defecation, incomplete evacuation, hard stools, pelvic heaviness, and the need for digital support [1, 2]. ODS is a common disorder affecting 18% of population and nearly 50% of patients with constipation [2–5]. Many of the patients are women, and the risk increases with parity and obesity [6]. Nerve damage from childbirth, chronic straining, and direct trauma can result in endopelvic fascia and pelvic support defects [7–10]. Abnormal function can cause poor pelvic muscle relaxation or rectal sensation.

History and Examination

Details regarding comorbidities, obstetric history, pelvic surgery, and conditions leading to chronic staining are obtained. Dietary habits, daily activities searching for modifiable behaviors, and current medications are elicited. Stool frequency and consistency are reported. On examination, a patulous anus may be present due to neurological injury, internal rectal prolapse (IRP) or external rectal prolapse (ERP). Digital exam can reveal masses, fecal impaction, rectocele, or levator

M.E. Carvalho e Carvalho (✉)
Division of Colorectal Surgery, Mater Dei Hospital, Belo Horizonte, MG, Brazil
e-mail: mariaeccarvalho@gmail.com

B.H. Gurland
Department of General Surgery, Division of Colorectal Surgery Stanford University, Palo Alto, CA, USA
e-mail: bgurland@stanford.edu

C.M. Schlachta, P. Sylla (eds.), *Current Common Dilemmas in Colorectal Surgery*,
https://doi.org/10.1007/978-3-319-70117-2_17

relaxation. Vaginal exam may reveal anterior (cystocele), middle (uterine), or posterior (rectocele, enterocele, sigmoidocele) compartment prolapse. Flattening of the perineum during Valsalva beyond the ischial tuberosity signifies perineal descent. Anoscopy is performed to evaluate patients for mucosal abnormalities, IRP, proctitis, or masses.

Testing

Blood testing should include thyroid function tests and ionized calcium. Screening colonoscopy is recommended to exclude obstructing lesions. Colon transit study distinguishes between functional and slow transit constipation. Anorectal physiology testing assesses pelvic floor muscle coordination, rectal sensation, and rectal anal inhibitory reflex (RAIR). RAIR excludes Hirschsprung's disease. Electromyography may reveal paradoxical muscle contractions. Balloon expulsion is an inexpensive method to assess the ability to evacuate [11].

Standard fluoroscopy and MRI defecography are radiologic tests to evaluate ODS. Defecography is performed with the patient on a radiopaque commode. Oral contrast opacifies the small bowel, a contrast-soaked tampon is inserted in the vagina, and rectal contrast fills the sigmoid and rectum. During evacuation, the ability to initiate and complete evacuation; the presence of a sigmoidocele, rectocele, intussusception, rectal prolapse, and perineal descent; and changes in the anorectal angle is recorded (Fig. 17.1). MRI involves less radiation and provides multicompartment images. Sitting and defecating MRI is not universally available, while supine is not physiologic nor as accurate [12].

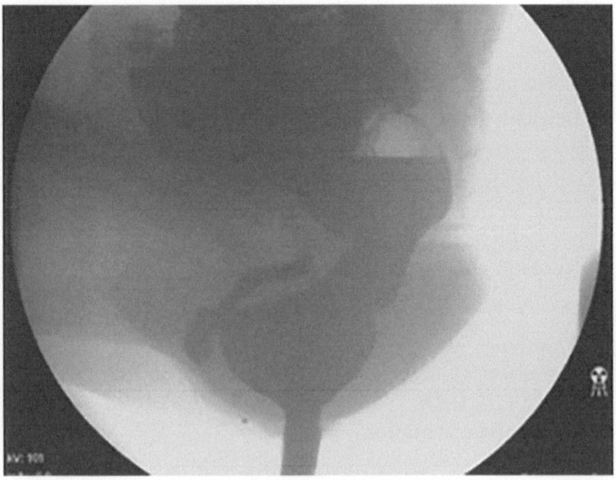

Fig. 17.1 Fluoroscopic defecography during the evacuation phase. An anterior rectocele is visualized. Reprinted with permission, Cleveland Clinic Center for Medical Art & Photography © 2009–2016. All Rights Reserved

Initial Therapy for ODS

Conservative treatments consist of high fiber diet, bulking agents, biofeedback, counseling, and relaxation techniques [13]. In the setting of slow transit constipation, a low-fiber diet and promotility agents are preferred. The low fermentable oligo-, di-, monosaccharides, and polyols (FODMAP) diet has emerged as an effective intervention for reducing symptoms of abdominal bloating and pain with IBS and can be recommended for patients with ODS [14].

Etiology and Treatment of ODS

Anatomic Defects

Rectocele

Rectocele is the herniation of the anterior rectal wall inside the vagina due to a defect of the rectovaginal fascia (Fig. 17.2). A rectocele can be classified on degree of protrusion relative to thc hymen or based on the size at maximal straining during defecography. Rectoceles are identified in up to 80% of women, and rectocele up to 2 cm is physiologic and does not warrant surgical repair. For women with a feeling of a bulge, stool trapping, fecal leakage, fecal digitation, or perineal support to evacuate, surgical correction can be effective.

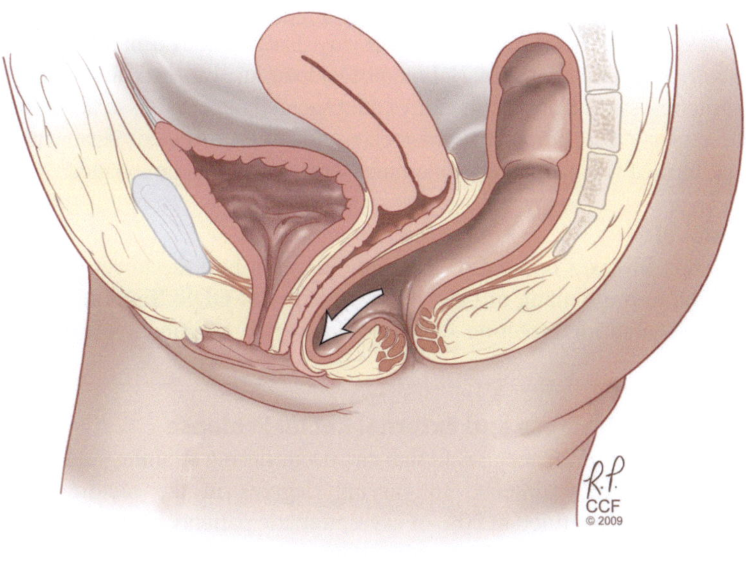

Fig. 17.2 Rectocele (white arrow). Reprinted with permission, Cleveland Clinic Center for Medical Art & Photography © 2009–2016. All Rights Reserved

Transvaginal Approach

The traditional technique for transvaginal rectocele repair involves a posterior colporraphy with vaginal mucosectomy and levator plication. The rectovaginal fascia defect is plicated (longitudinally) with suture of the puborectalis and perineal muscle. This technique corrects vaginal bulging in 80% and digitation in 67% with low complication rates [15–20]. Transvaginal repair with transverse closure of the RV septum defect has a low incidence of recurrence or need for digital assistance, but 25% of patients report dyspareunia [16, 21–24].

Transanal Approach

Transanal repair is associated with a lower incidence of dyspareunia compared to transvaginal repair. Randomized controlled trial (RCT) by Nieminen et al. [18] compared transanal and transvaginal repair. Symptoms were alleviated in 93 vs 73% of patients ($p < 0.08$). Decreased digital assist and improved rectal emptying occurred in both groups (66–27% vs 73–7% $p = 0.01$). The transanal technique was associated with higher rates of recurrent rectocele (40 vs 7% $p = 0.04$) and/or enterocele (4 vs 0% $p = 0.05$). Farid et al. [25] compared the functional outcome of perineal repair with and without levatorplasty versus transanal rectocele repair in a RCT of patients with ODS. ODS improved significantly in both groups undergoing transperineal but not transanal repair. Levatorplasty resulted in higher rates of dyspareunia and should be avoided in sexually active patients.

Enterocele

Enterocele is the descent of the small bowel into the rectovaginal space (Fig. 17.3). This may be an asymptomatic finding on defecography or may be associated with feelings of pressure and incomplete rectal emptying. Enterocele is usually found in individuals with other prolapse [26, 27]. Enterocele repair involves excision or obliteration of the peritoneal sac and approximation of uterosacral ligaments or sacral colpopexy or ventral rectopexy. Ligation of the enterocele sac and sacrospinous ligament fixation can be performed vaginally when abdominal surgery is not recommended.

Sigmoidocele

Sigmoidocele involves descent of the sigmoid colon into the lower pelvic cavity. This may be asymptomatic or can be associated with ODS. Sigmoidocele can be corrected via anterior resection or sigmoidopexy in conjunction with rectocele repair [28–30].

Internal Rectal Prolapse and External Rectal Prolapse

IRP is an infolding of the rectal wall that can occur during straining and defecation. The bowel wall may descend to varying degrees in the rectum and anus. Intussusception is identified in 30% of asymptomatic patients on defecography, and early studies suggested that IRP rarely progresses to ERP [31–33]. In the 1990s several publications discouraged surgery for IRP especially since posterior rectopexy can result in severe constipation [34–36]. More recently, there has been a reevaluation of surgery for IRP [37].

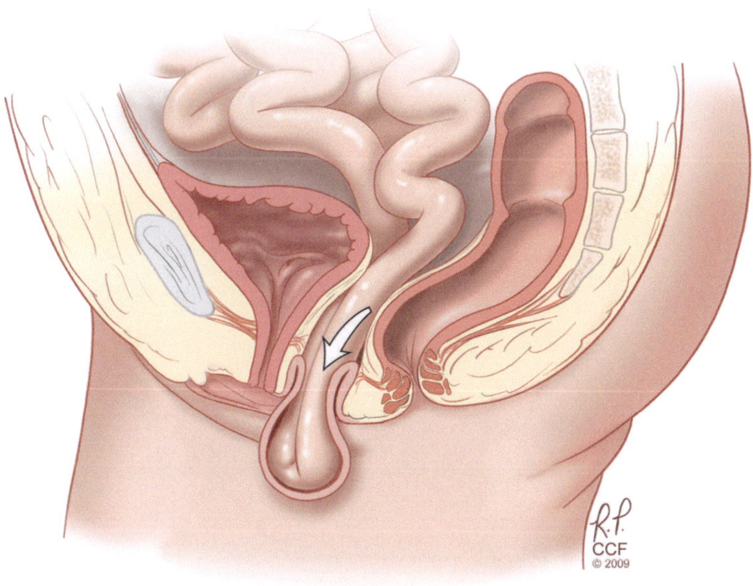

Fig. 17.3 Enterocele (white arrow). The small bowel is descending into the pelvis. The vagina cuff is prolapsing beyond the hymen. Reprinted with permission, Cleveland Clinic Center for Medical Art & Photography © 2009–2016. All Rights Reserved

Ventral Rectopexy

Laparoscopic ventral rectopexy (LVR) described by D'Hoore [38] corrects descent of the posterior and middle compartment by creating an anterior pocket down to the pelvic floor between the rectum and the vagina. The rectal-vaginal septum and anterior rectum are reinforced with mesh which is then fixed to the sacrum, thus elevating the pelvic floor (Fig. 17.4). LVR can correct ERP, rectoceles, IRP, and ODS and can be combined with vaginal prolapse procedures, such as sacrocolpopexy. Limiting dissection to the anterior rectum minimizes autonomic nerve damage which can occur with posterior dissection and division of the lateral rectal stalks. A meta-analysis of 789 patients in 12 published series of LVR reported recurrence rates for pelvic organ prolapse at 3.4% (95% CI 2.0–4.8) [39]. Complication rates varied from 14% to 47% with mesh-related issues at 2%. A significant decrease in ODS and fecal incontinence scores was reported with no new onset constipation.

STARR

Stapled transanal rectal resection (STARR) relieves ODS caused by rectocele and IRP. Boccasanta et al. [40] report ODS symptom improvement in 90%. Proctalgia, rectal bleeding, fecal urgency, rectovaginal fistula, hematoma, and pelvic sepsis are reported [41–45]. Boccasanta et al. [46] randomized 50 patients to STARR or stapled transanal prolapsectomy (STAPL) with levatorplasty. STAPL involves placing

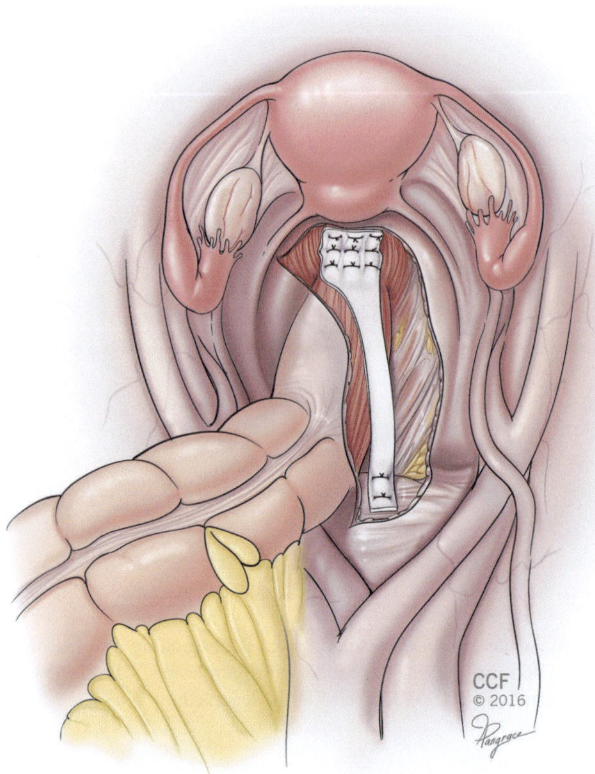

Fig. 17.4 Ventral rectopexy, mesh, or biological graft is sutured to the anterior rectum, and the material is fixed proximally to the sacrum to suspend the pelvic floor. Reprinted with permission, Cleveland Clinic Center for Medical Art & Photography © 2009–2016. All Rights Reserved

a purse-string suture above the hemorrhoid apex. A 33 circular stapler is placed above the suture, and the mucosa and submucosa are excised. A semicircular incision is performed along the perineal body to access the rectal-vaginal space for the levatorplasty. Constipation improved in both group. Dyspareunia was reported after STAPL ($p = 0.018$). Complications in the STARR group included bleeding (4%), urgency (16%), and flatus incontinence (8%) and in the STAPL group included delayed perineal wound healing (40%) and dyspareunia (20%). Renzi [47] randomized 63 patients to the procedure for prolapsing hemorrhoids (PPH) stapler vs Contour Star stapler. At 12 months ODS scores improved in both groups ($p < 0.0001$), but at 24 months, only the contour group maintained the improvement ($p < 0.03$). Shafik et al. [48] described stapled transvaginal rectal resection. A transverse incision is made at the mucocutaneous border of the vagina with dissection of the posterior vaginal wall. A PPH stapler is used to excise the rectocele. The redundant vaginal wall is excised and closed. ODS scores improved in 94% of patients at 12 months.

Descending Perineum Syndrome

Abnormal perineal descent results from the loss of pelvic floor fascia integrity and ballooning of the perineum. Patients may complain of rectal pain, incomplete evacuation, and incontinence. Renzi et al. [49] described a novel technique for suspension. A porcine graft is placed above the perineal superficial fascia through a 2 cm incision on either side of the ischial tuberosities, and the graft is fixed to the periosteal membrane of the ischial tuberosity. Out of 25 patients with failure of previous procedures (STARR, LVR, and Delorme), 12 reported significant improvement in ODS score (13.5 vs 7; $p < 0.0005$). Perineal descent improved on postoperative defecography ($p < 0.02$).

Functional Etiology

Pelvic Floor Dyssynergia

In normal defecation the puborectalis muscle relaxes to straighten the anorectal angle and facilitate the passage of stool. Paradoxical puborectalis occurs when the levator ani fails to relax or contract during defecation. Dyssynergic defecation is diagnosed by physical exam and confirmed with electromyography and defecography. Biofeedback is superior to laxatives, fiber, and education but inferior to botulinum toxin injection for improvement of ODS due to dyssynergic defecation [50, 51]. There is no consensus regarding the technique for biofeedback or number of biofeedback sessions needed. Chiarioni et al. [52] compared 14.6 g of PEG with weekly biofeedback sessions in patients who did not respond to conservative therapy. At 6 and 12 months, patients in the biofeedback arm improved compared to patients taking PEG (80 vs 22%). Biofeedback reduced straining, incomplete evacuation, the use of enemas, and abdominal pain ($p < 0.01$). A prospective randomized study [53] compared biofeedback with sham biofeedback or standard therapy (diet, exercise, and laxatives) in 77 patients. Dyssynergia was corrected in 79% of patients in the biofeedback group compared with 4% in the sham group.

Patients with dyssynergia can be considered for transrectal, vaginal, or perineal injection of botulinum toxin type A (Botox) into their pelvic floor muscles. Botox is a selective neuromuscular agent that produces a partial and reversible chemical denervation and paralysis of the muscle. Clinical effects are seen within 1 week, and benefits last from 3 to 6 months. Fecal incontinence or urgency can occur but usually resolves in 1–3 months. Several studies reported the efficacy of Botox injection with a success rate from 29 to 87% [54–57]. An observational study [57] with 56 patients with ODS and dyssynergia treated with Botox into the external sphincter and puborectalis muscle revealed response rates of 39% [16]. These patients were submitted to a reinjection of Botox and at a medium follow-up of 19.2 months, and 20 patients reported sustained improvement of ODS. Farid et al. [58] compared biofeedback training and Botox injection in 48 patients. In the biofeedback group, 50% of patients had an initial improvement, but long-term success was reported in 25%. In the Botox cohort, initial improvement was reported in 70.8%, but improvement only persisted in 33.3%.

Rectal Hyposensitivity

Rectal hyposensitivity is often seen concomitant with megarectum and frequent in patients with neurological and psychiatric disorders. The loss of perception of rectal contents or the rectal fullness sensation may lead to episodes of fecal impaction and distension of the rectum. Diagnosis is confirmed with anorectal manometry, defecography, and rectal biopsy to assess for ganglion cells. The absence of ganglion cells confirms the diagnosis of Hirschsprung's disease. Dietary and behavioral therapy, biofeedback using sensory training, rectal stimulation with suppository, and rectal irrigation with enemas can be helpful. Surgical treatment may include proctectomy and coloanal anastomosis with temporary diverting stoma.

Fecal Diversion

Fecal diversion may be considered as a last resort for the patients who fail other treatments and present with debilitating and refractory symptoms of ODS.

References

1. Ellis CN, Essani R. Treatment of obstructed defecation. Clin Colon Rectal Surg. 2012;25(01):024–33.
2. Khaikin M, Wexner SD. Treatment strategies in obstructed defecation and fecal incontinence. World J Gastroenterol. 2006;12(20):3168.
3. Drossman DA, Li Z, Andruzzi E, Temple RD, Talley NJ, Thompson WG, et al. US householder survey of functional gastrointestinal disorders. Dig Dis Sci. 1993;38(9):1569–80.
4. Everhart JE, Go VLW, Johannes RS, Fitzsimmons SC, Roth HP, White LR. A longitudinal survey of self-reported bowel habits in the United States. Dig Dis Sci. 1989;34(8):1153–62.
5. Stewart WF, Liberman JN, Sandler RS, Woods MS, Stemhagen A, Chee E, et al. Epidemiology of constipation (EPOC) study in the United States: relation of clinical subtypes to sociodemographic features. Am J Gastroenterol. 1999;94(12):3530–40.
6. Higgins PD, Johanson JF. Epidemiology of constipation in North America: a systematic review. Am J Gastroenterol. 2004;99(4):750–9.
7. Snooks S, Swash M, Setchell M, Henry M. Injury to innervation of pelvic floor sphincter musculature in childbirth. Lancet. 1984;324(8402):546–50.
8. Sultan AH, Monga AK, Stanton SL. The pelvic floor sequelae of childbirth. Br J Hosp Med. 1996;55(9):575–9.
9. DeLancey JO. Anatomie aspects of vaginal eversion after hysterectomy. Obstet Gynecol. 1992;166(6):1717–28.
10. Peschers UM, Schaer GN, DeLancey JO, Schuessler B. Levator ani function before and after childbirth. Int J Obstet Gynaecol. 1997;104(9):1004–8.
11. Barnett JL, Hasler WL, Camilleri M. American Gastroenterological Association medical position statement on anorectal testing techniques. American Gastroenterological Association. Gastroenterology. 1999;116(3):732–60.
12. Foti P, Farina R, Riva G, Coronella M, Fisichella E, Palmucci S, et al. Pelvic floor imaging: comparison between magnetic resonance imaging and conventional defecography in studying outlet obstruction syndrome. Radiol Med. 2013;118(1):23–39.
13. Podzemny V, Pescatori LC, Pescatori M. Management of obstructed defecation. World J Gastroenterol. 2015;21(4):1053–60.

14. Böhn L, Störsrud S, Liljebo T, Collin L, Lindfors P, Törnblom H, et al. Diet low in FODMAPs reduces symptoms of irritable bowel syndrome as well as traditional dietary advice: a randomized controlled trial. Gastroenterology. 2015;149(6):1399–407.
15. Mellgren A, Anzén B, Nilsson B, Johansson C, Dolk A, Gillgren P, et al. Results of rectocele repair. Dis Colon Rectum. 1995;38(1):7–13.
16. Kahn MA, Stanton SL. Posterior colporrhaphy: its effects on bowel and sexual function. Int J Obstet Gynaecol. 1997;104(1):82–6.
17. Harris MA, Ferrara A, Gallagher J, DeJesus S, Williamson P, Larach S. Stapled transanal rectal resection vs. transvaginal rectocele repair for treatment of obstructive defecation syndrome. Dis Colon Rectum. 2009;52(4):592–7.
18. Nieminen K, Hiltunen K, Laitinen J, Oksala J, Heinonen PK. Transanal or vaginal approach to rectocele repair: a prospective, randomized pilot study. Dis Colon Rectum. 2004;47(10):1636–42.
19. Tsujinaka S, Tsujinaka Y, Matsuo K, Akagi K, Hamahata Y. Changes in bowel function following transanal and transvaginal rectocele repair. Dig Surg. 2007;24(1):46–53.
20. Yamana T, Takahashi T, Iwadare J. Clinical and physiologic outcomes after transvaginal rectocele repair. Dis Colon Rectum. 2006;49(5):661–7.
21. Glavind K, Madsen H. A prospective study of the discrete fascial defect rectocele repair. Acta Obstet Gynecol Scand. 2000;79(2):145–7.
22. Cundiff GW, Weidner AC, Visco AG, Addison WA, Bump RC. An anatomic and functional assessment of the discrete defect rectocele repair. Obstet Gynecol. 1998;179(6):1451–7.
23. Kenton K, Shott S, Brubaker L. Outcome after rectovaginal fascia reattachment for rectocele repair. Obstet Gynecol. 1999;181(6):1360–4.
24. Porter WE, Steele A, Walsh P, Kohli N, Karram MM. The anatomic and functional outcomes of defect-specific rectocele repairs. Obstet Gynecol. 1999;181(6):1353–9.
25. Farid M, Madbouly KM, Hussein A, Mahdy T, Moneim HA, Omar W. Randomized controlled trial between perineal and anal repairs of rectocele in obstructed defecation. World J Surg. 2010;34(4):822–9.
26. Mellgren A, Johansson C, Dolk A, Anzen B, Bremmer S, Nilsson B, et al. Enterocele demonstrated by defaecography is associated with other pelvic floor disorders. Int J Color Dis. 1994;9(3):121–4.
27. Tulikangas PK, Piedmonte MR, Weber AM. Functional and anatomic follow-up of enterocele repairs. Obstet Gynecol. 2001;98(2):265–8.
28. Rickert A, Kienle P. Laparoscopic surgery for rectal prolapse and pelvic floor disorders. World J Gastroint Endosc. 2015;7(12):1045.
29. Maher C, Feiner B, Baessler K, Schmid C. Surgical management of pelvic organ prolapse in women. Cochrane Database Syst Rev. 2013;4:CD004014.
30. Miklos JR, Moore RD. The 26-minute laparoscopic sacral colpopexy: do we really need robotic technology? J Minim Invasive Gynecol. 2015;22(5):712.
31. MG F, Wald A, Caruana B, Bauman DH. Evacuation proctography in normal volunteers. Investig Radiol. 1991;26(6):581–5.
32. Mellgren A, Schultz I, Johansson C, Dolk A. Internal rectal intussusception seldom develops into total rectal prolapse. Dis Colon Rectum. 1997;40(7):817–20.
33. Shorvon PJ, McHugh S, Diamant NE, Somers S, Stevenson GW. Defecography in normal volunteers: results and implications. Gut. 1989;30(12):1737–49.
34. Yoshioka K, Heyen F, Keighley M. Functional results after posterior abdominal rectopexy for rectal prolapse. Dis Colon Rectum. 1989;32(10):835–8.
35. Christiansen J, Zhu B, Rasmussen O, Sørensen M. Internal rectal intussusception: results of surgical repair. Dis Colon Rectum. 1992;35(11):1026–9.
36. Orrom W, Bartolo D, Miller R, Mortensen NM, Roe A. Rectopexy is an ineffective treatment for obstructed defecation. Dis Colon Rectum. 1991;34(1):41–6.
37. Collinson R, Cunningham C, Lindsey I. Surgery for internal rectal prolapse. Color Dis. 2009;11(1):11–2.

38. D'Hoore A, Cadoni R, Penninckx F. Long-term outcome of laparoscopic ventral rectopexy for total rectal prolapse. Br J Surg. 2004;91(11):1500–5.
39. Samaranayake C, Luo C, Plank A, Merrie A, Plank L, Bissett I. Systematic review on ventral rectopexy for rectal prolapse and intussusception. Color Dis. 2010;12(6):504–12.
40. Boccasanta P, Venturi M, Stuto A, Bottini C, Caviglia A, Carriero A, et al. Stapled transanal rectal resection for outlet obstruction: a prospective, multicenter trial. Dis Colon Rectum. 2004;47(9):1285–97.
41. Dodi G, Pietroletti R, Milito G, Binda G, Pescatori M. Bleeding, incontinence, pain and constipation after STARR transanal double stapling rectotomy for obstructed defecation. Tech Coloproctol. 2003;7(3):148–53.
42. Bassi R, Rademacher J, Savoia A. Rectovaginal fistula after STARR procedure complicated by haematoma of the posterior vaginal wall: report of a case. Tech Coloproctol. 2006;10(4):361–3.
43. Naldini G, Martellucci J, Rea R, Lucchini S, Schiano di Visconte M, Caviglia A, et al. Tailored prolapse surgery for the treatment of haemorrhoids and obstructed defecation syndrome with a new dedicated device: TST STARR plus. Int J Color Dis. 2014;29(5):623–9.
44. Pescatori M. Troubleshooting the starr procedure. In: Reconstructive surgery of the rectum, anus and perineum. London: Springer; 2013. p. 305–13.
45. Pescatori M, Dodi G, Salafia C, Zbar AP. Rectovaginal fistula after double-stapled transanal rectotomy (STARR) for obstructed defaecation. Int J Color Dis. 2005;20(1):83–5.
46. Boccasanta P, Venturi M, Salamina G, Cesana BM, Bernasconi F, Roviaro G. New trends in the surgical treatment of outlet obstruction: clinical and functional results of two novel transanal stapled techniques from a randomised controlled trial. Int J Color Dis. 2004;19(4):359–69.
47. Renzi A, Brillantino A, Di Sarno G, Izzo D, D'Aniello F, Falato A. Improved clinical outcomes with a new contour-curved stapler in the surgical treatment of obstructed defecation syndrome: a mid-term randomized controlled trial. Dis Colon Rectum. 2011;54(6):736–42.
48. Shafik AA, El Sibai O, Shafik IA. Rectocele repair with stapled transvaginal rectal resection. Tech Coloproctol. 2016;20(4):207–14.
49. Renzi A, Brillantino A, Di Sarno G, d'Aniello F, Bianco P, Iacobellis F, et al. Transverse perineal support: a novel surgical treatment for perineal descent in patients with obstructed defecation syndrome. Dis Colon Rectum. 2016;59(6):557–64.
50. Rao SS. Dyssynergic defecation and biofeedback therapy. Gastroenterol Clin N Am. 2008;37(3):569–86.
51. Rao SS, Patcharatrakul T. Diagnosis and treatment of dyssynergic defecation. J Neurogastroenterol Motil. 2016;22(3):423–35.
52. Chiarioni G, Whitehead WE, Pezza V, Morelli A, Bassotti G. Biofeedback is superior to laxatives for normal transit constipation due to pelvic floor dyssynergia. Gastroenterology. 2006;130(3):657–64.
53. Rao SS, Seaton K, Miller M, Brown K, Nygaard I, Stumbo P, et al. Randomized controlled trial of biofeedback, sham feedback, and standard therapy for dyssynergic defecation. Clin Gastroenterol Hepatol. 2007;5(3):331–8.
54. Hallan R, Melling J, Womack N, Williams N, Waldron D, Morrison J. Treatment of anismus in intractable constipation with botulinum a toxin. Lancet. 1988;332(8613):714–7.
55. Joo JS, Agachan F, Wolff B, Nogueras JJ, Wexner SD. Initial north American experience with botulinum toxin type a for treatment of anismus. Dis Colon Rectum. 1996;39(10):1107–11.
56. Ron Y, Avni Y, Lukovetski A, Wardi J, Geva D, Birkenfeld S, et al. Botulinum toxin type-a in therapy of patients with anismus. Dis Colon Rectum. 2001;44(12):1821–6.
57. Hompes R, Harmston C, Wijffels N, Jones OM, Cunningham C, Lindsey I. Excellent response rate of anismus to botulinum toxin if rectal prolapse misdiagnosed as anismus ('pseudoanismus') is excluded. Color Dis. 2012;14(2):224–30.
58. Farid M, El Monem HA, Omar W, El Nakeeb A, Fikry A, Youssef T, et al. Comparative study between biofeedback retraining and botulinum neurotoxin in the treatment of anismus patients. Int J Color Dis. 2009;24(1):115–20.

Fecal Incontinence: Is Sacral Nerve Stimulation Always the Answer?

18

Teresa C. Rice and Ian M. Paquette

Abbreviations

ABS	Artificial bowel sphincter
FI	Fecal incontinence
SNS	Sacral nerve stimulator

Introduction

Fecal incontinence (FI) is defined as the involuntary or uncontrolled passage of solid or liquid stool. It is a common condition that affects 18 million US adults and up to 15% of individuals residing in the community [1]. Further, it afflicts nearly 50% of those residing in nursing homes [2] and is the second leading cause of nursing home placement [3], causing a significant burden on the health of patients [4]. The negative psychological effects, social stigma, and impaired quality of life can be debilitating for affected individuals. Accordingly, identifying effective management strategies for FI is necessary.

The etiology of FI is multifactorial, and there are a multitude of treatment options resulting in a complex treatment algorithm. Initial therapy should consist of conservative measures such as dietary alteration, fiber supplements, anti-motility agents

T.C. Rice
Department of Surgery, University of Cincinnati Medical Center, Cincinnati, OH, USA

I.M. Paquette (✉)
Division of Colon and Rectal Surgery, University of Cincinnati Medical Center, Cincinnati, OH, USA
e-mail: ian.paquette@uc.edu

C.M. Schlachta, P. Sylla (eds.), *Current Common Dilemmas in Colorectal Surgery*, https://doi.org/10.1007/978-3-319-70117-2_18

[5, 6], and possibly biofeedback [7–9]. When these initial modalities fail, consideration is given to surgical treatment strategies such as sacral nerve stimulation (SNS), sphincteroplasty, radiofrequency energy delivery [10, 11], and injectable bulking agents [12, 13]. SNS is an emerging surgical therapy that was first described for FI in 1995 [14]. Recent clinical practice guidelines by the American Society of Colon and Rectal Surgeons (ASCRS) recommend SNS as a first-line surgical option in patients with severe incontinence, with or without a sphincter defect [15]. Here, we aim to identify which patients with FI, refractory to medical management, would benefit from SNS and in whom other surgical modalities should be considered.

Results of Sacral Nerve Stimulation

SNS provides a significant advantage over other operative techniques in that it is a minimally invasive, two-stage procedure consisting of an initial trial phase followed by definitive implant. As such, efficacy of SNS can be ascertained during the trial phase, prior to permanent implantation. Success is defined as greater than 50% improvement in symptoms during the trial stimulation and is highly predictive of ultimate success with a permanent SNS [16]. Efficacy has consistently been demonstrated in the short and long term, as SNS reduces symptom severity and frequency of episodes [17–21]. On a per protocol pooled analysis (success of patients who receive a full-system implantation), patients demonstrating greater than 50% success in the short (<12 months), medium (12–36 months), and long term (>36 months) were 79, 80, and 84%, respectively [21]. When reported as an intention-to-treat analysis (inclusion of all patients, whether they had a successful test implantation or not), 63% of patients achieved success at short-term follow-up, and this effect was maintained in the long term [21]. Perfect continence was achieved in as many as 36% of patients at long-term follow-up [21, 22]. Maintenance of initial therapeutic effect has been shown to persist as long as 9 years after implantation [17, 23].

In addition to the high success achieved with SNS, this procedure has low morbidity and no reported mortality [24]. Hull et al. examined long-term durability of SNS and report the most common adverse events are implant site pain (32.5%), paresthesia (19.2%), change in sensation of stimulation (11.7%), and infection (10%) [22]. The majority of these adverse events occurred within the first 2 years of device implant and were managed noninvasively, with medication or reprogramming. Revision, replacement, or explant was required in 26.3% of patients who had a minimum of 5-year follow-up. This study demonstrates that while SNS is efficacious, there is a need for persistent long-term follow-up due to potential lead migration, battery depletion, and reprogramming.

Candidates for Sacral Nerve Stimulation

A trial of SNS should be considered in patients who have failed medical therapy and is recommended as a first-line surgical option [15]. A successful test, as defined by >50% improvement in FI severity, is achieved in 55–100% of patients (Table 18.1). These patients may then be offered a permanent device as a successful test phase is highly predictive of successful permanent device implantation [16]. Multiple studies have sought to identify preoperative factors indicative of success with definitive implant. Quezada et al. demonstrate that preoperative anal physiology testing and ultrasonography are not predictive of SNS success [25]. Some have suggested that three factors have been associated with failure during the test phase: increased age, defects in the external anal sphincter, and repeated percutaneous nerve evaluation (PNE) attempts [26]. However, a more recent study by Maeda et al. concludes that there is no preoperative predictor of PNE outcome [16]. While these factors may be associated with lower chance of success during the trial phase, they do not exclude patients form undergoing test stimulation. Further, the aforementioned factors were not associated with reduced success of a permanent implant [16, 26].

When SNS was first introduced, it was recommended for use in patients with an intact external anal sphincter. However, anorectal manometry studies demonstrate that SNS does not work by directly augmenting sphincter function [27]. As such, recent studies have confirmed that the presence of a sphincter defect up to 180° does not impact clinical outcome [28–31]. A recent study showed no reported difference between a group of 54 patients with an external anal sphincter defect and 91 patients with an intact sphincter following definitive implant [30]. Moreover, results did not differ between groups that had previously failed sphincteroplasty versus those who did not have a prior repair. While we conclude that SNS is a reasonable therapeutic option in patients with and without a sphincter defect, no direct comparison of SNS to sphincteroplasty has been conducted.

Few studies have been performed to evaluate efficacy of SNS in the setting of rectal prolapse [32, 33]. Though many patients present with incontinence associated with full thickness rectal prolapse, we recommend addressing the rectal prolapse surgically and reassessing bowel function 6–12 weeks after surgery. Prapasrivorakul et al. suggest that SNS is less efficacious in patients with high-grade internal rectal prolapse [33]. Since this data has yet to be reproduced, we believe that SNS should be attempted first, and if there is a failure, defecography can be performed to assess for internal rectal prolapse, which could be surgically addressed. A final emerging population is patients following LAR for rectal cancer. Initial prospective case series have had encouraging results in this setting [34, 35]; however, large prospective studies are necessary to validate the success of SNS in this select patient population.

There are relatively few contraindications to SNS. The device is thought to improve afferent transmission in the spinal cord, contributing to antegrade neuromodulation of the cerebral cortex [36]. This sensory response is thought to be more

Table 18.1 Outcomes following permanent implantation of SNS

Study	Study type	Temp/perm implant	Follow-up in months	% improvement		Wexner score		FI episodes		Sphincter defect
				>50%	100%	Baseline	F/U	Baseline	F/U	
Short (1–12 months)										
Mellgren et al. [62]	PS	133/120	3	86	40	39.9[a]	29[a]	9.4	1.7	
Leroi et al. [37]	RCT	34/28	6		26.3	16	8.5	7	1	
Quezada et al. [25]	R	60/55	12			15	4			Mean 113°
Chan et al. [63]	PS	21	12			15.7	1	13.8	5	<120°
		32						6.7	2	Intact
Johnson et al. [30]	PS	54	12	94.4		15	2			Mean 105°
		91	12	94.4		14	3			Intact
Tjandra et al. [38]	RCT	60/53	12	71	47.2	16	1	10	3	
Medium (13–36)										
Dueland-Jakobsen et al. [64]	PS	164/164	22			15	9	12	1	
Michelsen et al. [20]	PS	177/142	24	54		16	10			
Melenhorst et al. [65]	PS	134/100	25.5	81				31.3	4.8	
Wexner et al. [66]	PS	133/120	28	83	41	39[a]	30[a]	9.4	2.9	
Dudding et al. [67]	PS	81/58	29	56.9	15			9.9	1	
Melenhorst et al. [68]	R	A: 20/16	29.2	69				26.6	12.5	Post repair
		B: 20/14	22.6	79				24.9	4.1	<120°
Govaert et al. [26]	R	245/173	34.7	77						Mean 65°
Hong et al. [55]	R	33 Rs	31			17.5	11.5			
		11 abs	31	45		18.7	8.6			
		15 SNS	31	67		17.6	9.1			

Long (>36 months)										
Brouwer et al. [69]	PS	55/55	37	100		15	6			
Devroede [70]	PS	133/120	39	85.9	33.3	39.9[a]	28[a]	9.4	1.9	
Dueland-Jakobsen [71]	PS	129/129	46	75	36			19	2.5	
Faucheron et al. [72]	PS	123/87	48.5			13	8.2			
Ratto [31]	PS	14[b]	60	85.7		16.4	7.7			<180°
		10/10	33	100		18.3	9.7			<180°
Hull [22]	PS	133/120	60	88.9	36.1	38[a]	28[a]			
Altomare [73]	PS	407/272	84	85.1		16	7	7	0.25	

PS prospective, *R* retrospective, *RCT* randomized control trial, *ABS* artificial bowel sphincter, *A* treated with artificial bowel sphincter, *B* treated with SNS

[a]Fecal incontinence score index used to assess fecal severity

[b]Patients receiving sphincteroplasty as comparator

important than the muscle response of the anal sphincter [27]. As a result, SNS is not advised in patients with complete spinal cord transection. It is also contraindicated in patients that require spinal or pelvic MRI. In summary, SNS can be considered a first-line surgical option in most patients with refractory severe FI. Furthermore, the selection of patients should be based upon symptom improvement during the test phase as this is key to identifying patients who will ultimately have success with definitive implantation.

Comparison of SNS to Other Treatment Modalities

The majority of studies examining efficacy of SNS are prospective and limited by the lack of direct comparators. In a randomized double-blind crossover trial, the ability to postpone defecation, frequency of incontinent episodes, symptom severity score, and quality of life significantly improved during the “device on” versus “device off” phase [37]. When SNS is compared to optimal medical therapy in a randomized trial, the SNS group demonstrated significant improvement in quality of life, reduction in weekly incontinence episodes (from 9.5 to 3.1), and achievement of perfect continence in 47.2% [38]. In contrast, the medically managed group demonstrated no improvement in fecal incontinence or quality of life. Meurette et al. compared 15 patients with SNS to 15 matched patients who had received artificial bowel sphincter (ABS) [39]. While both groups demonstrated improvement in continence scores from baseline, SNS had higher postoperative incontinence scores (9.4 vs 5.7). However, constipation and symptoms of outlet obstruction were more frequent following ABS. Furthermore, there was no significant morbidity with SNS, while 53% of patients in the ABS group required additional surgical intervention due to mechanical failure, ulceration, or erosion of the anal canal. The FENIX magnetic sphincter augmentation (MSA) is a novel therapeutic option for FI that serves to increase anal sphincter tone. The SaFaRI trial is a randomized controlled, unblinded trial in Europe that seeks to compare efficacy of the FENIX MSA to SNS for moderate to severe incontinence [40]. Additional randomized trials comparing SNS to other therapies, such as the ongoing SaFaRI trial, may provide the clinical evidence required to design a definitive treatment algorithm.

Alternative Therapies

Sphincteroplasty

Traditionally, patients with FI secondary to sphincter injury were managed with sphincteroplasty, and good short-term results were achieved [47]. After 5–10 years, more than half of patients initially demonstrating success become incontinent again [48–50]. No single preoperative factor has been correlated with sphincteroplasty success. Unilateral or bilateral pudendal neuropathy was associated with poor outcome in some studies [51]. There is some thought that adjuvant biofeedback therapy may reduce the rate of deterioration and improve quality of life [52], although this study was limited by its small sample size and results have not been replicated. In patients who have recurrent incontinence after a repair, some suggest that a repeat sphincteroplasty can be considered and has similar short- and long-term results [53, 54].

Due to a loss of efficacy over time, the utility of sphincteroplasty has been questioned as SNS has emerged as a minimally invasive therapy that can be effective in patients with sphincter defects up to 180° (Table 18.1). Additionally, SNS has been proposed as a treatment option for patients following failed sphincteroplasty. In a study that compared SNS, artificial bowel sphincter (ABS), and repeat sphincteroplasty, no difference was found between incontinence scores or quality of life at follow-up [55]. Despite this evidence, no head-to-head comparison of SNS versus sphincteroplasty has been conducted to date. In a young patient with a recent sphincter injury, sphincteroplasty is a great first option. However, if a patient with a remote sphincter injury presents with new incontinence, the results of sphincter repair may not be ideal [47, 56]. Discussion of sphincter repair versus a trial stimulation with SNS should be considered.

Injection of Bulking Agents

Injection of bulking agents may benefit patients with mild incontinence as it aims to expand tissue in the anal canal and prevent passive FI. The majority of published studies on this topic are prospective and limited by the variety of implant materials, varying injection sites, and differing techniques. Evidence to support the use of injectables is also limited by the lack of comparison to alternative treatments. Currently, a non-animal stabilized hyaluronic acid/dextranomer gel (Solesta) is the only injectable agent approved by the FDA. In a randomized trial comparing Solesta to sham injection, Solesta led to a 50% reduction in frequency of episodes in 52% of patients as compared to 31% of sham patients, although incontinence scores were not different [41]. In another placebo-controlled study, there was no difference in symptomatic improvement between injectable and saline groups (23% vs 27%, respectively) [42]. A Cochrane review in 2013 describes modest improvements in short-term studies [13]. Mellgren et al. are the first to describe long-term results of injectables. A decrease in symptoms was achieved in 52% of patients at 6 months and was sustained at 36 months [43]. Overall, injectables are reported to be safe, with low rate of complications, and may provide benefit in patients with mild incontinence [15]. Injectable agents are contraindicated in pregnancy, inflammatory bowel disease, anorectal malformations, previous pelvic radiation, and full-thickness rectal prolapse [44]. Currently, these agents are very expensive and difficult to get covered by health insurance. They are likely reserved for patients with minor seepage rather than with severe incontinence.

Radiofrequency Energy Delivery

Radiofrequency energy delivery is thought to thicken the internal sphincter complex and increase outlet resistance via an increase in the muscularis propria and alter collagen fiber composition [45]. Studies reporting on efficacy in FI are limited with small cohorts. The largest cohort was a prospective trial with 50 patients that shows an improvement in incontinence scores from 14 to 11 at 6 months [46]. Some improvement in incontinence was observed in 55–80% of patients; however, most series failed to demonstrate >50% improvement, and none show complete continence [10, 46]. This procedure is contraindicated in patients with history of injectable agents or active fissure, fistula, or tumor [44]. Complications include pain, ulceration, infection, and bleeding. While this may be used in the management of FI, alternative therapies should be trialed prior to considering radiofrequency energy delivery.

Magnetic Sphincter Augmentation

Most recently, the FDA has approved the FENIX magnetic sphincter augmentation (MSA) system for management of FI. This device consists of a ring of magnetic titanium beads that is surgically placed around the anal sphincter, and continence is restored via passive resistance of the beads. To date, studies reporting on efficacy are limited, with small cohorts. Nonetheless, initial results demonstrate significant improvement in incontinence scores, from approximately 17 to 7, in the short term [57, 58]. In comparison to ABS, the FENIX MSA was able to achieve equivalent improvements in incontinence and quality of life [59]. However, complications occur in up to 20% of implanted patients, and explantation was required in nearly 10% [60]. There is an ongoing randomized clinical trial, SaFaRI, that seeks to compare the clinical effectiveness of FENIX MSA to SNS. Currently, MSA should be considered a third-line option for management of FI in the setting of a patient who has failed SNS, as it is labeled by the FDA as a humanitarian use device. Results from the SaFaRI trial may help provide evidence necessary to devise an optimal treatment plan.

Conclusion

Fecal incontinence is a common and debilitating condition that is frequently underreported due to the embarrassing nature of the disease. Once conservative measures have failed, the surgeon must develop a treatment plan to potentially improve quality of life. Based upon ASCRS clinical practice guidelines and the above data, we conclude that SNS is a first-line surgical option in patients with severe FI refractory to medical management. SNS is a relatively safe procedure with good efficacy in the short- and long-term, low morbidity, and no reported mortality. Importantly, the only reliable predictor of outcome with SNS is patient response to temporary stimulation [16, 25, 26, 61]. This is a significant advantage over other operative procedures in that it allows the patient and surgeon to trial the device to ensure that the treatment regimen will provide a successful outcome. We conclude that patients with severe FI may undergo SNS as first-line surgical management, though comparative studies to other modalities are lacking. The use of SNS to treat FI in subgroups of patients such as post-LAR for rectal cancer, or in patients with internal rectal prolapse, is inconclusive and requires additional studies in order to validate initial reports.

Currently, the main alternative treatment to SNS is sphincteroplasty. SNS outcomes are highly successful even with a sphincter defect. Sphincteroplasty is a reasonable approach in a young patient presenting with a sphincter defect, while SNS may be more appropriate for longer-term sphincter repair failures. SNS offers a lower morbidity profile and excellent long-term results. However, direct comparisons of SNS to other modalities is lacking in the literature. Direct comparisons to available modalities with regard to efficacy, long-term outcomes, and cost would benefit the development of an optimal treatment algorithm for this complex and chronic condition.

References

1. Nelson R, Norton N, Cautley E, Furner S. Community-based prevalence of anal incontinence. JAMA. 1995;274(7):559–61.
2. Nelson RL. Epidemiology of fecal incontinence. Gastroenterology. 2004;126(1 Suppl 1):S3–7.
3. Johanson JF, Lafferty J. Epidemiology of fecal incontinence: the silent affliction. Am J Gastroenterol. 1996;91(1):33–6.
4. Ng KS, Sivakumaran Y, Nassar N, Gladman MA. Fecal incontinence: community prevalence and associated factors--a systematic review. Dis Colon Rectum. 2015;58(12):1194–209.
5. Croswell E, Bliss DZ, Savik K. Diet and eating pattern modifications used by community-living adults to manage their fecal incontinence. J Wound Ostomy Continence Nurs. 2010;37(6):677–82.
6. Omar MI, Alexander CE. Drug treatment for faecal incontinence in adults. Cochrane Database Systemat Rev. 2013;6:CD002116.
7. Chiarioni G, Ferri B, Morelli A, Iantorno G, Bassotti G. Bio-feedback treatment of fecal incontinence: where are we, and where are we going? World J Gastroenterol. 2005;11(31):4771–5.
8. Norton C, Chelvanayagam S, Wilson-Barnett J, Redfern S, Kamm MA. Randomized controlled trial of biofeedback for fecal incontinence. Gastroenterology. 2003;125(5):1320–9.
9. Norton C, Cody JD, Hosker G. Biofeedback and/or sphincter exercises for the treatment of faecal incontinence in adults. Cochrane Database Systemat Rev. 2006;3:CD002111.
10. Frascio M, Mandolfino F, Imperatore M, et al. The SECCA procedure for faecal incontinence: a review. Color Dis. 2014;16(3):167–72.
11. Lam TJ, Visscher AP, Meurs-Szojda MM, Felt-Bersma RJ. Clinical response and sustainability of treatment with temperature-controlled radiofrequency energy (Secca) in patients with faecal incontinence: 3 years follow-up. Int J Color Dis. 2014;29(6):755–61.
12. Danielson J, Karlbom U, Wester T, Graf W. Efficacy and quality of life 2 years after treatment for faecal incontinence with injectable bulking agents. Tech Coloproctol. 2013;17(4):389–95.
13. Maeda Y, Laurberg S, Norton C. Perianal injectable bulking agents as treatment for faecal incontinence in adults. Cochrane Database Systemat Rev. 2013;2:CD007959.
14. Matzel KE, Stadelmaier U, Hohenfellner M, Gall FP. Electrical stimulation of sacral spinal nerves for treatment of faecal incontinence. Lancet. 1995;346(8983):1124–7.
15. Paquette IM, Varma MG, Kaiser AM, Steele SR, Rafferty JF. The American society of colon and rectal surgeons' clinical practice guideline for the treatment of fecal incontinence. Dis Colon Rectum. 2015;58(7):623–36.
16. Maeda Y, Norton C, Lundby L, Buntzen S, Laurberg S. Predictors of the outcome of percutaneous nerve evaluation for faecal incontinence. Br J Surg. 2010;97(7):1096–102.
17. George AT, Kalmar K, Panarese A, Dudding TC, Nicholls RJ, Vaizey CJ. Long-term outcomes of sacral nerve stimulation for fecal incontinence. Dis Colon Rectum. 2012;55(3):302–6.

18. Hollingshead JR, Dudding TC, Vaizey CJ. Sacral nerve stimulation for faecal incontinence: results from a single centre over a 10-year period. Color Dis. 2011;13(9):1030–4.
19. Lim JT, Hastie IA, Hiscock RJ, Shedda SM. Sacral nerve stimulation for fecal incontinence: long-term outcomes. Dis Colon Rectum. 2011;54(8):969–74.
20. Michelsen HB, Thompson-Fawcett M, Lundby L, Krogh K, Laurberg S, Buntzen S. Six years of experience with sacral nerve stimulation for fecal incontinence. Dis Colon Rectum. 2010;53(4):414–21.
21. Thin NN, Horrocks EJ, Hotouras A, et al. Systematic review of the clinical effectiveness of neuromodulation in the treatment of faecal incontinence. Br J Surg. 2013;100(11):1430–47.
22. Hull T, Giese C, Wexner SD, et al. Long-term durability of sacral nerve stimulation therapy for chronic fecal incontinence. Dis Colon Rectum. 2013;56(2):234–45.
23. Matzel KE, Lux P, Heuer S, Besendorfer M, Zhang W. Sacral nerve stimulation for faecal incontinence: long-term outcome. Color Dis. 2009;11(6):636–41.
24. Wong MT, Meurette G, Rodat F, Regenet N, Wyart V, Lehur PA. Outcome and management of patients in whom sacral nerve stimulation for fecal incontinence failed. Dis Colon Rectum. 2011;54(4):425–32.
25. Quezada Y, Whiteside JL, Rice T, Karram M, Rafferty JF, Paquette IM. Does preoperative anal physiology testing or ultrasonography predict clinical outcome with sacral neuromodulation for fecal incontinence? Int Urogynecol J. 2015;26(11):1613–7.
26. Govaert B, Melenhorst J, Nieman FH, Bols EM, van Gemert WG, Baeten CG. Factors associated with percutaneous nerve evaluation and permanent sacral nerve modulation outcome in patients with fecal incontinence. Dis Colon Rectum. 2009;52(10):1688–94.
27. Carrington EV, Knowles CH. The influence of sacral nerve stimulation on anorectal dysfunction. Color Dis. 2011;13(Suppl 2):5–9.
28. Abrams P, Andersson KE, Birder L, et al. Fourth international consultation on incontinence recommendations of the international scientific committee: evaluation and treatment of urinary incontinence, pelvic organ prolapse, and fecal incontinence. Neurourol Urodyn. 2010;29(1): 213–40.
29. Boyle DJ, Knowles CH, Lunniss PJ, Scott SM, Williams NS, Gill KA. Efficacy of sacral nerve stimulation for fecal incontinence in patients with anal sphincter defects. Dis Colon Rectum. 2009;52(7):1234–9.
30. Johnson BL, Abodeely A, Ferguson MA, Davis BR, Rafferty JF, Paquette IM. Is sacral neuromodulation here to stay? Clinical outcomes of a new treatment for fecal incontinence. J Gastrointest Surg. 2015;19(1):15–9. discussion 19–20.
31. Ratto C, Litta F, Parello A, Donisi L, Doglietto GB. Sacral nerve stimulation is a valid approach in fecal incontinence due to sphincter lesions when compared to sphincter repair. Dis Colon Rectum. 2010;53(3):264–72.
32. Mishra A, Prapasrivorakul S, Gosselink MP, et al. Sacral neuromodulation for persistent faecal incontinence after laparoscopic ventral rectopexy for high-grade internal rectal prolapse. Color Dis. 2016;18(3):273–8.
33. Prapasrivorakul S, Gosselink MP, Gorissen KJ, et al. Sacral neuromodulation for faecal incontinence: is the outcome compromised in patients with high-grade internal rectal prolapse? Int J Color Dis. 2015;30(2):229–34.
34. de Miguel M, Oteiza F, Ciga MA, Armendariz P, Marzo J, Ortiz H. Sacral nerve stimulation for the treatment of faecal incontinence following low anterior resection for rectal cancer. Color Dis. 2011;13(1):72–7.
35. Ratto C, Grillo E, Parello A, Petrolino M, Costamagna G, Doglietto GB. Sacral neuromodulation in treatment of fecal incontinence following anterior resection and chemoradiation for rectal cancer. Dis Colon Rectum. 2005;48(5):1027–36.
36. Lundby L, Moller A, Buntzen S, et al. Relief of fecal incontinence by sacral nerve stimulation linked to focal brain activation. Dis Colon Rectum. 2011;54(3):318–23.
37. Leroi AM, Parc Y, Lehur PA, et al. Efficacy of sacral nerve stimulation for fecal incontinence: results of a multicenter double-blind crossover study. Ann Surg. 2005;242(5):662–9.

38. Tjandra JJ, Chan MK, Yeh CH, Murray-Green C. Sacral nerve stimulation is more effective than optimal medical therapy for severe fecal incontinence: a randomized, controlled study. Dis Colon Rectum. 2008;51(5):494–502.
39. Meurette G, La Torre M, Regenet N, Robert-Yap J, Lehur PA. Value of sacral nerve stimulation in the treatment of severe faecal incontinence: a comparison to the artificial bowel sphincter. Color Dis. 2009;11(6):631–5.
40. Williams AE, Croft J, Napp V, et al. SaFaRI: sacral nerve stimulation versus the FENIX magnetic sphincter augmentation for adult faecal incontinence: a randomised investigation. Int J Color Dis. 2016;31(2):465–72.
41. Graf W, Mellgren A, Matzel KE, et al. Efficacy of dextranomer in stabilised hyaluronic acid for treatment of faecal incontinence: a randomised, sham-controlled trial. Lancet. 2011;377(9770):997–1003.
42. Siproudhis L, Morcet J, Laine F. Elastomer implants in faecal incontinence: a blind, randomized placebo-controlled study. Aliment Pharmacol Ther. 2007;25(9):1125–32.
43. Mellgren A, Matzel KE, Pollack J, et al. Long-term efficacy of NASHA Dx injection therapy for treatment of fecal incontinence. Neurogastroenterol Motil. 2014;26(8):1087–94.
44. Kaiser AM, Orangio GR, Zutshi M, et al. Current status: new technologies for the treatment of patients with fecal incontinence. Surg Endosc. 2014;28(8):2277–301.
45. Herman RM, Berho M, Murawski M, et al. Defining the histopathological changes induced by nonablative radiofrequency treatment of faecal incontinence--a blinded assessment in an animal model. Color Dis. 2015;17(5):433–40.
46. Efron JE, Corman ML, Fleshman J, et al. Safety and effectiveness of temperature-controlled radio-frequency energy delivery to the anal canal (Secca procedure) for the treatment of fecal incontinence. Dis Colon Rectum. 2003;46(12):1606–16. discussion 1616–1608
47. Glasgow SC, Lowry AC. Long-term outcomes of anal sphincter repair for fecal incontinence: a systematic review. Dis Colon Rectum. 2012;55(4):482–90.
48. Bravo Gutierrez A, Madoff RD, Lowry AC, Parker SC, Buie WD, Baxter NN. Long-term results of anterior sphincteroplasty. Dis Colon Rectum. 2004;47(5):727–31. discussion 731–722
49. Halverson AL, Hull TL. Long-term outcome of overlapping anal sphincter repair. Dis Colon Rectum. 2002;45(3):345–8.
50. Lamblin G, Bouvier P, Damon H, et al. Long-term outcome after overlapping anterior anal sphincter repair for fecal incontinence. Int J Color Dis. 2014;29(11):1377–83.
51. Gilliland R, Altomare DF, Moreira H Jr, Oliveira L, Gilliland JE, Wexner SD. Pudendal neuropathy is predictive of failure following anterior overlapping sphincteroplasty. Dis Colon Rectum. 1998;41(12):1516–22.
52. Davis KJ, Kumar D, Poloniecki J. Adjuvant biofeedback following anal sphincter repair: a randomized study. Aliment Pharmacol Ther. 2004;20(5):539–49.
53. Vaizey CJ, Norton C, Thornton MJ, Nicholls RJ, Kamm MA. Long-term results of repeat anterior anal sphincter repair. Dis Colon Rectum. 2004;47(6):858–63.
54. Giordano P, Renzi A, Efron J, et al. Previous sphincter repair does not affect the outcome of repeat repair. Dis Colon Rectum. 2002;45(5):635–40.
55. Hong KD, da Silva G, Wexner SD. What is the best option for failed sphincter repair? Color Dis. 2014;16(4):298–303.
56. Goetz LH, Lowry AC. Overlapping sphincteroplasty: is it the standard of care? Clin Colon and Rectal Surg. 2005;18(1):22–31.
57. Barussaud ML, Mantoo S, Wyart V, Meurette G, Lehur PA. The magnetic anal sphincter in faecal incontinence: is initial success sustained over time? Color Dis. 2013;15(12):1499–503.
58. Pakravan F, Helmes C. Magnetic anal sphincter augmentation in patients with severe fecal incontinence. Dis Colon Rectum. 2015;58(1):109–14.
59. Wong MT, Meurette G, Stangherlin P, Lehur PA. The magnetic anal sphincter versus the artificial bowel sphincter: a comparison of 2 treatments for fecal incontinence. Dis Colon Rectum. 2011;54(7):773–9.

60. Lehur PA, McNevin S, Buntzen S, Mellgren AF, Laurberg S, Madoff RD. Magnetic anal sphincter augmentation for the treatment of fecal incontinence: a preliminary report from a feasibility study. Dis Colon Rectum. 2010;53(12):1604–10.
61. Dudding TC, Hollingshead JR, Nicholls RJ, Vaizey CJ. Sacral nerve stimulation for faecal incontinence: patient selection, service provision and operative technique. Color Dis. 2011;13(8):e187–95.
62. Mellgren A, Wexner SD, Coller JA, et al. Long-term efficacy and safety of sacral nerve stimulation for fecal incontinence. Dis Colon Rectum. 2011;54(9):1065–75.
63. Chan MK, Tjandra JJ. Sacral nerve stimulation for fecal incontinence: external anal sphincter defect vs. intact anal sphincter. Dis Colon Rectum. 2008;51(7):1015–24. discussion 1024-1015
64. Duelund-Jakobsen J, Lehur PA, Lundby L, Wyart V, Laurberg S, Buntzen S. Sacral nerve stimulation for faecal incontinence-efficacy confirmed from a two-centre prospectively maintained database. Int J Color Dis. 2015;31(2):421–8.
65. Melenhorst J, Koch SM, Uludag O, van Gemert WG, Baeten CG. Sacral neuromodulation in patients with faecal incontinence: results of the first 100 permanent implantations. Color Dis. 2007;9(8):725–30.
66. Wexner SD, Coller JA, Devroede G, et al. Sacral nerve stimulation for fecal incontinence: results of a 120-patient prospective multicenter study. Ann Surg. 2010;251(3):441–9.
67. Dudding TC, Pares D, Vaizey CJ, Kamm MA. Predictive factors for successful sacral nerve stimulation in the treatment of faecal incontinence: a 10-year cohort analysis. Color Dis. 2008;10(3):249–56.
68. Melenhorst J, Koch SM, Uludag O, van Gemert WG, Baeten CGI. A morphologically intact anal sphincter necessary for success with sacral nerve modulation in patients with faecal incontinence? Color Dis. 2008;10(3):257–62.
69. Brouwer R, Duthie G. Sacral nerve neuromodulation is effective treatment for fecal incontinence in the presence of a sphincter defect, pudendal neuropathy, or previous sphincter repair. Dis Colon Rectum. 2010;53(3):273–8.
70. Devroede G, Giese C, Wexner SD, et al. Quality of life is markedly improved in patients with fecal incontinence after sacral nerve stimulation. Female Pelvic Med Reconst Surg. 2012;18(2):103–12.
71. Duelund-Jakobsen J, van Wunnik B, Buntzen S, Lundby L, Baeten C, Laurberg S. Functional results and patient satisfaction with sacral nerve stimulation for idiopathic faecal incontinence. Color Dis. 2012;14(6):753–9.
72. Faucheron JL, Voirin D, Badic B. Sacral nerve stimulation for fecal incontinence: causes of surgical revision from a series of 87 consecutive patients operated on in a single institution. Dis Colon Rectum. 2010;53(11):1501–7.
73. Altomare DF, Giuratrabocchetta S, Knowles CH, et al. Long-term outcomes of sacral nerve stimulation for faecal incontinence. Br J Surg. 2015;102(4):407–15.

Part V

Optimizing Outcomes in Laparoscopic Colorectal Surgery

Is There Still a Role for Hand-Assisted Laparoscopic Surgery (HALS)?

19

Nicholas Gerard Berger, Timothy J. Ridolfi, and Kirk A. Ludwig

Introduction

Laparoscopy was developed in the 1980s, with minimally invasive cholecystectomy quickly becoming the standard of care. Thereafter, laparoscopic techniques were applied to the performance of many intra-abdominal operations, in particular, foregut operations, gynecologic procedures, and inguinal hernia repair. However, adoption of minimally invasive techniques for colorectal surgery has proceeded at a slower pace, due in large part, to concerns related to relative difficulty and the long learning curve for complex multi-quadrant colorectal surgery. Since the most common indication for colon surgery is cancer, there were major concerns regarding the oncologic efficacy of these techniques as compared to standard open operations. Furthermore, early data did not report the same early postoperative advantages as had been demonstrated for other laparoscopic operations.

Initial efforts toward laparoscopic colectomy were targeted toward benign conditions such as Crohn's disease, ulcerative colitis, and diverticulitis, with malignant applications following. To address oncologic concerns, a series of prospective randomized trials were conducted which supported oncologic equivalency of minimally invasive colectomy compared to open techniques [1–6]. As the oncologic concerns were addressed, short-term patient benefits emerged as a result of minimally invasive techniques such as less pain, more rapid resolution of postoperative ileus, shorter hospitalization, a faster return to normal activities, and improved cosmetic outcome [7]. Furthermore, in an increasingly cost-conscious medical industry, the cost of laparoscopy has decreased over time given widespread adoption and the ability to get patients into and out of the hospital more efficiently [7, 8].

N.G. Berger • T.J. Ridolfi • K.A. Ludwig (✉)
Department of Surgery, Division of Colorectal Surgery, Medical College of Wisconsin, Froedtert Memorial Lutheran Hospital, Milwaukee, WI, USA
e-mail: nberger@mcw.edu; tridolfi@mcw.edu; kludwig@mcw.edu

C.M. Schlachta, P. Sylla (eds.), *Current Common Dilemmas in Colorectal Surgery*,
https://doi.org/10.1007/978-3-319-70117-2_19

Despite enthusiasm and advantages for these techniques, laparoscopic colorectal surgery is difficult. This single issue probably accounts for the fact that a large portion of colorectal surgery is still performed using open techniques [9]. Furthermore, while laparoscopic and open techniques are oncologically equivalent, in major trials, laparoscopic operations were longer than the open operations and the conversion rates to open surgery were not insignificant [1–4]. In this setting, hand-assisted laparoscopic surgery (HALS) for colorectal pathology was developed. Initially, HALS was considered an intermediate technique designed to help surgeons quickly gain experience and surmount the long learning curve of laparoscopy. Moreover, HALS could be applied to cases not progressing with straight laparoscopy to avoid conversion to a full laparotomy. With better hand-assisted devices, it became clear that HALS had some innate advantages over pure laparoscopic techniques that could make widespread adoption of these techniques a reasonable alternative while preserving the typical benefits of minimally invasive operations. As it stands, there have been no studies that show any short-term benefits of pure laparoscopic colorectal surgery over HALS, and in most reports the HALS approach saves time in the operating room and dramatically decreases conversion rates. All this while offering the surgeon the advantages of tactile feedback and multipoint retraction, one could only get using the most advanced, gentle, and sophisticated surgical instrument: the human hand.

The Troubles with Laparoscopy in Colorectal Surgery and Why a Hand-Assisted Approach Might Help

Laparoscopy has gained widespread application within general surgery, with cholecystectomy, appendectomy, Nissen fundoplication, inguinal hernia repair, hysterectomy, splenectomy, and even adrenalectomy being commonly performed with laparoscopic techniques. However, there are features of colorectal surgery that are intrinsically different that have major implications for any minimally invasive approach. In the authors' opinion, HALS techniques offer advantages in managing many of these issues over standard laparoscopic approaches.

First, when considering most non-colorectal laparoscopic operations, they are typically performed in a single abdominal quadrant, often in a very small area. Laparoscopic cholecystectomy takes place in an area a few square centimeters in size. Hiatal procedures such as Nissen fundoplication take place in a small confined area. Indeed, these small confined spaces and narrow working fields make laparoscopy advantageous. This is almost never the case with colon or rectal surgery, with the need to almost always access more than one abdominal quadrant and sometimes all four quadrants (Fig. 19.1). With multi-quadrant operations, proper placement of the camera and working ports is essential so that all parts of the organ can be approached properly. The large intra-abdominal area in which a typical colon or rectal operation is performed adds to the complexity. HALS techniques help conduct these multiquadrant operations efficiently. Bulky anatomic structures can be more easily manipulated with a hand inside which makes moving around the abdomen easier.

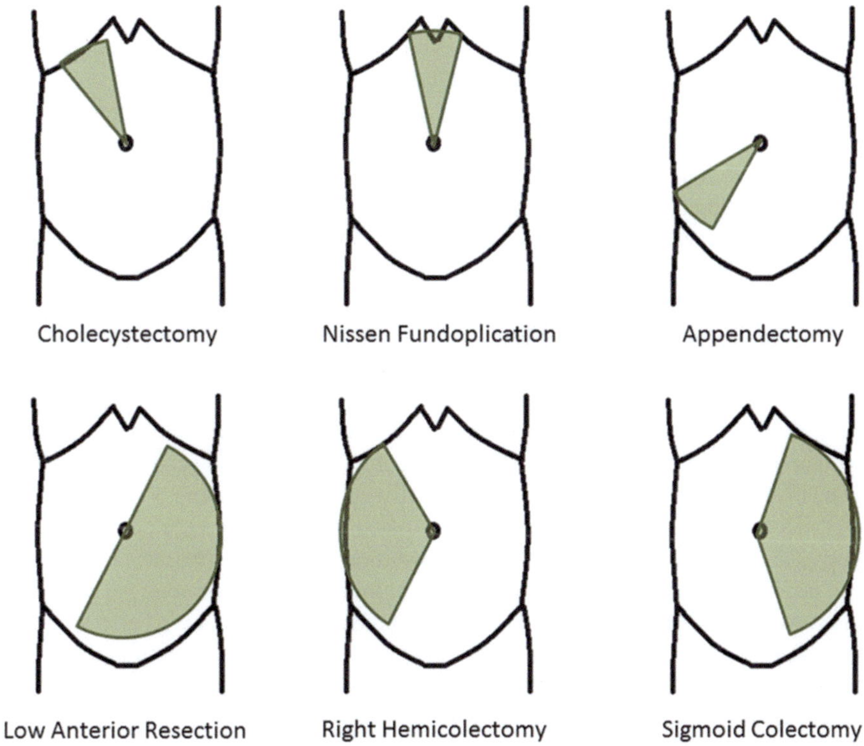

Fig. 19.1 Field of vision for key steps for various laparoscopic procedures. Laparoscopic cholecystectomy, Nissen fundoplication, and appendectomy have more narrow working fields of vision compared to various laparoscopic colectomy procedures

Secondly, the colon and rectum have a complex vascular anatomy, and each resection requires ligation of at least one (usually more) major vessel. For a right colon resection, the surgeon will need to manage the ileocolic artery at its origin off the superior mesenteric artery and the middle colic arteries and veins right over the pancreas. For a left-sided resection, the inferior mesenteric artery will be frequently taken off the aorta, and the inferior mesenteric vein taken at the inferior edge of the pancreas. These vessels can be relatively inaccessible at the base of the colonic mesentery. This mesentery is often thick and fatty, and it may be significantly inflamed, and exposing these vessels with colon and small bowel falling into the field can be very difficult. Changes in the position of the table, skilled assistance and experience can help, but proper exposure and management of multiple large vessels can be difficult. Inability to manage the anatomy at the root of either the right colon or the left colon mesentery often requires conversion to an open operation. Exposure is essential and the hand is the most precise retractor. Furthermore, should bleeding occur, it is much easier to manage confidently with HALS techniques than with straight laparoscopic techniques. With HALS techniques, the surgeon can calmly and confidently grab the bleeding vessel and take remedial steps to control the bleeding.

Third, unlike many of the usual laparoscopic operations, most colorectal operations are only half finished once the pathology is removed, as the surgeon still needs to reestablish GI tract continuity. This is arguably the most important part of the operation, and constructing a good anastomosis requires a keen eye and the utmost precision for technical success. In this regard, using a HALS technique for a right colectomy allows the surgeon to routinely obtain maximum mobilization of the transverse colon, so the ileocolic anastomosis can be constructed up on the abdominal wall and not deep within the extraction wound. For left colon resections, using the hand to manipulate the rectum and the stapler as it comes into the rectal stump from below gives the surgeon confidence that the circular stapled anastomosis is constructed with precision [10].

Colorectal surgery often differs in typical indications for surgery as well. Malignancy makes the fine details of colon and rectal resection critically important, while inflammatory disease distorts anatomy and tissue planes making even open surgery challenging. Again, the authors would argue that a HALS approach can help with precise manipulation of anatomic detail and the hand inside can certainly help with managing thick, inflamed, and bulky tissue. These challenges translate to a well-documented long learning curve associated with laparoscopic colorectal surgery. This learning curve increases operative time and conversion rates [1, 2, 4]. It can take 20–50 cases to reach proficiency and probably many more [11–13]. Given the colorectal surgery volume of the average general surgeon in a typical year, it can take many years to overcome this learning curve. A HALS operation can provide efficiency in the operating room and help shorten the time it takes for a surgeon to feel comfortable with these operations [14].

Similar to the familiar open experience, during a right or left HALS resection, the operation proceeds in a rather standard lateral to medial approach. Therefore, transitioning from open to HALS should be less difficult if the same process for colon mobilization is maintained. HALS operations carry a lower conversion rate than straight laparoscopic operations, and the operative times with a HALS operation are shorter than straight laparoscopy because of this transition [14–18]. Furthermore, some patients are marginal candidates for minimally invasive approaches to their colorectal disease, particularly patients with significant inflammation or obesity. As it stands, two thirds of Americans are either overweight or obese [19]. These are the types of patients that potentially stand to benefit the most from a minimally invasive operation. Using standard laparoscopic techniques, operating on obese patients can be very difficult, if not impossible. Moving heavy tissue around the abdomen with tiny instruments and gaining exposure in a viscerally obese man can be difficult if not dangerous. Having a hand inside the abdomen can help considerably.

A unique problem with techniques describing laparoscopic colorectal procedures involves having skilled assistants who usually control instruments through several ports. This can be a problem for the average surgeon. If an operation requires a team of people, it may not be possible or practical to have this team available for every operation. As we have described, whether doing a right colectomy of a left-sided resection, a HALS operation is a single-surgeon procedure which can be done with only one person needed to hold the laparoscope [20]. There is no need for a trained surgical assistant (Fig. 19.2).

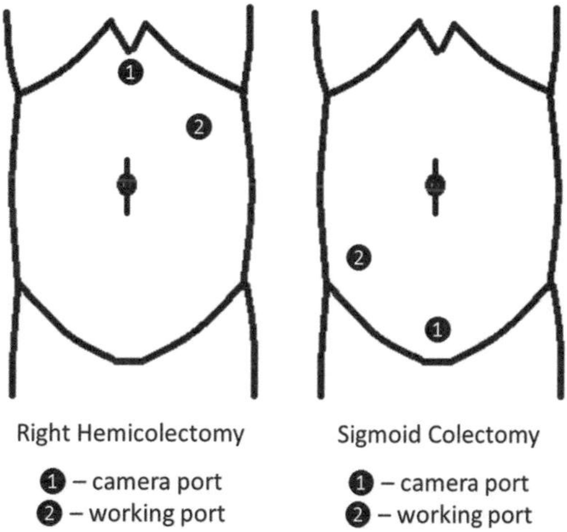

Fig. 19.2 Hand-assisted laparoscopic port placement for HALS right hemicolectomy and HALS sigmoid colectomy. In both cases, the hand port is placed in the center of the abdomen, typically centered on the umbilicus in an average size patient

Following any laparoscopic colon resection, there is just no getting around the fact that there will be a fairly large specimen that needs to be delivered through the abdominal wall. At some point toward the end of the operation, the surgeon will have to create a minilaparotomy incision and, at least for a right colectomy, use this incision to fashion an extracorporeal anastomosis. While there are techniques that have been described for delivering left-sided resection specimens through the open stump of the rectum or through a defect made in the vagina, these are not standard approaches. The standard is to make an incision. A not insignificant argument remains: why not make the minilaparotomy incision at the beginning of the procedure and use this incision for a hand port to facilitate a clean and efficient operation?

The Data on HALS Colorectal Surgery

HALS techniques in colorectal surgery were first reported in the mid-1990s. Through a 5–6 cm minilaparotomy, using either fascial ties or a pneumatic assistance device to provide adequate seal, the surgeon's left hand was inserted through a median or Pfannenstiel incision. A working port was placed to the right of the incision, with the camera port placed to the left with the assistant placed on the ipsilateral side of the surgeon. The working and camera ports are able to rotate on this axis to allow access to all four quadrants of the abdomen. These initial reports suggested that this HALS technique allowed for minimal learning curve, easy exposure, complete exploration, meticulous dissection, tactile feedback, and immediate hemostasis with short hospital stay and recuperation time and even improved cosmesis [21–24]. With essential tactile feedback and a dexterous hand, the surgeon was able to palpate lesions, retract the colon, and perform dissection in a manner very nearly replicating the open colectomy technique.

Several randomized controlled trials have demonstrated the superiority of HALS colonic surgery over traditional open techniques. In 2004, Kang et al. compared perioperative outcomes in 60 patients randomized to HAL or open colectomy. The study demonstrated shorter hospital stay, incision length, faster gastrointestinal function recovery, less analgesic use, and lower pain scores, with no differences in operative time or complications [25]. A similar study in 2007 examined 81 patients undergoing non-emergent colectomy for nonmetastatic right-sided lesions, demonstrating less blood loss, less pain and analgesia use, faster recovery, and shorter hospital stay but longer operative times (12.5 min) for HALS colectomy. Furthermore, long-term follow-up 28 months demonstrated no difference in disease recurrence or 5-year survival rates between HAL and open cohorts [26]. Finally, Sheng et al., in a report on 116 randomized patients, noted that HALS patients had a significantly shorter incision length, less blood loss, less pain, earlier passage of flatus, and shorter length of stay but longer operative time and higher costs compared to open cohorts. These three studies demonstrated improved perioperative outcomes for HALS over open colectomy, despite some reports of longer operative times and higher costs (Table 19.1) [27].

These outcomes are supported by retrospective National Surgical Quality Improvement Program (NSQIP) data reporting lower hospital stay and morbidity as defined as superficial surgical site infection (SSI), deep SSI, organ space SSI, wound disruption, sepsis, bleeding, and ileus [28]. As with previous comparisons of laparoscopic to open colectomy, HALS minimally invasive techniques provide improved perioperative outcomes, lower morbidity, and shorter hospital stay in the context of similar oncologic outcomes. An extensive review of the literature published in 2010 looking at studies comparing HALS versus open resection concluded that HALS has advantages over open surgery while reducing some of the disadvantages of laparoscopic surgery, and, overall, HALS provides an excellent treatment option for the management of colorectal disease [29].

In addition to offering advantages over open operation, HALS has also been demonstrated to have specific benefits over conventional laparoscopy. The HALS Study Group reported a series in which 40 patients were randomized to HALS versus straight laparoscopic operation for either benign or incurable malignant disease, reporting similar operative time, incision length, conversion rates, return of bowel function, length of stay, postoperative pain, and rate of functional recovery. The study concluded that HALS is safe and retains the perioperative benefits of minimally invasive laparoscopic colectomy and may allow a surgeon to perform complex operations more easily [30]. Marcello et al. reported a multicenter randomized trial examining HALS vs. laparoscopic sigmoid and total colectomy. Operative times were significantly decreased in the HALS group, though incision length was longer. There were no differences noted in perioperative parameters or conversion rates [17]. Examining long-term oncologic outcomes following right colectomy, Ng et al. demonstrated no difference in 5-year survival rates between HALS and laparoscopic groups, with no significant differences noted in operating time, length of stay, and morbidity [31]. Last, Targarona et al. examined clinical outcomes and inflammatory response of HALS vs. laparoscopic surgery, noting lower conversion

Table 19.1 Summarized outcomes of randomized trials comparing HALS colectomy to open colectomy

Reference	HALS approach	Open approach	No difference
Kang et al. [25]	Less operative blood loss		Operative time
	Shorter incision length		Overall complications
	Improved time to first oral intake		Time to resume normal activities
	Improved return of bowel function		
	Decreased length of stay		
Chung et al. [26]	Less operative blood loss	Shorter operative time	Lymph nodes harvested
	Improved time to first oral intake		Mortality
			Anastomotic leak
	Improved return of bowel function		Wound sepsis
			Oncologic survival
	Decreased length of stay		
	Improved pain scores		
	Decreased narcotic use		
Sheng et al. [27]	Less operative blood loss	Shorter operative time	Lymph nodes harvested
	Shorter incision length	Decreased overall costs	Overall complications
	Improved time to first oral intake		
	Improved return of bowel function		
	Decreased length of stay		
	Improved pain scores		

rate (7 vs. 23%) but increased interleuken-6 (IL-6) and C-reactive protein (CRP) during the postoperative period for HALS (Table 19.2) [32].

Clearly HALS is associated with equivalent perioperative outcome parameters and oncologic outcomes compared to purely laparoscopic approaches. A recent meta-analysis of the data concluded that compared to straight laparoscopic operations, HALS exhibited reduced operative times, a reduction in the likelihood of conversion to open operation, and no difference in hospital length of stay. The authors concluded that HALS approaches can provide a more efficient segmental colectomy compared to laparoscopic colectomy and the advantages for the HALS approach were particularly evident when the indication for operation was diverticulitis. They suggested that HALS must be considered a valuable addition to the laparoscopic armamentarium [14]. The reduced operative times and conversion rates demonstrating the effectiveness of HALS colectomy compared to laparoscopy are also supported by institutional reviews and nationwide database studies. The NSQIP targeted colectomy data set comparing HALS, and laparoscopy has demonstrated shorter operating times with similar hospital stay in HALS compared to laparoscopic cohorts. However, higher odds of SSI in the HALS group compared to straight laparoscopy was also reported. Other similar single-institution reviews of

Table 19.2 Summarized outcomes of randomized trials comparing HALS colectomy to laparoscopic colectomy

Reference	HALS approach	Laparoscopic approach	No difference
HALS Study Group [30]			Operative time
			Incision length
			Operative blood loss
			Conversion rates
			Postoperative pain
			Quality of life index
			Hospital length of stay
Marcello et al. [17]	Shorter operative time	Shorter incision length	Intraoperative
			Complications
			Conversion rates
			Operative blood loss
			Return of bowel function
			Hospital length of stay
Ng et al. [31]			Operative time
			Conversion rates
			Operative blood loss
			Postoperative pain
			Hospital length of stay
			Postoperative complications
			5-year survival
Targarona et al. [32]	Lower conversion rate	Lower postoperative IL-6	Operative time
		Lower postoperative CRP	Return of bowel function
			Overall complications
			Hospital length of stay

HAL vs. laparoscopic colectomy have demonstrated higher postoperative medical morbidity and similar costs in their HAL cohort, with one of these reviews demonstrating a higher lymph node yield for oncologic resections [18, 33, 34].

Conclusions

The surgical literature and practical considerations endorse HALS colon surgery as an appropriate, oncologically sound technique with many advantages over open surgery and several over laparoscopy. While HALS was initially considered an intermediate operation meant to encourage laparoscopic skill development, this is no longer the case. HALS colorectal surgery can be a destination operation that has advantages over open surgery and achieves the short-term benefits of straight laparoscopic operation while saving time in the operating room and minimizing conversion rates. Especially for complicated operations, extended resections, and operations conducted in overweight or obese patients, a HALS approach is a valuable technique for the minimally invasive surgeon to have at his or her disposal. The available data supports these contentions. So, to the question "is there still a role for hand-assisted laparoscopic surgery?" for colorectal disease, the authors would answer with an emphatic "yes."

References

1. Clinical Outcomes of Surgical Therapy Study Group, et al. A comparison of laparoscopically assisted and open colectomy for colon cancer. N Engl J Med. 2004;350(20):2050–9.
2. Colon Cancer Laparoscopic or Open Resection Study Group, et al. Survival after laparoscopic surgery versus open surgery for colon cancer: long-term outcome of a randomised clinical trial. Lancet Oncol. 2009;10(1):44–52.
3. Fleshman J, et al. Laparoscopic colectomy for cancer is not inferior to open surgery based on 5-year data from the COST study group trial. Ann Surg. 2007;246(4):655–62. discussion 662–4
4. Guillou PJ, et al. Short-term endpoints of conventional versus laparoscopic-assisted surgery in patients with colorectal cancer (MRC CLASICC trial): multicentre, randomised controlled trial. Lancet. 2005;365(9472):1718–26.
5. Jayne DG, et al. Randomized trial of laparoscopic-assisted resection of colorectal carcinoma: 3-year results of the UK MRC CLASICC trial group. J Clin Oncol. 2007;25(21):3061–8.
6. Lacy AM, et al. The long-term results of a randomized clinical trial of laparoscopy-assisted versus open surgery for colon cancer. Ann Surg. 2008;248(1):1–7.
7. Aly EH. Laparoscopic colorectal surgery: summary of the current evidence. Ann R Coll Surg Engl. 2009;91(7):541–4.
8. Franks PJ, et al. Short-term costs of conventional vs laparoscopic assisted surgery in patients with colorectal cancer (MRC CLASICC trial). Br J Cancer. 2006;95(1):6–12.
9. Kang CY, et al. Laparoscopic colorectal surgery: a better look into the latest trends. Arch Surg. 2012;147(8):724–31.
10. Hyman N. How much colorectal surgery do general surgeons do? J Am Coll Surg. 2002;194(1):37–9.
11. Senagore AJ, Luchtefeld MA, Mackeigan JM. What is the learning curve for laparoscopic colectomy? Am Surg. 1995;61(8):681–5.
12. Simons AJ, et al. Laparoscopic-assisted colectomy learning curve. Dis Colon Rectum. 1995;38(6):600–3.
13. Wishner JD, et al. Laparoscopic-assisted colectomy. The learning curve. Surg Endosc. 1995;9(11):1179–83.
14. Aalbers AG, et al. Hand-assisted or laparoscopic-assisted approach in colorectal surgery: a systematic review and meta-analysis. Surg Endosc. 2008;22(8):1769–80.
15. Benlice C, et al. Comparison of straight vs hand-assisted laparoscopic colectomy: an assessment from the NSQIP procedure-targeted cohort. Am J Surg. 2016;212(3):406–12.
16. Chang YJ, et al. Hand-assisted laparoscopic sigmoid colectomy: helping hand or hindrance? Surg Endosc. 2005;19(5):656–61.
17. Marcello PW, et al. Hand-assisted laparoscopic vs. laparoscopic colorectal surgery: a multicenter, prospective, randomized trial. Dis Colon Rectum. 2008;51(6):818–26. discussion 826–8
18. Ringley C, et al. Comparison of conventional laparoscopic and hand-assisted oncologic segmental colonic resection. Surg Endosc. 2007;21(12):2137–41.
19. Flegal KM, et al. Prevalence of obesity and trends in the distribution of body mass index among US adults, 1999-2010. JAMA. 2012;307(5):491–7.

20. Hata J, et al. Laparoscopic colectomy and abdominal perineal resection. In: Pappas TN, Harnisch M, Pryor AD, editors. Atlas of laparoscopic surgery. 3rd ed. Philadelphia: Current Medicine; 2007.
21. Bemelman WA, et al. Laparoscopic-assisted colectomy with the dexterity pneumo sleeve. Dis Colon Rectum. 1996;39(10 Suppl):S59–61.
22. Mooney MJ, et al. Hand-assisted laparoscopic sigmoidectomy for diverticulitis. Dis Colon Rectum. 1998;41(5):630–5.
23. O'Reilly MJ, et al. Technique of hand-assisted laparoscopic surgery. J Laparoendosc Surg. 1996;6(4):239–44.
24. Ou H. Laparoscopic-assisted mini laparatomy with colectomy. Dis Colon Rectum. 1995;38(3):324–6.
25. Kang JC, et al. Hand-assisted laparoscopic colectomy vs open colectomy: a prospective randomized study. Surg Endosc. 2004;18(4):577–81.
26. Chung CC, et al. Hand-assisted laparoscopic versus open right colectomy: a randomized controlled trial. Ann Surg. 2007;246(5):728–33.
27. Sheng QS, et al. Hand-assisted laparoscopic versus open right hemicolectomy: short-term outcomes in a single institution from China. Surg Laparosc Endosc Percutan Tech. 2012;22(3):267–71.
28. Benlice C, et al. Hand-assisted laparoscopic vs open colectomy: an assessment from the American college of surgeons national surgical quality improvement program procedure-targeted cohort. Am J Surg. 2016;212(5):808–13.
29. Aalbers AG, et al. Hand-assisted laparoscopic versus open approach in colorectal surgery: a systematic review. Color Dis. 2010;12(4):287–95.
30. HALS Study Group. Hand-assisted laparoscopic surgery vs standard laparoscopic surgery for colorectal disease: a prospective randomized trial. Surg Endosc. 2000;14(10):896–901.
31. Ng LW, et al. Hand-assisted laparoscopic versus total laparoscopic right colectomy: a randomized controlled trial. Color Dis. 2012;14(9):e612–7.
32. Targarona EM, et al. Prospective randomized trial comparing conventional laparoscopic colectomy with hand-assisted laparoscopic colectomy: applicability, immediate clinical outcome, inflammatory response, and cost. Surg Endosc. 2002;16(2):234–9.
33. Ozturk E, et al. Hand-assisted laparoscopic colectomy: benefits of laparoscopic colectomy at no extra cost. J Am Coll Surg. 2009;209(2):242–7.
34. Ozturk E, et al. Hand-assisted laparoscopic surgery may be a useful tool for surgeons early in the learning curve performing total abdominal colectomy. Color Dis. 2010;12(3):199–205.

20 Intracorporeal Anastomosis for Right Colon Resection: Should This Be the Preferred Method?

Barry Salky

Abbreviations

BMI	Body mass index
EC	Extracorporeal
IBD	Inflammatory bowel disease
IC	Intracorporeal
LLQ	Left lower quadrant
LUQ	Left upper quadrant

Definitions

Laparoscopic-assisted extracorporeal anastomosis: (EC) The bowel is mobilized intracorporeally with division of the blood vessels inside the abdomen. An incision is then made in the abdominal wall with extraction of the mobilized segment. The two ends of the bowel are anastomosed outside the abdomen, and the completed anastomosis is put back into the abdomen. The extraction incision is closed.

Laparoscopic intracorporeal anastomosis: (IC) The bowel is mobilized intracorporeally with division of the blood vessels inside the abdomen. The bowel is transected laparoscopically with laparoscopic stapling instruments. The two ends of the bowel are then anastomosed inside the abdomen. The specimen is then extracted through an incision in the abdominal wall. The extraction site is closed.

B. Salky (✉)
Department of Surgery, Mount Sinai Health System, New York, NY, USA
e-mail: barry.salky@mountsinai.org

C.M. Schlachta, P. Sylla (eds.), *Current Common Dilemmas in Colorectal Surgery*,
https://doi.org/10.1007/978-3-319-70117-2_20

Introduction

I began laparoscopic colectomy in late 1992, and I have now performed about 1300 colorectal procedures. At the beginning, all procedures were laparoscopic-assisted with extracorporeal anastomoses. While early procedures were performed with a lateral to medial dissection, almost all are now performed medial to lateral. At the beginning, all blood vessels were divided with clips and ties (or endoloop); now every blood vessel is divided with either an energy source or vascular-loaded stapling devices. I began to switch to an intracorporeal technique in 2007; the reason why is an interesting, short story. I was performing a demonstration right colectomy for cancer at a teaching conference in Europe. I was getting ready to extract the specimen in my usual way when Professor Jacques Perrisat asked me, "Why don't you make the anastomosis intracorporeally?" He then said, "It's sitting right in front of you, and you know how to use staplers and you can sew." He was correct. So, my first intracorporeal anastomosis was on closed circuit television to more than 100 surgeons. It went beautifully. As the patient had a body mass index (BMI) of 36, I was able to make a relatively short Pfannenstiel incision for extraction (my usual incision was transverse midline). The postoperative pain difference was dramatic, and I have not done an extracorporeal anastomosis for a right colon since then.

Advantages of IC Anastomosis

It was difficult to change after having already performed more than 500 right colectomies in an extracorporeal fashion. I couldn't believe that there was a better way. Therefore, I began a prospective study of my own cases, comparing consecutive cases [1]. Tables 20.1 and 20.2 list the patient demographics and intraoperative findings in these two, consecutive groups of patients. There were no statistical differences in any category except that it took longer in the intracorporeal group, but the blood loss was more in the extracorporeal group. The clinical differences in the post-op course are listed in Table 20.3, and they were dramatic, all in favor of intracorporeal anastomosis group.

The study clearly demonstrated less morbidity with the IC vs EC anastomosis, all statistically significant. As a side benefit, the time to flatus was shorter, time to

Table 20.1 Demographics

	Intracorporeal (n = 54)	Extracorporeal (n = 51)	P value
Age (years)	45	50	0.181
Male to female (n)	19(35)	28(23)	0.042
BMI (kg/m^2)	23.8	23.4	0.705
ASA class (mean)	2.1	2.2	0.242
Prior operation	21	23	0.519
Indication for surgery			0.167
IBD	33	30	
Neoplasm	19	16	
Other	2	5	

Table 20.2 Intraoperative

Operation performed	Intracorporeal ($n = 54$)	Extracorporeal ($n = 51$)	p value
Ileocolic	33	33	0.583
R hemi	14	15	
L hemi	6	3	
Subtotal	1	0	
Fistula takedown	14	16	0.537
OR time (min)	190	156	0.001
EBL (mL)	85.4	164	0.014
Intraop narcotics (mg) morphine equivalents	49	48	0.826
Intraop complications	0	0	

Table 20.3 Postoperative

	Intracorporeal	Extracorporeal	P value
Narcotic use (mg)	16	49	0.001
Time to flatus (days)	2.0	2.4	0.017
Time to BM (days)	2.2	2.5	0.167
Length of stay (days)	3.2	3.8	0.019
Periop morbidity (n)	6	15	0.019
Anastomotic leak	0	1	
Enterotomy	1	0	
GI bleed	0	2	
Obstruction	1	4	
Intra-abd abscess	0	2	
Wound infection	0	2	
Cardiac	2	0	
Blood transfusion	1	3	
Urinary retention	0	1	
Hematuria	0	2	
Other	0	2	
Mortality	0	0	

bowel movement shorter, and length of stay shorter as well (all statistically significant). There was three-quarter *less* morphine equivalent usage as well. All extraction sites were Pfannenstiel, which is a cosmetic bonus. When setting up the anastomosis, the base of the mesentery is clearly seen, so that twisting the anastomosis is really impossible (I have twisted three EC anastomoses).

Disadvantages of IC Anastomosis

The only disadvantage I can think of is that the surgeon has to be comfortable with intracorporeal suturing and knot-tying techniques. I would argue that this should be a prerequisite for advanced laparoscopic cases anyway. It does require a change in the thought process of the surgeon used to doing an extracorporeal anastomosis. It's hard to believe that an IC anastomosis can lead to less morbidity and a nicer cosmetic result unless the surgeon actually sees it.

Technique for Laparoscopic Ileocolic or Right Hemicolectomy

The patient is prepared for surgery according to modern guidelines and positioned supine, unless a known ileosigmoid fistula is present, and first trocar access is obtained. (I was trained to mechanically bowel prep patients having colon resection. I have not seen any deleterious effects of bowel prepping a patient over the 40 years of performing colon surgery, and I am familiar with the literature). In my own study quoted above, the only infectious complications were in the extracorporeal patients, and the bowel prep was the same in both groups. Four trocars are placed. The 5 mm epigastric port is used for retraction, the midline 5 mm for the 30-degree optic, and the surgeon uses the suprapubic 5 mm and the left lower quadrant (LLQ) 12 mm port to work. A 12 mm port is necessary for placement of the stapling instruments. I prefer bipolar energy and a medial to lateral approach to the dissection, but other energy sources are okay, and a lateral to medial approach is fine too. Because I have a 12 mm port for the stapling instruments, I use a 10 mm bipolar energy instrument. It is possible to use a 5 mm bipolar device, but there is too much "play" within the trocar for me with a 5 mm instrument.

Identify the Anatomy

The first step is identifying the anatomy, which includes the ileocolic vessels, the duodenum and the right transverse mesocolon (Fig. 20.1). The assistant uses the epigastric port to grasp the cecum and elevate it. This will put tension on the IC vessels. In the vast majority of cases (even obese patients), the second portion of the duodenum will be visible with this maneuver. Depending on the pathology, the anastomosis could be as low as the ascending colon or as high as the right mid-transverse colon. If the anastomosis is lower, then the 12 mm port is in the LLQ. If the anastomosis is going to be into the transverse colon, then the 12 mm port is placed in the left upper quadrant (LUQ). This will make it much easier to place the laparoscopic GIA into the ileum and colon.

Intracorporeal Resection

Once the proper anatomy has been identified, traction is placed on the cecum with the epigastric port grasper. (It is easier to use a self-locking grasper here). The peritoneum over the ileocolic vessels. If this is an inflammatory bowel disease (IBD)

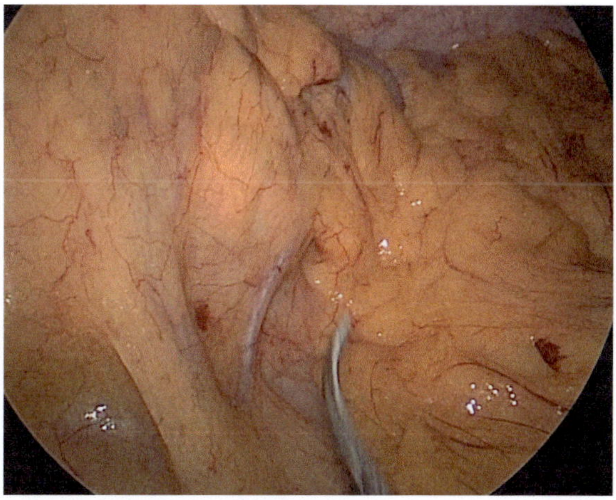

Fig. 20.1 A prominent ileocolic blood vessel is seen in the foreground. The second portion of the duodenum is seen just below the scissor tip. This patient has a right colic vessel as well

patient, the division of the peritoneum is higher on the mesentery. If this is for cancer, the division is lower in order to encompass a complete lymphadenectomy. I like to use an electrocautery scissor to score the mesentery. It is important to not get into the mesenteric fat (bleeding) doing this scoring of the mesentery. I use 20 watts of current on the electrocautery. The main reason for scoring the mesentery is to allow the energy source that is going to divide the vessels to be placed directly on the vessel, not the peritoneum over the vessel. This will decrease the risk of bleeding from use of the energy device. The proper surgical plane between the mesentery and the retroperitoneal fascia is developed here. The ureters and gonadal vessels are below this fascial plane. It is common to see vermiculation of the ureter through the fascia, but I don't make an effort to actually see the ureter. I do insist on seeing an intact retroperitoneal fascia. If the fascia has been breached (or if this is a secondary ileocolic resection), the ureter is identified. In my mind, this would be a reason for conversion to open if the ureter (or fascia) could not be identified with certainty. This is an avascular plane between the mesentery and the retroperitoneal fascia. If bleeding occurs here, it should alert the surgeon that the proper plane has not been entered. If in the correct plane, the medial to lateral dissection should be very quick and bloodless. Depending on the pathology, the actual number of blood vessels to be divided can be different, but the principles are the same. There is also an avascular plane just next to the bowel wall. I like to dissect all the tissues off so that I have only bowel wall to transect with the laparoscopic linear cutting stapler. It is important to transect at right angle to the bowel wall (Fig. 20.2). This will reduce the incidence of ischemia of the bowel wall. I must say it is encouraging to see a little bleeding from the staple line to confirm good blood supply. Once the proximal and distal bowel segments have been divided, the specimen is placed in the pelvis for extraction later on in the surgery. If this is cancer or there was a fistula, the bowel is stored in a nonporous retrieval bag until extracted.

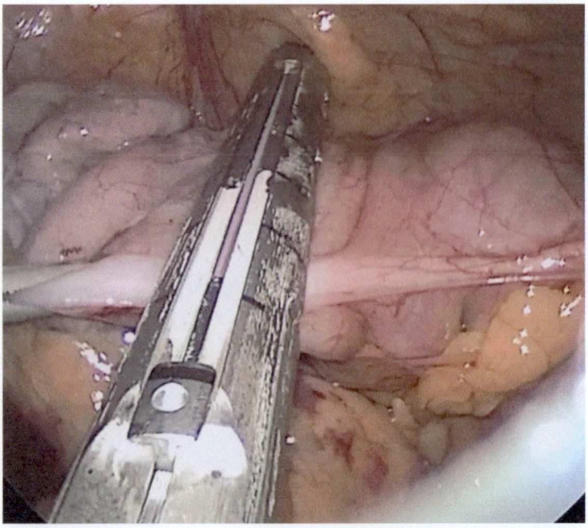

Fig. 20.2 The base of the mesentery is visualized to make sure it is not twisted before making the isoperistaltic anastomosis

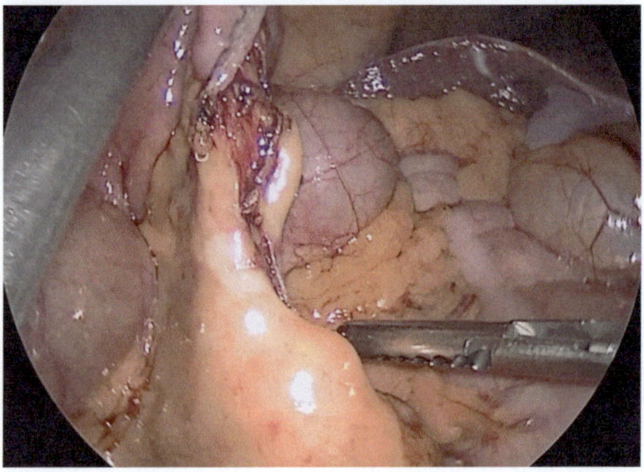

Fig. 20.3 Stapler applied at a right angle to the colon wall. Notice the clear difference in vascularity. It is important to make sure the stapler is in the well-vascularized portion

Anastomosis

The next step is to align the two ends of the bowel properly. The base of the mesentery is identified, and the mesentery on each side is traced back to the bowel wall. This will prevent a twist of the mesentery prior to the anastomosis (Fig. 20.3). I prefer an isoperistaltic anastomosis, but I know that many surgeons use a reverse peristaltic configuration. It just seems to me that we should try to restore bowel continuity as close to the original position as possible (no science behind that). Enterotomies are made with hook electrode on 30 watts of cutting current. I use cutting current, as the waveform is much less traumatic to the tissues than coagulation current. It is important to make sure the enterotomy is all the way into the bowel lumen, and I confirm that by either seeing the mucosa or placing a Maryland-type grasper into the opening (Fig. 20.4). It is not impossible to make a false lumen with the stapling instruments. It is important to make the enterotomies large enough to admit the profile of each side of the stapler.

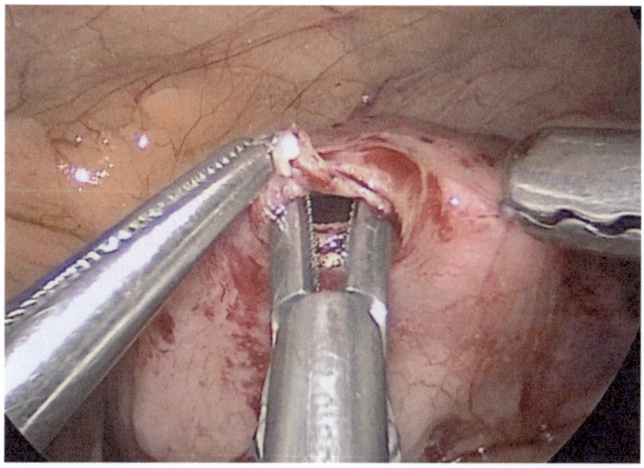

Fig. 20.4 Confirmation that the small enterotomy is actually into the lumen is important. I prefer a 5 mm Maryland-type grasper for this, but this is purely the surgeon's preference

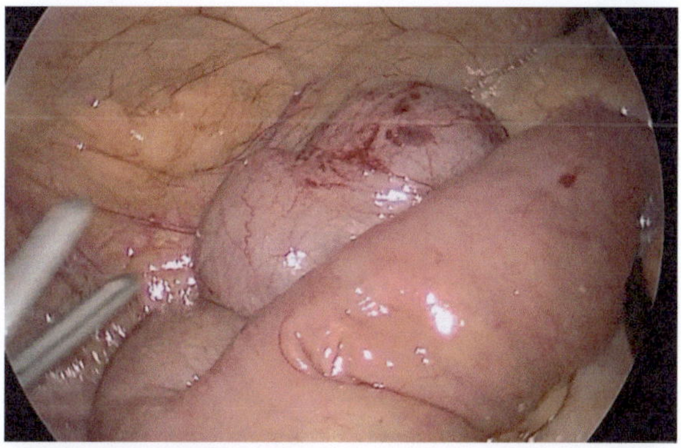

Fig. 20.5 I prefer an isoperistaltic anastomosis. Both the small bowel (foreground) and the colon (background) are aligned. Good vascularity is seen, and there is no tension on either piece of intestine

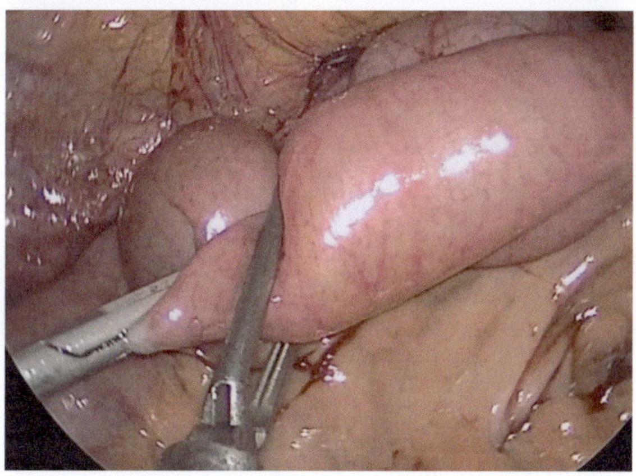

Fig. 20.6 Bulldog clamp is applied to proximal distended small bowel to prevent spillage

Special Considerations

A special note about obstructed small bowel as commonly seen in Crohn's disease cases: I apply a laparoscopic bulldog to the dilated bowel to prevent abdominal cavity contamination in these cases (Figs. 20.5 and 20.6). I use a linear cutting stapler instrument to construct a side-to-side, functional end-to-end, isoperistaltic anastomosis. It is easier to apply the first profile of the stapler into the bowel that is closest to the surgeon. In general, this is the ileum. Once the ileum is cannulated with one arm of the stapler, it is held in place by the assistant's grasper (epigastric port). Next, the other arm is inserted into the colonic enterotomy. The surgeon should try to make each limb of the bowel equal in length on each arm of the stapler (Fig. 20.7). This will facilitate closure of the common enterotomy when the stapler is closed, fired, and removed.

A trick I have learned over the years is to have the assistant's grasper hold the distal part of the anastomosis up after the stapler is removed (Fig. 20.8). This will prevent any spillage of intestinal material while preparing for closure of the enterotomy. Another "trick" is to position the stapler (after firing it) inside the 12 mm trocar and remove the trocar from the abdominal wall. I then wash and clean the inside of the stapler and the trocar before reinsertion. (I replace the trocar with a new one only if I can't clean the first one well). Have the assistant or scrub nurse put a finger into the trocar incision to maintain pneumoperitoneum while the trocar cleaning/exchange occurs.

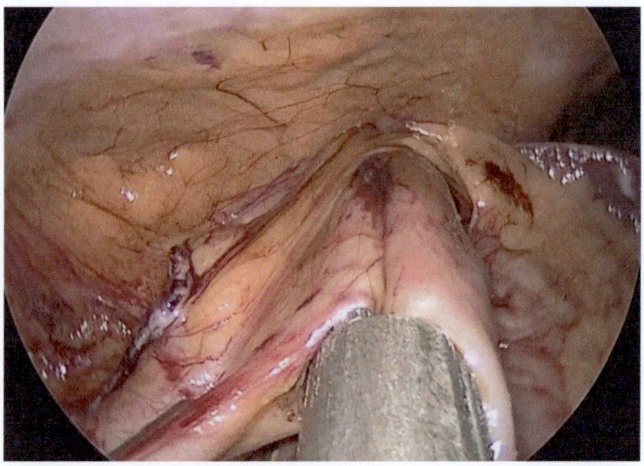

Fig. 20.7 The 60 mm linear cutting stapler is inserted onto both limbs of the intestine, closed and activated

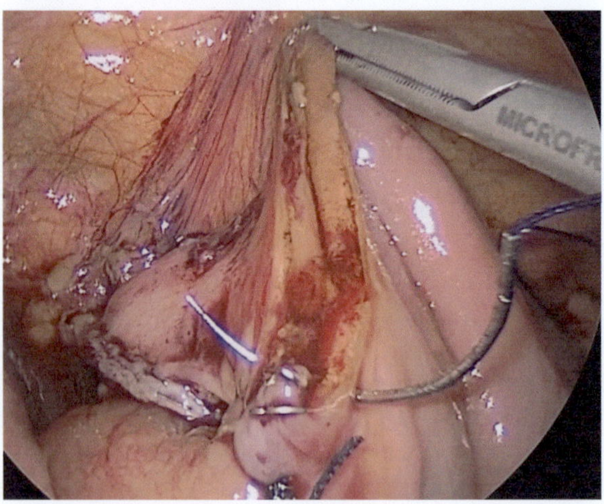

Fig. 20.8 The intestine is aligned so that the suture will pass through the bowel wall at 90° angles. Notice the assistant's grasper elevating the bowel away from the surgeon. This will help in preventing any intestinal content from escaping from the lumen while suturing or closing the defect

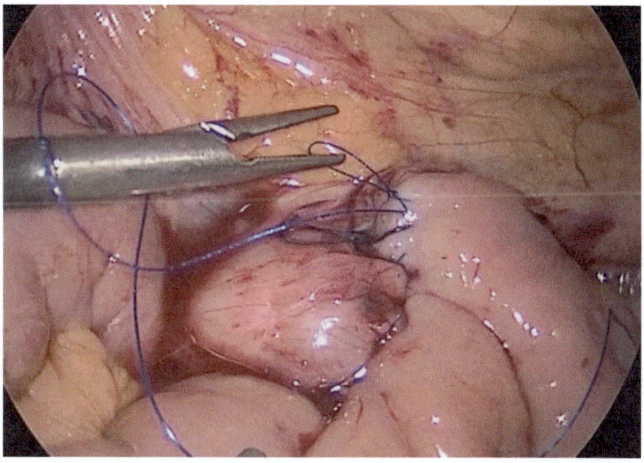

Fig. 20.9 This is a picture of the final 3-0 Prolene® suture being tied to complete the closure of the common enterotomy. Ileum is to the right and colon to the left

Enterotomy Closure

After the trocar has been reinserted, the enterotomy is ready for closure. I was trained in a two-layer closure, but I know that some surgeons do this in one layer. I use 2-0 polyglactin continuous sutures for the inner layer and 3-0 polypropylene continuous seromuscular sutures for the outer layer. I try to place the latter in between the former. I also sew away from myself. I have found over the years that it is much simpler to sew away from than toward yourself, as it allows easier positioning of the sutures in the bowel (Fig. 20.9). Barbed sutures have recently been introduced. For those surgeons performing a single-layer anastomosis, they are an option. They seem inherently more traumatic to the bowel wall than a smooth suture, but I don't know of any data to show a higher leak rate with their use.

Closure of the mesenteric defect has always been controversial. I do not close it, and to my knowledge, I have not had any patient present with an internal hernia with obstruction in more than 700 ileocolic resections. However, I do not have 100% follow-up. I do cover the defect with omentum.

Once the anastomosis is completed, the area is irrigated with saline (no science here), and a thorough check for hemostasis is made. I have not had any take backs for postoperative hemorrhage with the use of the bipolar energy device.

The specimen is extracted through a relatively small, muscle-splitting Pfannenstiel incision. As the specimen can now be extracted on end, the incision size is solely dictated by the diameter of the bowel to be removed. In laparoscopic-assisted surgery, a loop of bowel has to be removed which necessitates a larger incision. No matter how it is extracted, the wound is protected with plastic sleeve to help prevent infectious contamination or implantation of malignant cells.

The fascia of the 12 mm port is sutured closed.

Results

We published our initial results on comparing intracorporeal to extracorporeal anastomoses in 2010 [1]. It was a consecutive series, single surgeon (me). As Tables 20.1 and 20.2 show, the demographics and the operative events were similar, respectively, with the only difference being a longer operative time for the intracorporeal patients. Table 20.3 details the morbidity in this series. The results were so overwhelming in favor of intracorporeal anastomoses that it became the standard procedure for all of these cases.

Since switching to an intracorporeal anastomosis in 2007, I have had experience with more than 200 intracorporeal anastomoses for ileocolic, right hemicolectomy, left hemicolectomy, and high ileosigmoid both for benign and malignant disease. All extractions have been muscle-splitting Pfannenstiel incisions. While my experience is heavily weighted toward right-sided disease, few patients undergoing left hemicolectomy for cancer in this series and subtotal colectomy with a high ileosigmoid anastomosis had similar outcomes as right-sided intracorporeal cases. To date, there have been no incisional hernias and no postoperative obstructions from internal hernia, twisting, or adhesions. In patients who have had both extracorporeal and intracorporeal anastomoses (previous IBD patients), the difference in pain management and overall feeling is dramatically better in the intracorporeal group. There have been two leaks (0.9%). Similar results have been obtained in a recently published series as well [2]. A recent meta-analysis also confirms the advantage of intracorporeal anastomoses with the addition of a decreased incisional hernia rate compared to extracorporeal anastomosis [3].

Conclusion

Laparoscopic intracorporeal anastomosis has been found to have advantages over the extracorporeal anastomotic method in both the short-term (decreased pain and shorter LOS) and the long-term (incisional hernia). This technique does require suturing and knot-tying skills. There will be an increase in the initial operative time with the first few cases, but this will dissipate as suturing and knot-tying skills are acquired. From a patient perspective, this should be the preferred approach.

References

1. Grams J, Tong W, Greenstein AJ, Salky B. Comparison of intracorporeal versus extracorporeal anastomosis in laparoscopic-assisted hemicolectomy. Surg Endosc. 2010;24(8):1886–91.
2. Shapiro R, Keler U, Segev L, Sarna S, Hatib K, Hazzan D. Laparoscopic right hemicolectomy with intracorporeal anastomosis: short- and long-term benefits in comparison with extracorporeal anastomosis. Surg Endosc. 2015;30(9):3823–9.
3. Carnuccio P, Jimeno J, Pares D. Laparoscopic right colectomy: a systematic review and meta-analysis of observational studies comparing two types of anastomosis. Tech Coloproctol. 2014;18(1):5–12.

Transrectal Specimen Extraction: Should This Be Catching On?

21

Albert M. Wolthuis

Introduction

Over the last 20 years, laparoscopic colorectal surgery has shown equal efficacy in cancer treatment as open surgery [1]. In comparison to open colorectal surgery, a laparoscopic approach reduces postoperative morbidity and shortens hospital stay [2]. With the introduction of enhanced recovery protocols, hospital stay after a laparoscopic colorectal resection has been further reduced [3–5]. Fast-track programs or so-called enhanced recovery after surgery protocols, pioneered by Kehlet, were developed to reduce the surgical stress response, organ dysfunction, and morbidity. Postoperative recovery is enhanced by a multimodality set of measures proposed by the various stakeholders in postoperative care [3]. However, a laparoscopic approach still has inherent drawbacks, such as incision-related complications (wound infection/incisional hernia). Moreover, incision-related pain and long-term cosmetic outcomes are important issues regarding the laparoscopic (assisted) approach. In the quest to optimize outcomes after laparoscopic colorectal surgery, reduction of access trauma by means of laparoscopic natural orifice specimen extraction (NOSE) colectomy is a possible way to improve recovery. NOSE could be the key to reducing access trauma in laparoscopic colorectal surgery, with the subsequent reduction of postoperative pain, improvement of patient recovery, and positive long-term outcomes including cosmesis and incisional hernia rates. Because the length of the abdominal incision is directly related to the incisional hernia rate [6], avoiding laparotomy might influence the rate of postoperative wound complications. In NOSE, the specimen is delivered via a natural orifice, and the anastomosis is created intracorporeally. Different methods are used to extract the specimen and to create a bowel anastomosis. Currently, specimens can be delivered transcolonically, transrectally, transanally, or transvaginally.

A.M. Wolthuis (✉)
Abdominal Surgery, University Hospital Leuven, Leuven, Belgium
e-mail: albert.wolthuis@uzleuven.be

C.M. Schlachta, P. Sylla (eds.), *Current Common Dilemmas in Colorectal Surgery*,
https://doi.org/10.1007/978-3-319-70117-2_21

Each of these NOSE procedures raises specific issues with regard to operative technique and application. Transrectal specimen extraction could be performed during a sigmoid or high anterior resection, in contrast to transanal specimen extraction, which is performed after a TME [7]. The aim of this chapter is to discuss laparoscopic NOSE colectomy with transrectal specimen extraction and its current position in the armamentarium of minimally invasive surgery.

Background

Franklin et al. developed the concept of a totally laparoscopic approach for a sigmoid resection in the early 1990s, and Darzi et al. described the technique of a laparoscopic sigmoid resection with transrectal extraction in 1994 [8–10]. However, the technique of a laparoscopic NOSE colectomy did not gain widespread popularity. With recent advances in minimally invasive surgery, a new era has dawned to further minimize access trauma and to explore the surgical possibilities in bridging conventional laparoscopic colorectal surgery and true human natural orifice transluminal endoscopic surgical (NOTES) procedures. NOSE [11] could be the answer to avoid small laparotomy for specimen extraction leading to a totally laparoscopic sigmoid resection. NOSE in laparoscopic colorectal surgery has the potential advantage of decreasing surgical trauma to the abdominal wall, resulting in a lower complication rate, faster recovery, and shorter length of hospital stay. A review performed in 2012 showed lack of evidence (level IV–V) for NOSE colectomy [12]. Because of the heterogeneity and the bias of the studies included, no recommendations could be made, and clear answers to questions about postoperative recovery, cosmesis, and functional outcomes could not be given. Standardization of technique and terminology and comparison with conventional laparoscopic resection are necessary to solve the problems mentioned above. We reported our technique in a step-by-step approach in 2011 and some modifications in 2015 [13–15].

Indications

Previously, we reported that standardized laparoscopic left-sided NOSE colectomy is feasible and safe [16]. Laparoscopic NOSE colectomy for left-sided disease involves transrectal specimen extraction and intracorporeal colorectal anastomosis formation. A specimen retrieval pouch can be used to extract the specimen. However, positional changes of the specimen and air trapping in the bag can hamper extraction. Extraction of lengthy and voluminous specimens could be problematic. Therefore, we propose the use of a laparoscopic camera sleeve through the anorectum to extract the specimen longitudinally [15]. This modification may expand the indications and feasibility for left-sided NOSE colectomy to extract larger specimens or to perform subtotal colectomy. To date, indications for laparoscopic NOSE colectomy are benign or malignant sigmoid colon diseases, such as diverticular disease (elective sigmoid resections for recurrent diverticulitis), endometriosis, a benign adenoma or lipoma, or a non-transmural carcinoma smaller than 4 cm in diameter. Some criteria to exclude patients from NOSE relate to specific patient and pathologic features. Patient-specific exclusion criteria are pregnancy, body mass index (BMI) >35 kg/m^2, being on immunosuppressive medication or immunocompromised, abnormal blood coagulation, undergoing peritoneal dialysis, and history of anal surgery. Pathology-specific exclusion criteria are diverticulitis of the proximal sigmoid colon, acute diverticulitis including Hinchey stages 1 to 4, and advanced colon carcinoma, defined as clinically staged T3 or T4 tumors.

Technical Aspects

The patient is placed in a modified Lloyd-Davies position on a moldable beanbag and a standardized four-port laparoscopic approach is used. First, vessel ligation by conventional medial-to-lateral approach and isolation of the specimen was performed. After the proximal and distal margins have been established, the sigmoid mesentery is divided. The devascularized specimen is isolated, and both the proximal sigmoid colon and proximal rectum are tied off. The anvil of a 28 or 29 mm circular stapler was delivered into the peritoneal cavity via proximal rectotomy (Figs. 21.1 and 21.2). The spike with a monofilament suture is mounted onto the

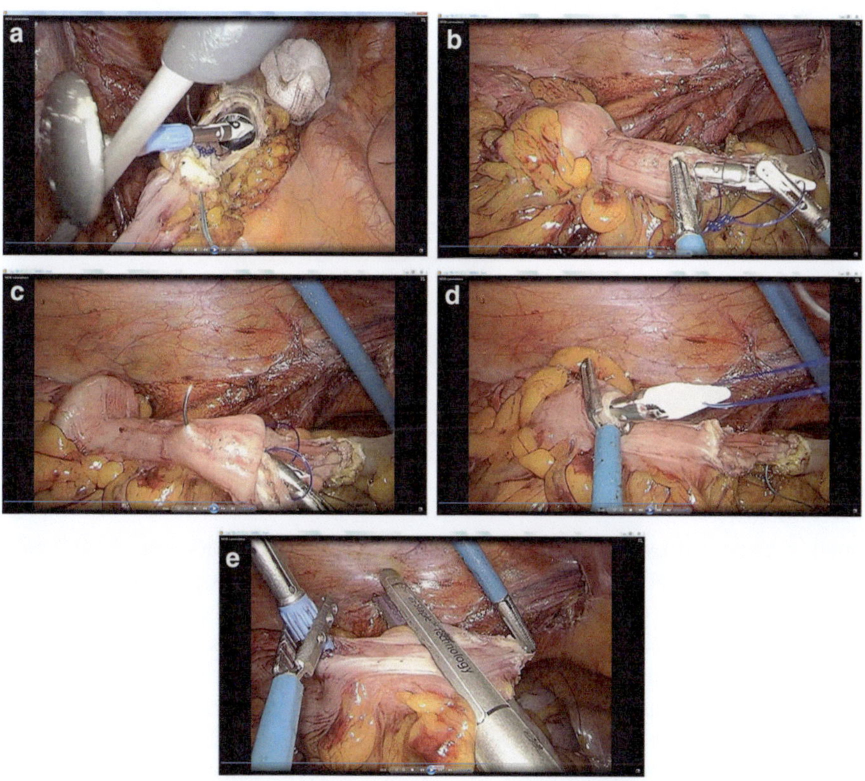

Fig. 21.1 Operative view: critical steps of laparoscopic transrectal NOSE colectomy. (**a**) Anvil insertion into the abdominal cavity via proximal rectotomy. Note the spike and the monofilament suture already mounted onto the anvil. (**b**) Anvil insertion into the descending colon. (**c**, **d**) Anvil retrieval by pulling on the anti-mesenteric placed stitch. (**e**) The proximal bowel is divided with a 60-mm endoscopic linear stapler

a b c d e

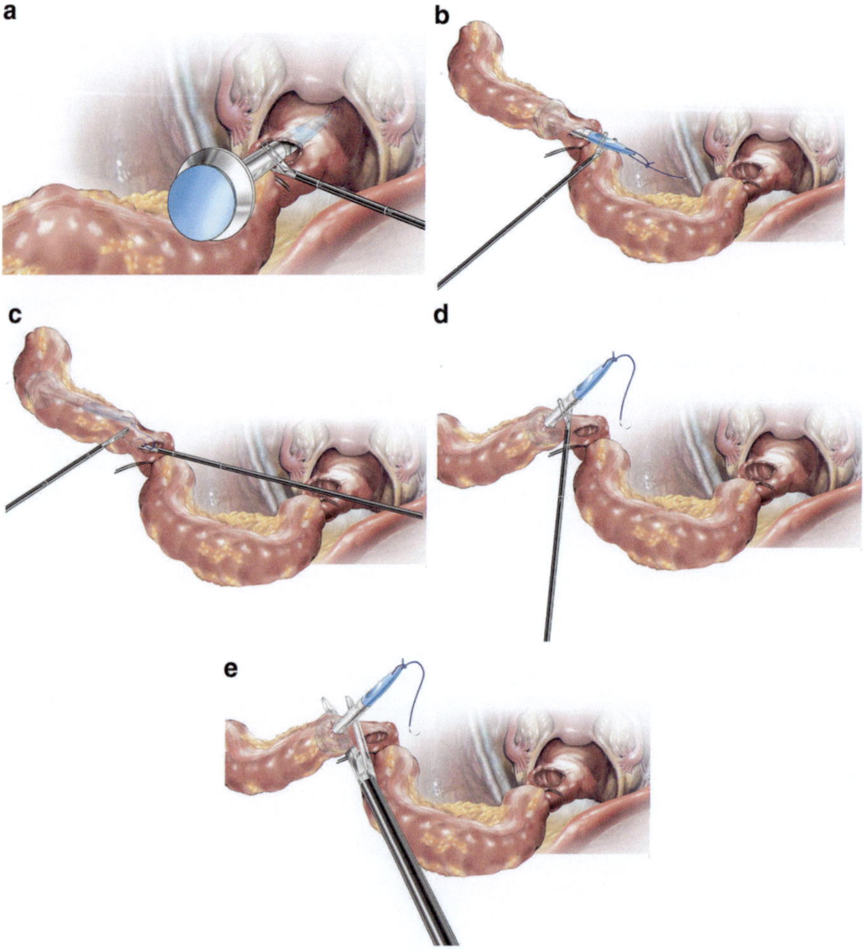

Fig. 21.2 Schematic drawing of the first steps of laparoscopic transrectal NOSE colectomy. Preparation of the proximal part of the anastomosis (**a**–**e**)

anvil. A camera sleeve is inserted through the anorectum to protect the rectal lumen and to facilitate specimen extraction. A proximal colotomy is performed, and the anvil is inserted into the descending colon. The needle attached to the suture and the spike is used to place an anti-mesenterical stitch. This stitch is placed from within the bowel lumen to the outside. Thereafter, gentle pulling on the mounted spike and suture retrieves the anvil through the colon. Now, the anvil is in place for the future circular anastomosis. The colotomy is closed and cross-stapled with an endoscopic linear stapler, so that the proximal part of the colorectal anastomosis is ready for use. The rectum is transected and the isolated specimen is extracted transrectally in a longitudinal way (Figs. 21.3 and 21.4). The rectum is closed with an endoscopic linear stapler, and a circular stapled colorectal anastomosis is completed.

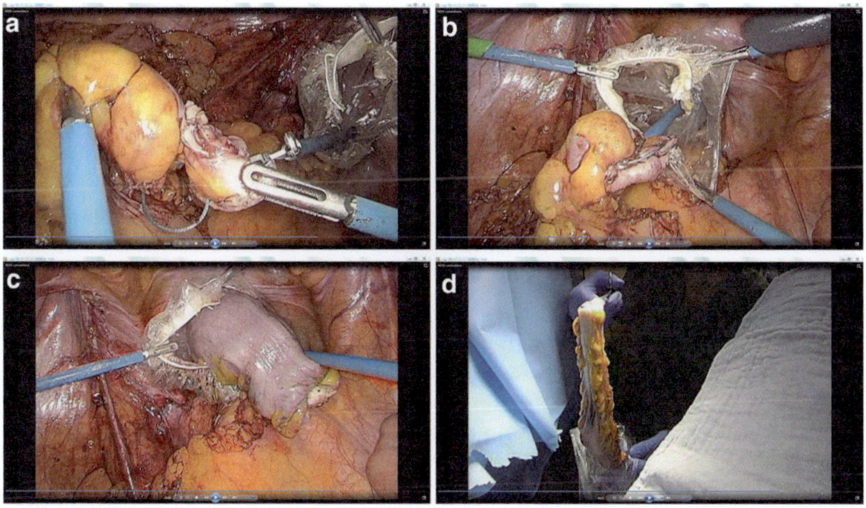

Fig. 21.3 Operative view: critical steps of laparoscopic transrectal NOSE colectomy. A plastic camera sleeve was inserted to protect the rectum. The specimen was extracted transrectally in a longitudinal way by pulling on the grasping forceps (**a**–**d**)

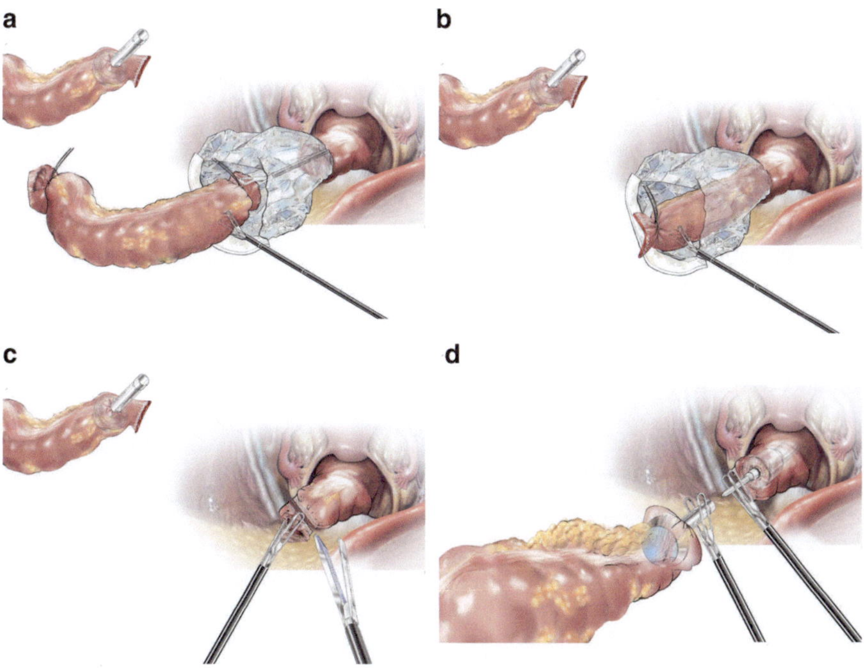

Fig. 21.4 Schematic drawing of the final steps of laparoscopic transrectal NOSE colectomy. Transrectal longitudinal specimen extraction via a protected rectum with a camera sleeve (**a** and **b**). The rectum was closed with an endoscopic linear stapler and a circular stapled colorectal anastomosis was made (**c** and **d**)

Advantages and Disadvantages

To date, a variety of transrectal NOSE techniques have been described by different authors (Table 21.1). There is heterogeneity among studies with regard to the number of operating ports, the use of rectal sleeves for extraction, and anastomotic technique (double stapled versus tripled stapled). The main advantage of the present technique is the extraction of a colonic specimen in a longitudinal way via a protected rectum. In contrast, in a specimen-retrieval pouch, the specimen will form into a ball by winding, which could hamper extraction. Although the current technique can be used in patients with the same clinical characteristics as those who had laparoscopic NOSE colectomy with a specimen retrieval pouch, it remains to be shown that it is appropriate for use in left-sided colonic disease [15]. Compared to conventional laparoscopic colectomy, one study failed to show any benefit from transrectal NOSE [17], while there was a significantly lower analgesic requirement in the transrectal NOSE colectomy groups in two other papers [13, 18]. Moreover, a significantly shorter operative time was observed when comparing transrectal NOSE colectomy with conventional laparoscopic colectomy [13]. Presumed advantages such as less postoperative pain and improved cosmetic outcome have also been evaluated [19, 20]. A single-blind randomized controlled trial showed a significant difference in morphine analogue requirements: 5% in the NOSE group versus 50% in the conventional group ($P = 0.003$) [19]. The strength of this study is that randomization was done during the operation as close to the time of the intervention as possible to reduce the chance that the allocated intervention would not have been delivered [21]. A case-matched study comparing conventional laparoscopic colectomy with laparoscopic NOSE colectomy could demonstrate better cosmetic outcome in the NOSE group [20]. Possible drawback of this technique is the intraperitoneal opening of both the colon and rectum, which could potentially increase infectious complications. Another disadvantage is that it cannot be implemented in the general population. Indeed, patient selection is key for this procedure. Factors limiting the applicability of this technique are patients with a BMI >35 kg/m^2 and a bulky mesocolon, large (voluminous) tumors >4 cm, the presence of a rectal stricture, and proximal diverticulosis. Because the colorectal anastomosis is created using a triple-stapling technique, diverticular disease present on the proximal colon could possibly lead to an anastomotic leak, due to inadvertent diverticulum cross stapling.

Difficulties and Complications

Laparoscopic NOSE colectomy for left-sided colonic disease involves transrectal specimen extraction. To protect the rectum and facilitate specimen extraction, several authors have reported different specimen extraction techniques. Specimen extraction without rectal protection is an option for benign disease, but this can be difficult, because the specimen can become blocked in the rectum, causing an obstruction [22, 23]. Moreover, there are no data on oncological safety regarding tumor extraction through an unprotected rectum. Most authors recommend rectal protection during specimen extraction, especially when resections are performed for malignant disease. This can be accomplished with a specimen retrieval pouch [13, 14, 24] or by inserting a rigid rectoscope [25, 26] normally used during transanal endoscopic microsurgery or a camera sleeve [17]. Insertion of a rigid rectoscope requires anal dilation, and the inner diameter of the rectoscope will determine the size of the retrieval specimen. Therefore, larger specimens should be extracted in a retrieval pouch, which is impermeable for fluids, thus minimizing the risk of tumor cell dissemination. We have used a specimen retrieval pouch for over 100 transrectal NOSE colectomies [16]. Although conversion rate was only 1%, specimen extraction can be difficult with large and voluminous specimens. We also evaluated the feasibility of longitudinal specimen extraction using a camera sleeve. This is the technique shown in the present chapter and that has become the technique of choice. Specimen extraction is either performed with a long laparoscopic grasper or a long sponge-holding forceps [15]. In the literature, other studies have shown equivalent results with regard to postoperative morbidity and length of hospital stay for laparoscopic NOSE colectomy (Table 21.1) [13, 14, 17, 18, 22–30]. Intraoperative complications include peritoneal spillage of stool, leading to bacterial contamination. However, one study showed polybacterial growth in all peritoneal culture samples, without any impact on incidence of infectious complications [23]. Moreover, in a series of over 100 laparoscopic NOSE colectomies, there were no wound infections, and incidence of nosocomial infections was only 4% [16]. Postoperatively, anastomotic leakage is the most feared complication, but the safety of a triple-stapled anastomosis was previously demonstrated. Intraluminal bleeding remains a concern and its incidence is around 4.5% [16]. If anastomotic bleeding occurs, it can be controlled by bedside flexible endoscopy, and it does not compromise patients' recovery.

Discussion

Conventional treatment for both benign and malignant left-sided colonic disease is via laparoscopic approach. Major disruptive change occurred when laparoscopic colectomy was first introduced in the early 1990s. Short-term benefits compared to open colorectal surgery immediately became clear. Randomized controlled trials have shown the same effectiveness, better short-term outcome, shorter length of hospital stay, less morbidity, higher pregnancy rate, and comparable oncological outcome when laparoscopic colectomy was compared with open colectomy [31–36]. However, when development of new surgical techniques aims to further minimize minimally invasive surgery, it is very difficult to prove any benefit from these new approaches. Reduction of access trauma surgery aims to avoid any abdominal wall incision >1 cm. Hence, alternatives must be searched to extract the specimen and to perform a safe bowel anastomosis. Technically, the leap from conventional laparoscopic colectomy to laparoscopic NOSE colectomy is substantial in comparison to the presumed benefit. Transrectal NOSE colectomy appears to be a valid option for specimen extraction and the creation of a colorectal anastomosis because of its applicability in both sexes and its frequent indications in left-sided colonic disease. Moreover, the straightness of the rectum and relatively easy access to the

Table 21.1 Studies reporting on NOSE colectomy with transrectal specimen extraction

Author, year	Type of study	No. of patients	Indication	No. of ports	Protection	Anastomosis	Duration of surgery	Morbidity (No., Dindo)	LOS (days)
Akamatsu et al., 2009	Case series	16	Malignant	4	None	TS	Mean 180 (137–257)	Wound infection (1, 1)	Mean 11 (8–14)
Cheung et al., 2009	Case series	10	Malignant	5	TEO	TS	Median 127.5 (105–170)	None	Median 7 (4–18)
Christoforidis et al., 2013	Case matched	11	Benign	4	Camera sleeve	TS	Median 200 (120–360)	Abscess (1, 3a), leakage (3b), and trocar hernia (3b)	Median 6 (4–33)
Costantino et al., 2012	Case matched	17	Benign	3	None	TS	Mean 122 (std 36.5)	Bleeding (1, 1), fever (2, 2), abscess (1, 2), leakage (1, 3b)	Mean 7.2 (std 4.9)
Franklin et al., 2013	Case series	277	Benign and malignant	4	Retrieval bag	TS	Mean 164.7 ± 47.5	Leakage (3, 3b)	Mean 6.9 ± 2.8
Fuchs et al., 2013	Case series	15	Benign	3	TEA	TS	Mean 131 (55–184)	Bleeding(1, 1), ileus(1, 2)	NA
Han et al., 2013	Case series	34	Malignant	5	TEM and bag	DS	Mean 151.6 (125–185)	Leakage (6, 3b)	Median 9 (7–66)
Leroy et al., 2011	Case series	16	Diverticulitis	3	None	TS	Mean 120.9 (std 41.9)	Epigastric pain (1, 1) and transient fever (3, 2)	Mean 6.1 (std 2.4)
Nishimura et al., 2011	Case series	16	Malignant	5	Wound retractor	DS	Mean 241 (188–309)	Leakage (1, 2)	Median 6 (4–16)
Saad et al., 2010	Case series	8	Benign and malignant	4	McCartney tube	TS	95–180	None	4–8 days
Wolthuis et al., 2011	Case matched	21	Endometriosis	4	Retrieval bag	TS	Median 90 (85–105)	UTI (1, 2)	Median 6 (5–7)
Wolthuis et al., 2011	Case series	21	Benign and malignant	4	Retrieval bag	TS	Median 105 (90–110)	Leakage (1, 3b)	Median 6 (5–7)

DS double stapled, *LOS* length of stay, *NA* not available, *No.* number, *std.* standard deviation, *TEA* transanal endoscopic applicator, *TEM* transanal endoscopic microsurgery, *TEO* transanal endoscopic operation, *TS* triple stapled, *UTI* urinary tract infection.

peritoneal cavity further contribute to the feasibility of the procedure. In addition to the abovementioned technical difficulties, the bacteriological impact on the peritoneal cavity secondary to intraoperative colo- and rectotomy with possible intracorporeal soiling might be a concern. Although an increased incidence of intraperitoneal abscesses was not demonstrated [18, 23], this complication has not yet been studied in a large prospective controlled study. It has been shown however that after NOSE colectomy, a higher inflammatory response was observed [37]. Intuitively, one would expect a higher CRP level and more positive cultures in a group of patients who underwent NOSE colectomy, because both colon and rectum are opened intracorporeally during this procedure. This leads to bacterial contamination of the peritoneal cavity, but its impact on clinical outcomes remains unclear.

Conclusion

A new era has dawned to further minimize access trauma and to explore new surgical strategies in bridging conventional laparoscopic surgery to pure human NOTES procedures. NOSE could be the next step in minimizing minimally invasive surgery. Although NOSE theoretically has the potential to improve outcome in laparoscopic colorectal surgery, its implementation in daily practice and its assumed benefits have yet to be studied in prospective controlled trials.

References

1. Kuhry E, Schwenk WF, Gaupset R, Romild U, Bonjer HJ. Long-term results of laparoscopic colorectal cancer resection. Cochrane Database Syst Rev. 2008;2:CD003432.
2. Schwenk W, Haase O, Neudecker J, Muller JM. Short term benefits for laparoscopic colorectal resection. Cochrane Database Syst Rev. 2005;3:CD003145.
3. Kehlet H. Fast-track colorectal surgery. Lancet. 2008;371:791–3.
4. Spanjersberg WR, Reurings J, Keus F, van Laarhoven CJ. Fast track surgery versus conventional recovery strategies for colorectal surgery. Cochrane Database Syst Rev. 2011;2:CD007635.
5. Vlug MS, Wind J, Hollmann MW, Ubbink DT, Cense HA, Engel AF, Gerhards MF, van Wagensveld BA, van der Zaag ES, van Geloven AA, Sprangers MA, Cuesta MA, Bemelman WA, Group Ls. Laparoscopy in combination with fast track multimodal management is the best perioperative strategy in patients undergoing colonic surgery: a randomized clinical trial (LAFA-study). Ann Surg. 2011;254:868–75.
6. Laurent C, Leblanc F, Bretagnol F, Capdepont M, Rullier E. Long-term wound advantages of the laparoscopic approach in rectal cancer. Br J Surg. 2008;95:903–8.
7. D'Hoore A, Wolthuis AM. Laparoscopic low anterior resection and transanal pull-through for low rectal cancer: a natural orifice specimen extraction (NOSE) technique. Color Dis. 2011;13(Suppl 7):28–31.
8. Darzi A, Super P, Guillou PJ, Monson JR. Laparoscopic sigmoid colectomy: total laparoscopic approach. Dis Colon Rectum. 1994;37:268–71.
9. Franklin ME, Diaz-E JA. Laparoscopic left hemicolectomy with transanal extraction of the specimen. In: Ballantyne GH, editor. Atlas of laparoscopic surgery. Philadelphia: W.B. Saunders; 2000. p. 386–404.

10. Franklin ME Jr, Ramos R, Rosenthal D, Schuessler W. Laparoscopic colonic procedures. World J Surg. 1993;17:51–6.
11. Palanivelu C, Rangarajan M, Jategaonkar PA, Anand NV. An innovative technique for colorectal specimen retrieval: a new era of "natural orifice specimen extraction" (N.O.S.E). Dis Colon Rectum. 2008;51:1120–4.
12. Wolthuis AM, Van Geluwe B, Fieuws S, Penninckx F, D'Hoore A. Laparoscopic sigmoid resection with transrectal specimen extraction: a systematic review. Color Dis. 2012;14:1183–8.
13. Wolthuis AM, Meuleman C, Tomassetti C, D'Hooghe T, Fieuws S, Penninckx F, D'Hoore A. Laparoscopic sigmoid resection with transrectal specimen extraction: a novel technique for the treatment of bowel endometriosis. Hum Reprod. 2011;26:1348–55.
14. Wolthuis AM, Penninckx F, D'Hoore A. Laparoscopic sigmoid resection with transrectal specimen extraction has a good short-term outcome. Surg Endosc. 2011;25:2034–8.
15. Wolthuis AM, De Buck Van Overstraeten A, D'Hoore A. Laparoscopic NOSE colectomy with a camera sleeve: a technique in evolution. Color Dis. 2015;17:O123–5.
16. Wolthuis AM, de Buck van Overstraeten A, Fieuws S, Boon K, D'Hoore A. Standardized laparoscopic NOSE-colectomy is feasible with low morbidity. Surg Endosc. 2014;29:1167–73.
17. Christoforidis D, Clerc D, Demartines N. Transrectal specimen extraction after laparoscopic left colectomy: a case-matched study. Color Dis. 2013;15:347–53.
18. Costantino FA, Diana M, Wall J, Leroy J, Mutter D, Marescaux J. Prospective evaluation of peritoneal fluid contamination following transabdominal vs. transanal specimen extraction in laparoscopic left-sided colorectal resections. Surg Endosc. 2012;26:1495–500.
19. Wolthuis AM, Fieuws S, Van Den Bosch A, de Buck van Overstraeten A, D'Hoore A. Randomized clinical trial of laparoscopic colectomy with or without natural-orifice specimen extraction. Br J Surg. 2015;102:630–7.
20. Wolthuis AM, Meuleman C, Tomassetti C, D'Hooghe T, Fieuws S, de Buck van Overstraeten A, D'Hoore A. How do patients score cosmesis after laparoscopic natural orifice specimen extraction colectomy? Color Dis. 2015;17:536–41.
21. Pocock S. Methods of randomisation. In: Clinical trials: a practical approach. New York: Wiley; 1983. p. 66–90.
22. Akamatsu H, Omori T, Oyama T, Tori M, Ueshima S, Nakahara M, Abe T, Nishida T. Totally laparoscopic sigmoid colectomy: a simple and safe technique for intracorporeal anastomosis. Surg Endosc. 2009;23:2605–9.
23. Leroy J, Costantino F, Cahill RA, D'Agostino J, Morales A, Mutter D, Marescaux J. Laparoscopic resection with transanal specimen extraction for sigmoid diverticulitis. Br J Surg. 2011;98:1327–34.
24. Franklin ME Jr, Liang S, Russek K. Natural orifice specimen extraction in laparoscopic colorectal surgery: transanal and transvaginal approaches. Tech Coloproctol. 2013;17(Suppl 1):S63–7.
25. Cheung HY, Leung AL, Chung CC, Ng DC, Li MK. Endo-laparoscopic colectomy without mini-laparotomy for left-sided colonic tumors. World J Surg. 2009;33:1287–91.
26. Han Y, He YG, Zhang HB, Lv KZ, Zhang YJ, Lin MB, Yin L. Total laparoscopic sigmoid and rectal surgery in combination with transanal endoscopic microsurgery: a preliminary evaluation in China. Surg Endosc. 2013;27:518–24.
27. Fuchs KH, Breithaupt W, Varga G, Schulz T, Reinisch A, Josipovic N. Transanal hybrid colon resection: from laparoscopy to NOTES. Surg Endosc. 2013;27:746–52.
28. Leung AL, Cheung HY, Fok BK, Chung CC, Li MK, Tang CN. Prospective randomized trial of hybrid NOTES colectomy versus conventional laparoscopic colectomy for left-sided colonic tumors. World J Surg. 2013;37:2678–82.
29. Nishimura A, Kawahara M, Suda K, Makino S, Kawachi Y, Nikkuni K. Totally laparoscopic sigmoid colectomy with transanal specimen extraction. Surg Endosc. 2011;25:3459–63.
30. Saad S, Hosogi H. Natural orifice specimen extraction for avoiding laparotomy in laparoscopic left colon resections: a new approach using the McCartney tube and the tilt top anvil technique. J Laparoendosc Adv Surg Tech A. 2010;20:689–92.
31. Darai E, Dubernard G, Coutant C, Frey C, Rouzier R, Ballester M. Randomized trial of laparoscopically assisted versus open colorectal resection for endometriosis: morbidity, symptoms, quality of life, and fertility. Ann Surg. 2010;251:1018–23.

32. Fleshman J, Sargent DJ, Green E, Anvari M, Stryker SJ, Beart RW Jr, Hellinger M, Flanagan R Jr, Peters W, Nelson H, Clinical Outcomes of Surgical Therapy Study Group. Laparoscopic colectomy for cancer is not inferior to open surgery based on 5-year data from the COST study group trial. Ann Surg. 2007;246:655–62. discussion 662–654
33. Guillou PJ, Quirke P, Thorpe H, Walker J, Jayne DG, Smith AM, Heath RM, Brown JM, Group MCt. Short-term endpoints of conventional versus laparoscopic-assisted surgery in patients with colorectal cancer (MRC CLASICC trial): multicentre, randomised controlled trial. Lancet. 2005;365:1718–26.
34. Jayne DG, Thorpe HC, Copeland J, Quirke P, Brown JM, Guillou PJ. Five-year follow-up of the Medical Research Council CLASICC trial of laparoscopically assisted versus open surgery for colorectal cancer. Br J Surg. 2010;97:1638–45.
35. Lacy AM, Garcia-Valdecasas JC, Delgado S, Castells A, Taura P, Pique JM, Visa J. Laparoscopy-assisted colectomy versus open colectomy for treatment of non-metastatic colon cancer: a randomised trial. Lancet. 2002;359:2224–9.
36. van der Pas MH, Haglind E, Cuesta MA, Furst A, Lacy AM, Hop WC, Bonjer HJ, Group COcLoORIS. Laparoscopic versus open surgery for rectal cancer (COLOR II): short-term outcomes of a randomised, phase 3 trial. Lancet Oncol. 2013;14:210–8.
37. Wolthuis AM. New strategies to improve outcome after colorectal surgery. PhD thesis. Katholieke Universiteit Leuven, Leuven. 2015.

Part VI

Parastomal Hernia

Parastomal Hernia: An Ounce of Prevention

22

Kristina L. Guyton and Neil H. Hyman

Abbreviations

APCM	Acellular porcine collagen matrix
CT	Computed tomography
DLI	Diverting loop ileostomy
EC	End colostomy
EI	End ileostomy
Lap	Laparoscopic
PD	Polydioxanone
PG	Poliglecaprone
PP	Polypropylene
PSH	Parastomal hernia
PTFE	Polytetrafluoroethylene
PVDF	Polyvinylidene fluoride
US	Ultrasound

Introduction

Parastomal hernia (PSH) is generally a late but unfortunately common consequence following the creation of an intestinal stoma. Though many patients with parastomal hernias are asymptomatic, complications from a PSH can be life threatening. Symptomatic patients may present with a wide range of symptoms, including abdominal pain, cramping, difficulty with appliance seating, obstructive symptoms, and hernia strangulation [1]. Parastomal hernia negatively impacts patient psychological

K.L. Guyton • N.H. Hyman (✉)
Department of Surgery, The University of Chicago Hospitals, Chicago, IL, USA
e-mail: kristina.guyton@uchospitals.edu; nhyman@surgery.bsd.uchicago.edu

C.M. Schlachta, P. Sylla (eds.), *Current Common Dilemmas in Colorectal Surgery*,
https://doi.org/10.1007/978-3-319-70117-2_22

well-being and quality of life and increases healthcare utilization [1, 2]. Numerous methods of PSH repair have been proposed and practiced, but the results have been historically quite poor, with recurrence seen in over 50% of patients after suture repair or resiting and in 10–30% of patients after mesh repair [3]. In light of the high recurrence rates after repair, increased focus has been placed on preventative measures.

Definition

There is no universally accepted definition for parastomal hernia [3]. Broadly, a PSH is an incisional hernia at, or immediately adjacent to, a stoma. PSH are classically detectable on physical examination as a parastomal bulge which may be accentuated by a Valsalva maneuver. CT imaging may identify smaller parastomal hernias not detected on exam. Classification of PSH based on CT findings includes type I (hernia sac containing stoma loop), type II (hernia sac containing omentum), and type III (hernia sac containing a loop other than the stoma) parastomal hernias [4].

Incidence

Parastomal hernias occur in as many as 78% of patients with a stoma [3]. Typically a late complication of stoma creation, PSH frequently occurs within the first 2 years after surgery but may occur as late as 30 years from the index operation. It has been suggested that a parastomal hernia may be an inevitable consequence of stoma creation, given enough time to develop. The marked heterogeneity in reported incidence can be explained by varied definitions, methods of detection, and length of follow-up [3]. Some studies define hernias based on patient symptoms alone, some include palpation on physical exam, and others add identification on imaging studies in asymptomatic patients. The incidence may be underestimated by studies with a 1–2-year follow-up, failing to capture late PSH occurrence. Retrospective studies suggest that stoma type impacts the incidence of parastomal hernia occurrence, end colostomy having the highest incidence (Table 22.1) [1, 3, 5–7].

Table 22.1 Parastomal hernia incidence by stoma type [1, 3, 5–7]

Stoma type	Incidence
End colostomy	4–57% [1, 5], 13.3–17.8% [6, 7]
Extraperitoneal end colostomy	6.4% [6, 7]
Loop colostomy	0–30.8% [5]
End ileostomy	1.8–28.3% [5]
Loop ileostomy	0–6.2% [5]
Urostomy	5–28% [3], 17% [36]

Impact of Parastomal Hernias on Patients

While many patients with PSH are asymptomatic, those who are symptomatic may present with peristomal bulging, abdominal pain, cramping, distension, diarrhea, ostomy appliance leakage and subsequent dermatitis, obstructive symptoms, hernia strangulation, or life-threatening sepsis from bowel perforation or necrosis [1, 3]. Stoma creation and abdominal wall hernia have separately been shown to be predictors of decreased quality of life. In a study of patients with parastomal hernias, van Dijk et al. found that the presence of a PSH significantly decreased reported quality of life and that a higher proportion of patients felt ashamed of their scars compared to those with a colostomy without herniation [1].

Risk Factors

Numerous risk factors have been proposed to contribute to PSH development. Decreased tissue strength, poor wound healing, increased intra-abdominal pressure, immunosuppression, and infection are common characteristics among the risk factors that have been identified (Table 22.2) [3, 8].

Table 22.2 Patient risk factors for subsequent parastomal hernia development [3, 8]

Risk factors	Impact on healing
Age	Decreased tissue strength
Connective tissue disorder	
Poor nutritional status	
Diabetes mellitus	
Prior abdominal wall surgeries	
Smoking status	Poor wound healing
Corticosteroid use	
Poor nutritional status	
Diabetes mellitus	
Elevated BMI/waist circumference	Increased intra-abdominal pressure
Respiratory comorbidity	
Chronic cough	
Constipation	
Benign prostatic hypertrophy	
Ascites	
Emergency surgery	Infection
Postoperative wound infection	
Corticosteroid use	

Recurrence After Repair is High

Repair of parastomal hernias is a challenging surgical problem that will be addressed in the subsequent chapter. Simple fascial repair and stoma translocation both have high rates of hernia recurrence. Synthetic and biologic mesh repairs are associated with decreased hernia recurrence rates, ranging from 6.9% to 30%, depending on mesh and technique [3, 9]. Laparoscopic techniques offer a less invasive alternative to open repair of parastomal hernia repair and may have lower rates of recurrent herniation [10, 11]. The high incidence, potentially debilitating symptoms, and suboptimal outcomes associated with repair of these defects have led to increased interest in measures to prevent initial parastomal hernia occurrence.

Parastomal Hernia Prevention

Stoma construction requires creation of a fascial defect and therefore provides the opportunity for herniation of additional abdominal contents. In fact, one might argue that simply having an intestinal stoma represents a "hernia" as there is a surgically created abdominal wall defect with a loop of bowel protruding through it. Holes tend to get bigger, and over time and as ostomates age and stress their abdominal walls, the requisite abdominal defect tends to enlarge. Early stoma reversal, which may be an underutilized safe practice [12], is by far the most effective method of hernia prevention. However, for those patients who require permanent ostomies, practices to reduce hernia formation are highly desirable.

Stoma Placement

Traditional teaching includes placing the stoma through the rectus muscle and a flat segment of abdominal wall that is 5 cm away from bony prominences, the umbilicus, prior surgical scars, and skinfolds. Often this is at the site of the infraumbilical bulge; however, obese patients with a large pannus may need placement in the thinner upper abdominal wall to facilitate self-care and prevent retraction [13, 14]. While often presented as dogma, the evidence for many of our common practices is often quite scant. For example, the evidence for the standard practice of maturing a stoma through the rectus abdominis muscle instead of lateral to it is supported by a small observational study [15]. Interestingly, other studies have not replicated this finding, and a 2013 Cochrane review concluded that there was no statistically significant difference in rates of parastomal herniation or stomal prolapse between the two techniques [8, 16]. Nonetheless, the site of ostomy placement is important both for stoma function and ease of use for the patient. Retrospective analyses have demonstrated that preoperative siting and education by an enterostomal therapist are unequivocally beneficial in reducing stoma-related complications and improving postoperative quality of life and independence [13, 14].

Stoma Creation Technique

In addition to external stoma location, surgeons have investigated different ways of bringing the intestine through the abdominal wall. Goligher and Stames first reported extraperitoneal stoma formation in 1958 [3, 17]. This technique involves tunneling the bowel outside the parietal peritoneum prior to bringing it through the abdominal wall (Fig. 22.1a). Several studies have reported that this technique decreases the risk of PSH, but thus far no randomized trials have demonstrated superiority [6, 7]. This technique requires additional time and expertise and tends to increase bowel angulation and may be difficult using a laparoscopic approach [8].

During stoma creation, a fascial defect, known as a trephine, is created just large enough to allow passage of the bowel and its mesentery, but not so large as to enable bowel herniation. The ideal aperture size is often described as less than 25 mm. Most surgeons are taught that the trephine should be large enough to allow entry of

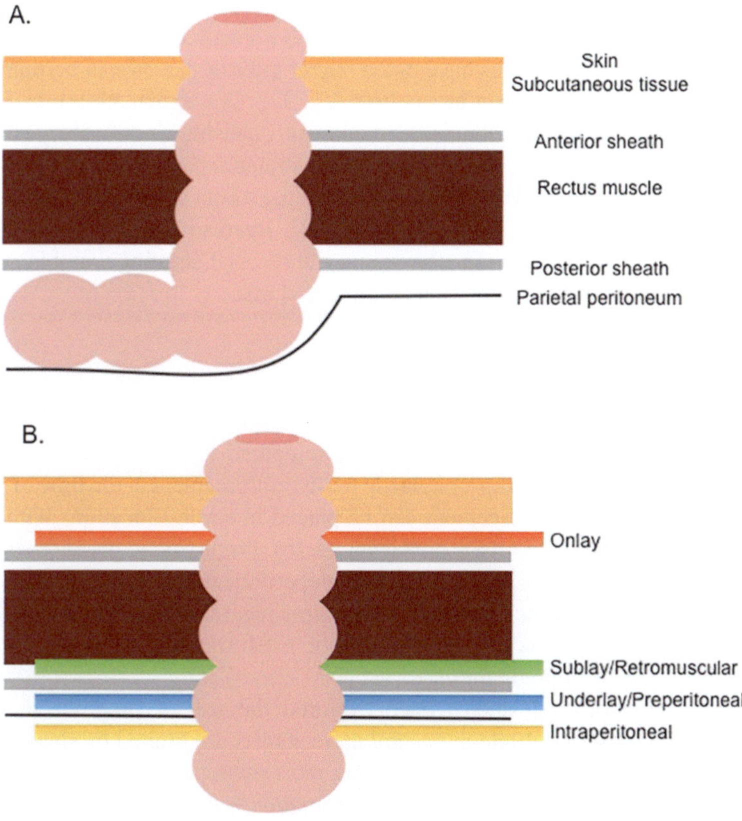

Fig. 22.1 Prophylactic measures to prevent parastomal herniation: extraperitoneal tunneling and prophylactic mesh. (**a**) The bowel may be tunneled extraperitoneally prior to traversing the abdominal wall. (**b**) Prophylactic mesh may be placed between various layers of the abdominal wall to reinforce the fascial layers and prevent enlargement of the abdominal wall defect

two of the surgeon's fingers. However, this principle will result in significant variation based on surgeon hand size, with a 35 mm trephine created by a surgeon who wears glove size 7.5 [8]. One study demonstrated that for every millimeter increase in the aperture diameter, the potential herniation risk increased by 10% [18]. Devices have been developed to accurately size the aperture during surgery, but have not been tested in a randomized manner [8].

Several other common techniques intended to reduce hernia formation have been passed on as good surgical practice without definitive level 1 evidence of efficacy. Placement of the ostomy below the arcuate line of Douglas may increase rates of parastomal herniation [19]. Many surgeons sew the bowel mesentery to the peritoneum with the intent of fixing it in place [5]. Others endorse spreading the muscle fibers bluntly as opposed to cutting through muscle when creating the tunnel for the stoma. The depth and surgical management of the subcutaneous tissue may also play a role in hernia formation [20].

Increasing use of laparoscopy in colorectal procedures offers advantages and disadvantages for stoma creation. Laparoscopy allows for confirmation of bowel and mesenteric orientation after fascial closure and immediately prior to stoma maturation. However, some studies have noted higher rates of parastomal herniation in laparoscopic compared to open procedures [21, 22]. One explanation may be the use of the stoma site as the specimen extraction site, causing an obligatory enlargement of the fascial defect. Another study demonstrated a parastomal hernia rate of 10.1% when the specimen was extracted through the stoma site as opposed to 4.2% when extracted through a separate incision [23]. Interestingly, there was not an increased rate of recurrent hernia after stoma site reversal, arguing that this may be a reasonable option in the setting of a temporary stoma.

Use of Foreign Body Reinforcement

Increased efficacy of PSH repair with mesh compared to primary repair led surgeons to investigate the use of prophylactic mesh reinforcement at the time of initial stoma creation. Mesh reinforcement can be placed in several locations within the abdominal wall surrounding the stoma (Fig. 22.1b). Prophylactic parastomal mesh is most frequently placed in the sublay and preperitoneal locations. Initial studies were performed with synthetic mesh [3]. Concerns regarding the risk of bowel wall erosion and delayed obstruction due to synthetic mesh shrinkage have led to investigation of the use of biologic mesh.

Numerous randomized studies have explored the use of prophylactic mesh (Table 22.3) [20, 24–32]. While in general these studies are limited by small patient numbers and various mesh types and locations, most support the safety of prophylactic mesh and suggest decreased rates of PSH formation with placement of prophylactic mesh, at least with permanent materials [3, 33, 34]. A large multicenter randomized trial suggested no benefit with the use of biologic mesh [22]. Prophylactic parastomal mesh may be cost-effective for patients who undergo permanent end colostomy creation by decreasing subsequent healthcare utilization [2]. Multiple studies are

Table 22.3 Randomized controlled trials in prophylactic parastomal mesh placement [20, 24–32]

Trial	Study size	Approach, stoma type	Mesh type, fixation method, and position	Follow-up (months)	Rate of PSH: mesh vs. control	Reoperation for PSH: mesh vs. control
Brandsma et al., 2016	150	Open EC	PP, absorbable sutures, sublay	12[a]	Clinical (CT confirmation): 24 vs. 4.5%	0/72 vs. 0/78
López-Cano et al., 2016	52	Lap EC	PP/PD/PG, tacks, intraperitoneal onlay	26[a]	CT: 25 vs. 64%	1/24 vs. 0/28
Vierimaa et al., 2015	70	Lap EC	PP/PVDF, tacks, intraperitoneal onlay	12[b]	CT: 51 vs. 53% Clinical: 14 vs. 32%	0/35 vs. 1/32
Lambrecht et al., 2015	58	Open EC	PP, absorbable sutures, sublay	40[a]	Clinical: 6 vs. 46%	Not reported
Fleshman et al., 2014	113	Mixed EC and EI	APCM, no fixation, sublay	24[b]	Clinical: 12 vs.13%	3/55 vs. 6/58
López-Cano et al., 2012	36	Lap EC	PD/PP, tacks, intraperitoneal onlay	10.4[a]	CT: 50 vs. 93%	1/18 vs. 3/16
Serra-Aracil et al., 2009	55	Open EC	PG/PP, absorbable sutures, sublay	29[a]	CT/US: 22 vs. 44% Clinical: 14 vs. 40%	Not reported
Hammond et al., 2008	20	Open DLI	APCM, Prolene sutures, preperitoneal	6.5[a]	Clinical/US: 0 vs. 30%	None
Jänes et al., 2004, 2009	54	Open EC	Polyglactin/PP, absorbable sutures, sublay	12[b] 60[b]	Clinical: 0 vs. 44% Clinical: 13 vs. 81%	Not reported 0/15 vs. 5/21

EC end colostomy, *EI* end ileostomy, *DLI* diverting loop ileostomy, *Lap* laparoscopic, *PTFE* polytetrafluoroethylene, *PP* polypropylene, *PVDF* polyvinylidene fluoride, *PG* poliglecaprone, *PD* polydioxanone, *US* ultrasound, *CT* computed tomography, *APCM* acellular porcine collagen matrix

[a]Median

[b]Mean

ongoing to more robustly test various prophylactic mesh designs and surgical techniques to optimize hernia prevention.

Evaluation by CT scan is often utilized as a more sensitive indicator of hernia presence than clinical exam; however, one study demonstrated poor correlation between CT findings and hernia detection on clinical exam [26]. The rate and course of progression from an asymptomatic CT-detected hernia to clinically significant hernia are poorly understood. Use of CT scan has demonstrated that prophylactic parastomal mesh decreases the gradual fascial defect enlargement over time [26].

Despite increasing evidence for the efficacy of prophylactic mesh in preventing or delaying the progression to PSH, use of prophylactic mesh has been slow to be incorporated into widespread practice presumably related to concerns about mesh erosion. In a 2014 email survey, only 17% of authors recently contributing to colorectal journals reported using or observing the use of prophylactic mesh during the most recent elective permanent colostomy at which they had been present [35]. While 43% would consider the use of prophylactic mesh when creating an emergency end colostomy for which the patient was unlikely to undergo reversal, 73% stated they personally would not choose to use prophylactic mesh.

Conclusions

Parastomal hernia remains a persistent problem for colorectal patients. While many patients with parastomal hernias are asymptomatic, the development of a symptomatic PSH significantly impacts patient quality of life and puts patients at risk for major surgical complications. Methods of repair have improved, but recurrence rates remain around 20% with mesh [3]. By far, the most effective method of PSH prevention is the avoidance of stoma creation entirely or the early reversal of temporary stomas. The decrease in recurrence after PSH repair with mesh prompted an interest in utilizing similar mesh techniques for PSH prevention, especially when creating permanent stomas. Prophylactic mesh appears to reduce the incidence of radiologically detected and clinically detected parastomal hernias. The optimal mesh types and position within the abdominal wall have not yet been determined, and studies are currently underway testing a variety of methods. Although surgeons remain skeptical and this technique is not yet practiced extensively, increasing evidence supports use of prophylactic mesh to prevent parastomal herniation.

References

1. van Dijk SM, Timmermans L, Deerenberg EB, Lamme B, Kleinrensink G-J, Jeekel J, et al. Parastomal hernia: impact on quality of life? World J Surg. 2015;39(10):2595–601.
2. Lee L, Saleem A, Landry T, Latimer E, Chaudhury P, Feldman LS. Cost effectiveness of mesh prophylaxis to prevent parastomal hernia in patients undergoing permanent colostomy for rectal cancer. J Am Coll Surg. 2014;218(1):82–91.
3. Aquina CT, Iannuzzi JC, Probst CP, Kelly KN, Noyes K, Fleming FJ, et al. Parastomal hernia: a growing problem with new solutions. Dig Surg. 2014;31(4-5):366–76.

4. Moreno-Matias J, Serra-Aracil X, Darnell-Martin A, Bombardo-Junca J, Mora-Lopez L, Alcantara-Moral M, et al. The prevalence of parastomal hernia after formation of an end colostomy. A new clinico-radiological classification. Color Dis. 2009;11(2):173–7.
5. Carne PWG, Robertson GM, Frizelle FA. Parastomal hernia. Br J Surg. 2003;90(7):784–93.
6. Lian L, Wu X-R, He X-S, Zou Y-F, Wu X-J, Lan P, et al. Extraperitoneal vs. intraperitoneal route for permanent colostomy: a meta-analysis of 1,071 patients. Int J Color Dis. 2012;27(1):59–64.
7. Kroese LF, de Smet GHJ, Jeekel J, Kleinrensink G-J, Lange JF. Systematic review and meta-analysis of extraperitoneal versus transperitoneal colostomy for preventing parastomal hernia. Dis Colon Rectum. 2016;59(7):688–95.
8. Hotouras A, Murphy J, Thaha M, Chan CL. The persistent challenge of parastomal herniation: a review of the literature and future developments. Color Dis. 2013;15(5):e202–14.
9. Hansson BME, Slater NJ, van der Velden AS, Groenewoud HMM, Buyne OR, de Hingh IHJT, et al. Surgical techniques for parastomal hernia repair: a systematic review of the literature. Ann Surg. 2012;255(4):685–95.
10. DeAsis FJ, Lapin B, Gitelis ME, Ujiki MB. Current state of laparoscopic parastomal hernia repair: a meta-analysis. World J Gastroenterol. 2015;21(28):8670–7.
11. DeAsis FJ, Linn JG, Lapin B, Denham W, Carbray JM, Ujiki MB. Modified laparoscopic Sugarbaker repair decreases recurrence rates of parastomal hernia. Surgery. 2015;158(4):954–9.
12. Danielsen AK, Park J, Jansen JE, Bock D, Skullman S, Wedin A, et al. Early closure of a temporary ileostomy in patients with rectal cancer: a multicenter randomized controlled trial. Ann Surg. 2016;265:284.
13. Person B, Ifargan R, Lachter J, Duek SD, Kluger Y, Assalia A. The impact of preoperative stoma site marking on the incidence of complications, quality of life, and patient's independence. Dis Colon Rectum. 2012;55(7):783–7.
14. Bass EM, Del Pino A, Tan A, Pearl RK, Orsay CP, Abcarian H. Does preoperative stoma marking and education by the enterostomal therapist affect outcome? Dis Colon Rectum. 1997;40(4):440–2.
15. Sjödahl R, Anderberg B, Bolin T. Parastomal hernia in relation to site of the abdominal stoma. Br J Surg. 1988;75(4):339–41.
16. Hardt J, Meerpohl JJ, Metzendorf M-I, Kienle P, Post S, Herrle F. Lateral pararectal versus transrectal stoma placement for prevention of parastomal herniation. Cochrane Database Syst Rev. 2013;11:CD009487.
17. Goligher JC. Extraperitoneal colostomy or ileostomy. Br J Surg. 1958;46(196):97–103.
18. Pilgrim CHC, McIntyre R, Bailey M. Prospective audit of parastomal hernia: prevalence and associated comorbidities. Dis Colon Rectum. 2010;53(1):71–6.
19. Al-Momani H, Miller C, Stephenson BM. Stoma siting and the "arcuate line" of Douglas: might it be of relevance to later herniation? Color Dis. 2014;16(2):141–3.
20. López-Cano M, Lozoya-Trujillo R, Quiroga S, Sánchez JL, Vallribera F, Martí M, et al. Use of a prosthetic mesh to prevent parastomal hernia during laparoscopic abdominoperineal resection: a randomized controlled trial. Hernia. 2012;16(6):661–7.
21. Randall J, Lord B, Fulham J, Soin B. Parastomal hernias as the predominant stoma complication after laparoscopic colorectal surgery. Surg Laparosc Endosc Percutan Tech. 2012;22(5):420–3.
22. Mishra A, Keeler BD, Maxwell-Armstrong C, Simpson JA, Acheson AG. The influence of laparoscopy on incisional hernia rates: a retrospective analysis of 1057 colorectal cancer resections. Color Dis. 2014;16(10):815–21.
23. Li W, Benlice C, Stocchi L, Kessler H, Gorgun E, Costedio M. Does stoma site specimen extraction increase postoperative ileostomy complication rates? Surg Endosc. 2017;31:3552.
24. López-Cano M, Serra-Aracil X, Mora L, Sánchez-García JL, Jiménez-Gómez LM, Martí M, et al. Preventing parastomal hernia using a modified Sugarbaker technique with composite mesh during laparoscopic abdominoperineal resection: a randomized controlled trial. Ann Surg. 2016;264:923.
25. Vierimaa M, Klintrup K, Biancari F, Victorzon M, Carpelan-Holmström M, Kössi J, et al. Prospective, randomized study on the use of a prosthetic mesh for prevention of parastomal hernia of permanent colostomy. Dis Colon Rectum. 2015;58(10):943–9.

26. Lambrecht JR, Larsen SG, Reiertsen O, Vaktskjold A, Julsrud L, Flatmark K. Prophylactic mesh at end-colostomy construction reduces parastomal hernia rate: a randomized trial. Color Dis. 2015;17(10):O191–7.
27. Fleshman JW, Beck DE, Hyman N, Wexner SD, Bauer J, George V, et al. A prospective, multicenter, randomized, controlled study of non-cross-linked porcine acellular dermal matrix fascial sublay for parastomal reinforcement in patients undergoing surgery for permanent abdominal wall ostomies. Dis Colon Rectum. 2014;57(5):623–31.
28. Serra-Aracil X, Bombardo-Junca J, Moreno-Matias J, Darnell A, Mora-Lopez L, Alcantara-Moral M, et al. Randomized, controlled, prospective trial of the use of a mesh to prevent parastomal hernia. Ann Surg. 2009;249(4):583–7.
29. Hammond TM, Huang A, Prosser K, Frye JN, Williams NS. Parastomal hernia prevention using a novel collagen implant: a randomised controlled phase 1 study. Hernia. 2008;12(5):475–81.
30. Jänes A, Cengiz Y, Israelsson LA. Randomized clinical trial of the use of a prosthetic mesh to prevent parastomal hernia. Br J Surg. 2004;91(3):280–2.
31. Jänes A, Cengiz Y, Israelsson LA. Preventing parastomal hernia with a prosthetic mesh: a 5-year follow-up of a randomized study. World J Surg. 2009;33(1):118–21.
32. Brandsma H-T, Hansson BME, Aufenacker TJ, van Geldere D, Lammeren FMV, Mahabier C, et al. Prophylactic mesh placement during formation of an end-colostomy reduces the rate of parastomal hernia: short-term results of the Dutch PREVENT-trial. Ann Surg. 2017;265:663.
33. Cornille JB, Pathak S, Daniels IR, Smart NJ. Prophylactic mesh use during primary stoma formation to prevent parastomal hernia. Ann R Coll Surg Engl. 2017;99:2–11.
34. Wang S, Wang W, Zhu B, Song G, Jiang C. Efficacy of prophylactic mesh in end-colostomy construction: a systematic review and meta-analysis of randomized controlled trials. World J Surg. 2016;40:2528.
35. Parkinson F, Dafydd L, Singh R, Wood S, Williams GL, Stephenson BM. Preventing parastomal herniation in 2014 and beyond. Color Dis. 2014;16(5):390.
36. Narang SK, Alam NN, Campain NJ, Pathak S, McGrath JS, Daniels IR, et al. Parastomal hernia following cystectomy and ileal conduit urinary diversion: a systematic review. Hernia. 2017;21:163.

Parastomal Hernia: Optimal Strategies for Repair

23

Birgitta M.E. Hansson

Introduction

A parastomal hernia is an incisional hernia related to the stoma site. It is the most frequent complication after stoma formation; 50% of all patients with a stoma develop a symptomatic parastomal hernia over time [1–3]. Parastomal hernias are observed in all types of stomas. However, patients with a colostomy are most likely to develop a parastomal hernia [4, 5]. Symptoms may range from mild abdominal discomfort to severe abdominal pain due to stretching of the abdominal wall. Patients may suffer from a poor fitting stoma appliance resulting in leakage and subsequent skin problems. Moreover, life-threatening complications may occur in case of obstruction or strangulation. Bulging around the stoma can also cause cosmetic complains and impair the quality of life of the patient.

Diagnosis

Physical examination with the patient in upright position performing a Valsalva manoeuvre is often sufficient to diagnose a parastomal hernia. When in doubt, additional radiological imaging can be performed. A CT scan with oral contrast and Valsalva manoeuvre or a CT scan in prone position can reveal the diagnosis [6]. Ultrasonography is a good alternative, especially in experienced hands [7]. Once diagnosed, the hernia can be classified according to the EHS classification system [8].

In this system, the parastomal hernia size and the presence of a concomitant incisional hernia matter (Table 23.1).

B.M.E. Hansson (✉)
Department of Surgery, Canisius-Wilhelmina Hospital Nijmegen, Nijmegen, The Netherlands
e-mail: b.hansson@cwz.nl

C.M. Schlachta, P. Sylla (eds.), *Current Common Dilemmas in Colorectal Surgery*,
https://doi.org/10.1007/978-3-319-70117-2_23

Table 23.1 EHS classification

			Primary	Recurrent
EHS parastomal hernia classification		Largest size of hernia defect	Small ≤5 cm	Large >5 cm
Concomitant incisional hernia?	No		I	III
	Yes		II	IV

The use of a classifications system is encouraged by the European Hernia Society in order to report and compare surgical outcome [9].

Treatment

Conservative Treatment

When a patient is asymptomatic, a wait-and-see policy can be sufficient. In case of obesity, advise the patient to lose weight. When a patient is symptomatic, his or her complaints should be analysed carefully [10]. If the main complaint is leakage, advice from the stoma care therapist can be crucial. A slight change is stoma care can be sufficient to solve the problem, and surgery can be postponed or even cancelled (e.g. using convex appliances, wearing a stoma belt, stoma irrigation). A parastomal hernia bandage can be useful to reduce the pain from the stretched abdominal wall and give comfort and support to the patient. Nevertheless, conservative treatments will not treat the hernia itself and only relieve hernia-related symptoms.

Surgical Treatment

When conservative treatment fails, surgery will be the next step. Prior to surgery it is advised to perform a CT scan. A CT scan can diagnose concomitant incisional hernias, and the size of the hernia can be measured precisely. One can classify the patient according to the EHS classification system [8, 9]. Moreover, recurrent malignancy must be ruled out. This is important because recurrent malignancy or a concomitant incisional hernia can alter your surgical strategy. Various surgical techniques to repair a parastomal hernia have been described in the literature [11]. Which surgical technique to use depends on patient-related factors and surgeon-related factors, the so-called tailored surgery. One by one, the most important techniques will be described, and advice will be given on when to use or not use this technique.

Local Suture Repair

A peristomal incision is made, the hernia contents are reduced, and the fascia is closed with sutures (Fig. 23.1). Reviewing the literature shows a recurrence rate of 70% (Table 23.2). Therefore, the advice is not to use this technique anymore [11].

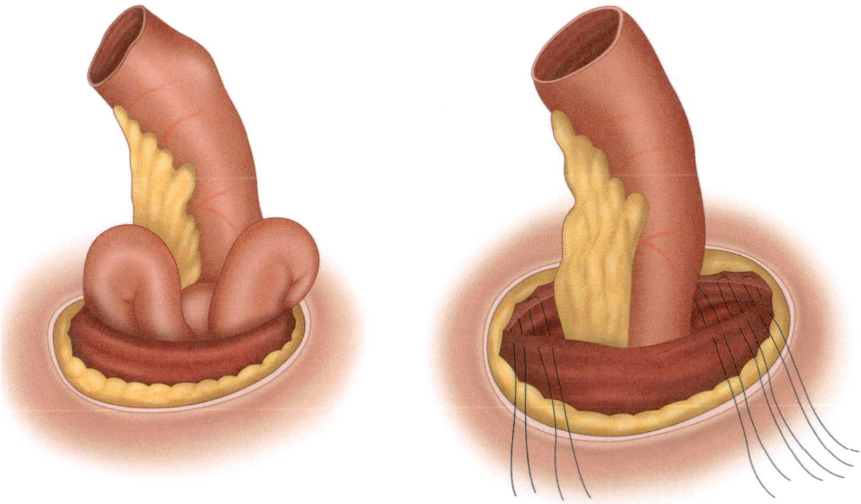

Fig. 23.1 Local suture repair

Local Repair With Mesh

Rosin and Bonardi were the first to report on this technique in 1977 [12]. After peristomal incision and closure of the fascia, the abdominal wall is reinforced by a synthetic mesh (Fig. 23.2). Review of the literature shown in Table 23.3 shows a recurrence rate of 17.2% after a follow-up of 2 years and a mesh infection rate of 2.6% (Table 23.3) [11]. This technique may be indicated in patients who are not fit for laparotomy or laparoscopy.

Laparoscopic Repair

The laparoscopic approach is associated with minimal additional damage to the abdominal wall, an abdominal wall that is already at risk for herniation. Another potential benefit is a superior view of the defect allowing a more precise repair. Moreover, concomitant incisional hernias can be detected and repaired at the same time [13]. The disadvantage of laparoscopy is the learning curve, especially the adhesiolysis and reduction of the hernia content. This may lead to iatrogenic bowel injury and severe complications [13, 14]. There are three different ways to reinforce the abdominal wall with a mesh and thus repair the hernia. With the keyhole technique, a mesh with a hole is used (Fig. 23.3). The Sugarbaker technique uses a mesh without a hole (Fig. 23.4), whereas the Sandwich technique uses two meshes [15–17].

Reviewing the literature on the Keyhole technique revealed a high recurrence rate (34%) [10].

When operating on patients with a recurrence, the mesh was everted, and the central opening of the mesh was enlarged leading to recurrence [23]. This can be

Table 23.2 Study characteristics and outcomes of suture repair of parastomal hernia

Reference	Time period	Mod. MINORS index	No. repairs	Type of stoma	Type of sutures	No. complications (%)		Mortality	Recurrence (%)[a]	Follow-up[b]
						Infection	Other			
Rubin et al. [10]	1983–1991	10	36	EC, LC, EI	>85% nonabsorbable	5	2	0	29 (80.6)	31
Cheung et al. [11]	1990–1999	11	16	EC, LC	Nonabsorbable	0	5	3	6 (46.2)	38
Rieger et al. [12]	1990–2002	10	14	EC, El, LI, LC	NS	4	3	1	7 (53.8)	7[b]
Riansuwan et al. [13]	1999–2005	11	27	10 C, 17 IC	Nonabsorbable	2	0	0	20 (74.1)	23
Pastor et al. [14]	1999–2006	11	13	9 C, 4 IC	91% nonabsorbable	NS	NS	0	7 (53.8)	14
Weighted pooled % (95% CI)	–		106	–	–	11.8% (6.1–20.2)	10.8% (5.3–18.9)	3.8% (1.0–9.4)	69.4%[c], (59.7–78.3)	Median[d]: 27

C indicates colostomy, *EC* end colostomy, *EI* end ileostomy, *IC* ileal conduit, *LC* loop colostomy, *LI* loop ileostomy, *NS* not specified
[a]Excluding in-hospital deaths
[b]Values are mean months follow-up unless otherwise stated
[c]Weighted pooled proportion (fixed effects model) using only studies with >12 months mean follow-up
[d]Median of reported follow-up of studies with >12 months follow-up

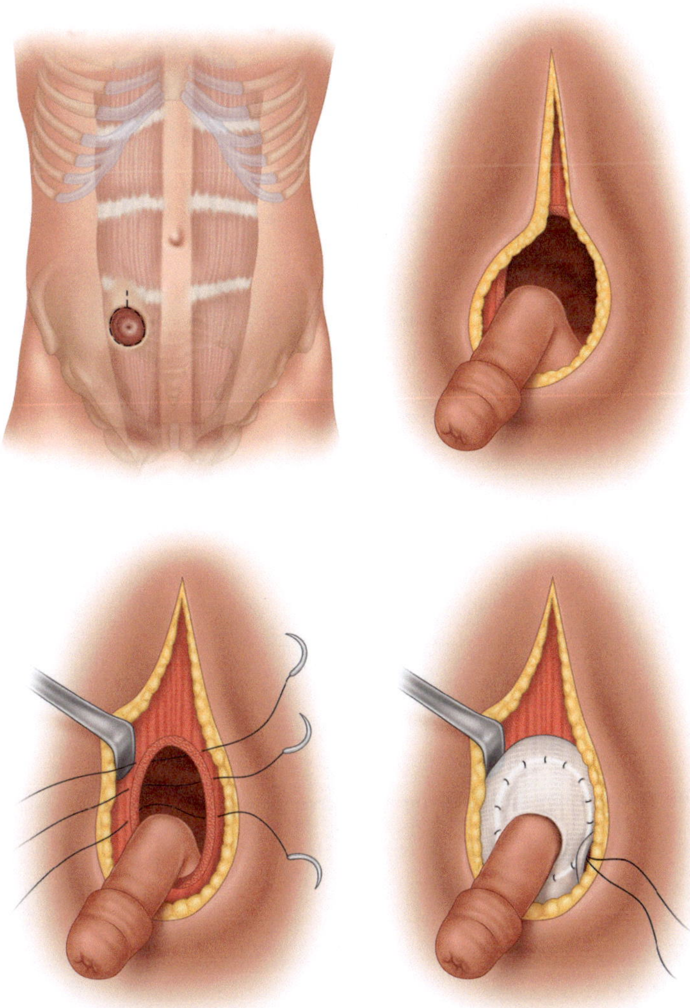

Fig. 23.2 Local repair with mesh

explained by the intra-abdominal pressure and the tangential forces working on the abdominal wall leading to ongoing widening of the keyhole according to Laplace's law ($T = P \times R/2$) [17]. Therefore, the Keyhole technique is no longer advised.

With the Sugarbaker technique, a mesh without a hole is used after lateralization of the bowel.

The technique was first described by Sugarbaker in 1985 [16]. At that time, the mesh was only sutured to the fascial edges. As we have learned from incisional hernia repair, an overlap of 3–5 cm between the mesh and the adjacent fascia is mandatory to prevent recurrent hernias [18]. Therefore, the Sugarbaker technique was modified according to Fig. 23.4.

Table 23.3 Study characteristics and outcomes of onlay mesh repair of parastomal hernia

Reference	Time period	Mod. MINORS index	No. repairs	Type of stoma	Material; technique	No. complications (%)			Mortality	Recurrence (%)	Follow-up[a]
						Wound infection	Mesh infection	Other			
Ho and Fawcett [15]	1982–2001	11	15	IC	PPM; KH	0	0	2	0	1 (6.7)	15
De Ruiter and Bijnen [16]	1988–2002	11	46	C	CRE-PPM	0	3	1	0	7 (15.2)	51
Steele et al. [17]	1988–2002	11	58	31 EC, 24 EI, 3 LI	PPM; 'Stove pipe hat'	2	0	9	0	15 (25.9)	51
Venditti et al. [18]	1993–1996	9	8	EC	PPM; KH	1	0	0	0	0 (0)	38
Lüning and Spillenaar-Bilgen [19]	1997–2006	11	16	12 C, 3 IC	PPM (7), PE (6), Vicryl (1); KH (14), CRE-PPM (2)	0	1	1	NS	3 (18.8)	33
Amin et al. [20]	1999	9	9	1 C, 8 EI	PPM; KH	0	0	0	0	0 (0)	7
Kald et al. [21]	1999–2000	10	5	4 C, 1 EI	PPM; KH	0	0	0	0	1 (20.0)	12
Weighted pooled% (95-CI)	–		157	–	–	1.9% (0.4–5.5)	2.6% (0.7–6.4)	8.3% (4.5–13.7)	0% (0.0–2.3)	17.2%[b] (11.9–23.4)	Median[c]: 36

C indicates colostomy, *CRE-PPM* central ring enforced polypropylene mesh, *EC* end colostomy, *EI* end ileostomy, *IC* ileal conduit, *LC* loop colostomy, *LI* loop ileostomy, *NS* not specified

[a]Values are mean months follow-up unless otherwise stated

[b]Weighted pooled proportion (fixed effects model) using only studies with >12 months mean follow-up

[c]Median of reported follow-up of studies with >12 months follow-up

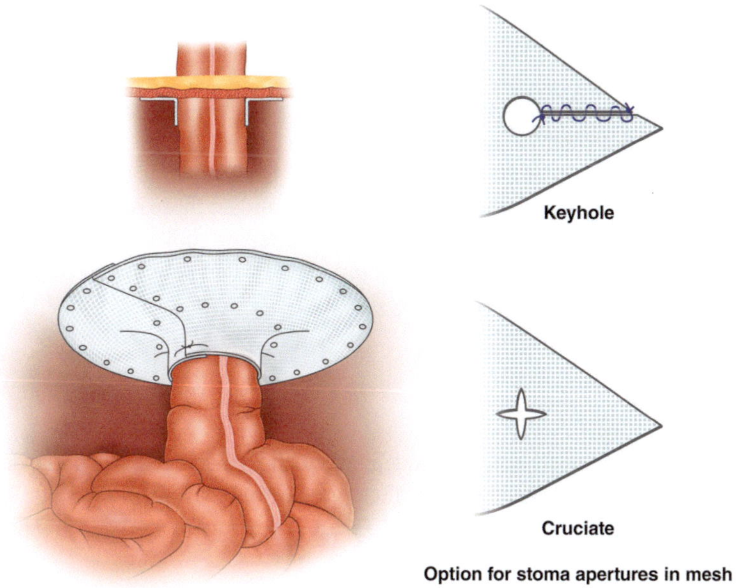

Fig. 23.3 Keyhole technique

Fig. 23.4 Sugarbaker technique

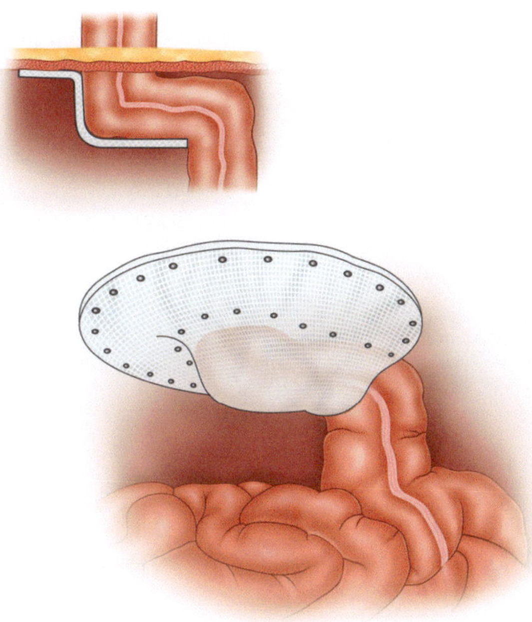

The Sugarbaker technique has a recurrence rate of 10.2% when repaired with a ePTFE mesh [11, 13, 19]. No publications on long-term outcome of other meshes are available so far.

Berger and coworkers reported on the use of a Sandwich technique, which combines both Keyhole and Sugarbaker techniques using PVDF-PP mesh (Dynamesh®) [17]. After a follow-up of 20 months, one out of 47 (2.1%) had a recurrence. While outcome is positive, more studies are needed to validate these results [19].

Meta-analysis of all studies on laparoscopic repair shows that the Sugarbaker technique has the best results and is recommended when patient and surgeon are fit for laparoscopy [11, 13, 20–22].

Open Repair

The open modified Sugarbaker technique is an excellent alternative when a laparoscopic approach is not suitable. Reviewing the literature showed only one study reporting on 20 repairs. No mesh infections occurred and 3 out of 20 hernias recurred (15%) [22].

Conclusion

Parastomal hernia continues to be a common complication of stoma surgery that can have a significant impact on quality of life and may even carry life-threatening risk. An organized approach to these patients with multidisciplinary management is essential. Choice of surgical repair depends on patient factors; however, a minimally invasive approach is feasible in many circumstances (Fig. 23.5).

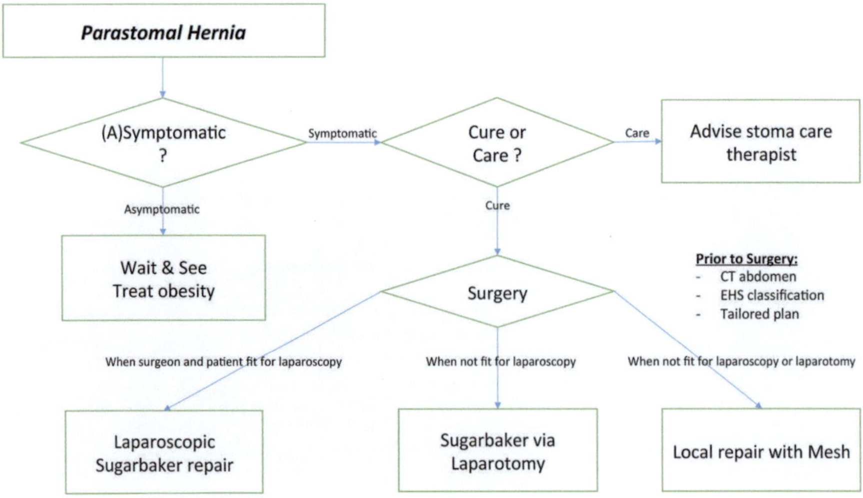

Fig. 23.5 Flowsheet

References

1. Pearl RK. Parastomal hernias. World J Surg. 1989;13:569–72.
2. Cingi A, Carik T, Sever A, Aktan AO. Enterostomy site hernias: a clinical and computerized tomographic evaluation. Dis Colon Rectum. 2006;49:1559–63.
3. Moreno-Matias J, Serra-Aracil X, Darnell-Martin A, Bonbardo- Junca J, Mora-Lopez L, Alcantara-Moral M, Ayguavives-Garnica I, Navarro-Soto S. The prevalence of parastomal hernia after formation of an end colostomy. Color Dis. 2009;11:173–7.
4. Pilgrim CHC, McIntyre R, Bailey M. Prospective audit of parastomal hernia: prevalence and associates comorbidities. Dis Colon Rectum. 2010;53:71–6.
5. Nastro P, Knowles CH, McGrath A, Porrett TRC, Lunniss PJ. Complications of intestinal stomas. Br J Surg. 2010;97:1885–9.
6. Janes A, Weisby L, Israelsson LA. Parastomal hernia: clinical and radiological definitions. Hernia. 2011;15:189–92.
7. Nasvall P, Wikner F, Gunnarsson U, Rutegard J, Stringard K. A comparision between 3D ultrasonography, CT scanning and findings at surgery in patients with stomal complaints. Int J Color Dis. 2014;29:1263–6.
8. Smietanski M, Szczepkowski M, Alexandre JA, Berger D, Bury K, Conze J, Hansson B, Janes A, Miserez M, Mandala V, Montgamery A, Morales-Conde S, Muysoms F. European Hernia Society classification of parastomal hernias. Hernia. 2014;18:1–6.
9. Stravos AA, Muysoms F et al. EHS parastomal hernia guidelines. Submitted in Hernia.
10. Krogsgaard M, Pilsgaard B, Borglit TB, Bentzen J, Balleby L, Krarup PM. Symptom load and individual symptoms before and after repair of parastomal hernia: a prospective single centre study. Color Dis. 2017;19:200.
11. Hansson BME, Slater NJ, Schouten van der Velden AP, Groenewoud HMM, Buyne OR, de Hingh IJT, Bleichrodt RP. Surgical techniques for parastomal hernia repair: a systematic review of the literature. Ann Surg. 2012;255:685–95.
12. Rosin JD, Bonardi RA. Paracolostomy hernia repair with Marlex mesh: a new technique. Dis Colon Rectum. 1977;20:299–302.
13. Hansson BME, Morales-Conde S, Mussack T, Valdes J, Muysoms FE, Bleichrodt RP. Laparoscopic modified Sugarbaker technique is safe and has a low recurrence rate: a multicenter cohort study. Surg Endosc. 2013;27:494–500.
14. Hansson BME, de Hingh IHJT, Bleichrodt RP. Laparoscopic parastomal hernia repair is feasible and safe: early results of a prospective clinical study including 55 consecutive patients. Surg Endosc. 2007;21:989–93.
15. Hansson BME, van Nieuwenhoven EJ, Bleichrodt RP. Promising new technique in the repair of parastomal hernia. Surg Endosc. 2003;17:1789–91.
16. Sugarbaker PH. Peritoneal approach to prosthetic mesh repair of paraostomy hernias. Ann Surg. 1985;201:344–6.
17. Berger D, Bientzle M. Polyvinylidene fluoride: a suitable mesh material for laparoscopic incisional and parastomal hernia repair! A prospective, observational study with 344 patients. Hernia. 2009;13:167–72.
18. de Vries Reilingh TS, van Geldere D, Langenhorst B, de Jong D, van der Wilt GJ, van Goor H, Bleichrodt RP. Repair of large midline incisional hernias with polypropylene mesh: comparison of three operative techniques. Hernia. 2004;8:56–9.
19. Stelzner S, Hellmich G, Ludwig K. Repair of paracolostomy hernias with a prosthetic mesh in the intraperitoneal onlay position: modified Sugarbaker technique. Dis Colon Rectum. 2004;47:185–91.
20. Levy S, Plymale MA, Miller MT, Davenport DL, Roth JS. Laparoscopic parastomal hernia repair: no different than a laparoscopic ventral hernia repair? Surg Endosc. 2016;30:1542–6.
21. DeAsis F, Lapin B, Gitelis M, Ujiki M. Current state of laparoscopic parastomal hernia repair: a meta-analysis. World J Gastroenterol. 2015;21:8670–7.
22. DeAsis FJ, Linn JG, Lapin B, Denham W, Carbray JM. Modified laparoscopic Sugarbaker repair decreases recurrence rates of parastomal hernia. Surgery. 2015;158:954–9.
23. Hansson BME, Bleichrodt RP, De Hingh IH. Laparoscopic parastomal hernia repair using a keyhole technique results in a high recurrence rate. Surg Endosc. 2009;23:1456–9.

Part VII

Optimizing Pelvic Dissection for Rectal Cancer

Proctectomy for Advanced Rectal Cancer: APE or ELAPE?

24

Torbjörn Holm

Introduction

Ernest Miles' paper "A method of performing abdomino-perineal excision for carcinoma of the rectum and of the terminal portion of the pelvic colon" was published in The Lancet in 1908 [1]. This description of an abdominoperineal excision of the rectum has since been called "the Miles' operation" and had a strong impact on rectal cancer surgery. In the original description of the procedure, the rectum was bluntly mobilized down to the sacrococcygeal articulation, to the prostate, and to "the upper surface of the levatores ani" laterally, thus leaving the mesorectum attached to the pelvic floor. After mobilization of the rectum, a colostomy was created, and the abdominal wall was closed. The patient was turned over and placed in the right lateral and semi-prone position. Miles emphasized that the levator muscles should be divided "as far outwards as their origin from the white line so as to include the lateral zone of spread," and as a result the perineal part of the operation included a wide excision of skin, fat, and pelvic floor (levator muscles).

The Lancet paper had an enormous impact on the surgical community, and for many decades, the "Miles operation" was the gold standard procedure for all rectal carcinomas. However, the concept of removing the entire rectum, the anus, and the perineum in all patients with rectal cancer was gradually abandoned. An increasing experience with bowel reconstruction, including developments of stapling instruments, led to a new concept of anterior resection (AR) and low anterior resection (LAR), which became the standard procedures for tumors of the upper and mid-rectum [2–6].

For tumors of the lower rectum, most surgeons continued to perform abdominoperineal excision (APE), although the extensive perineal approach described by Miles was more or less neglected and the synchronous combined APE was

T. Holm (✉)
Section of Coloproctology, Department of Surgical Gastroenterology,
Karolinska University Hospital, Stockholm, Sweden
e-mail: torbjorn.holm@ki.se

C.M. Schlachta, P. Sylla (eds.), *Current Common Dilemmas in Colorectal Surgery*,
https://doi.org/10.1007/978-3-319-70117-2_24

introduced as a feasible procedure which became popular and gained widespread use in the treatment of low rectal cancer [7]. During the synchronous combined operation, the perineal part is carried out simultaneously with the pelvic part of the abdominal procedure, with the patient in the supine lithotomy or Lloyd-Davies position; the rectum with its mesorectum is first mobilized down to the pelvic floor, and the perineal surgeon then enters the pelvic cavity just in front of the coccyx, the levator muscles are divided on both sides, and finally the rectum is dissected off the prostate or the vagina, and the specimen is delivered through the perineum.

Although there were gradual improvements in the treatment of rectal cancer during the twentieth century, local control remained a major problem after surgery, with local recurrence rates of up to 40% after potentially curative resections [8] (Fig. 24.1).

With the development of total mesorectal excision (TME), as described by Bill Heald, treatment results improved dramatically, both concerning local control and survival. Heald reported a local recurrence rate around 5% and a cancer-specific survival around 70% at 5 years, without radiotherapy [9, 10]. During the recent two decades, the TME technique has been introduced in many countries, and subsequently the results with regard to local control and cancer survival have improved significantly. Local recurrence rates are now reported to be less than 10% in population-based studies [11, 12].

Consequently, teaching rectal cancer surgery has mainly focused on the operative technique of TME and AR. Although the technique used for the abdominal part of an APE was modified along the lines of TME, little attention was given to the perineal part of the procedure. Thus, most surgeons adopted the technique of sharp dissection under direct vision outside the mesorectal fascia down to the pelvic floor, with the aim to save autonomic nerves and to create a perfect specimen with an

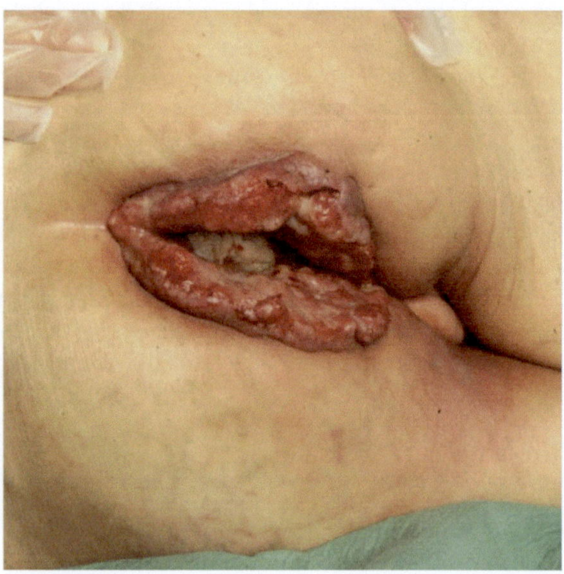

Fig. 24.1 Patient with a large local recurrence growing in the perineum after a standard APR

intact mesorectal fascia. The perineal part, however, was often completed in the conventional way, with dissection close to the external sphincter and with the division of the levator muscles close to the rectal wall. With the patient in the supine lithotomy position, it is difficult to achieve an optimal view, especially anteriorly, and therefore parts of the perineal dissection are often done with blunt dissection when this approach is used.

Problems Related to the Conventional APE

With an increasing focus on oncological outcomes and improved audit, several authors have acknowledged the fact that local control and survival after APE have not improved to the same degree as that seen after AR. In one study based on 561 patients from Leeds, UK, it was reported that patients undergoing APE had a higher local failure rate (22.3 vs. 13.5%) and a poorer survival (52.3 vs. 65.8%) compared with patients who had an AR during the same time period [13].

In another paper based on data from five different European trials, it was reported that the APE procedure was associated with an increased risk of circumferential resection margin (CRM) involvement, an increased local recurrence rate, and a decreased cancer-specific survival [14]. A large cohort study from Norway also reported a higher local recurrence rate (15 vs. 10%) and a poorer 5-year survival (55 vs. 68%) after APE than after AR [12].

These differences in oncological outcomes between the two procedures may be explained by several factors, including anatomical difficulties and the surgical technique associated with standard APE surgery. In the lower rectum, the surrounding mesorectum is reduced in size and disappears at the top of the sphincters. Below this level, the sphincter muscle forms the circumferential resection margin (CRM). As mentioned above, the abdominal dissection during a conventional APE is often carried out along the mesorectum, all the way down to the pelvic floor and the top of the puborectalis muscle, with the mesorectum being mobilized off the levator muscles. The perineal dissection then follows the external sphincter to meet the pelvic dissection at the top of the anal canal (Fig. 24.2). With this technique the retrieved specimen often has a typical "waist" at 3–5 cm from the distal end, corresponding to the top of the external sphincter at the level of the puborectalis muscle and the lowest part of the mesorectum (Fig. 24.3).

The inward coning at the pelvic floor carries the dissection close to the rectal wall, and several studies have reported higher rates of bowel perforation and tumor involvement of the CRM after APE as compared with AR. Nagtegaal et al. assessed 846 AR specimens and 373 APE specimens from the Dutch TME trial and found that the plane of resection was within the sphincter muscle, the submucosa or lumen in more than 1/3 of the APE cases, and in the remainder was on the sphincter muscles. This resulted in a positive CRM rate of 30.4% after APE versus 10.7% after AR and a perforation rate of 13.7% after APE versus 2.5% after AR [15]. Similarly, population-based reports from Sweden, Norway, and Holland have shown a threefold increase in perforation rates after APE compared to AR (14–15% vs. 3–4%)

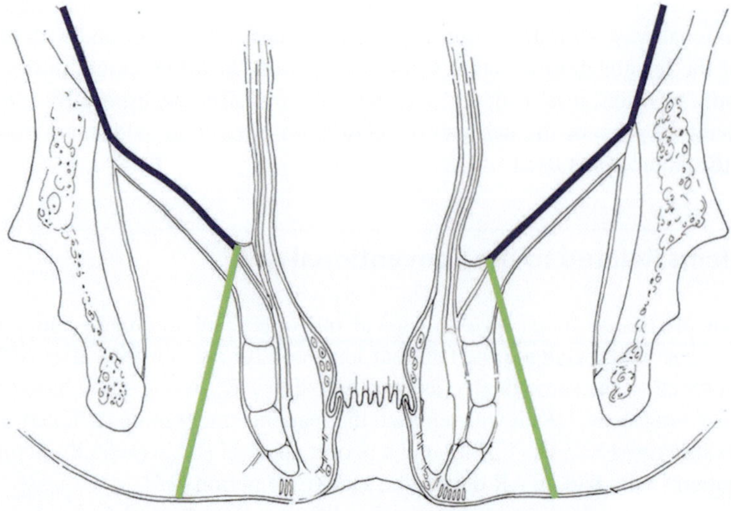

Fig. 24.2 The pelvic dissection in a conventional APE is carried along outside the mesorectal fascia down to the top of the anal canal (blue line), and the perineal dissection is carried along the external sphincter (green line). The two dissection planes meet at the level of the puborectal muscle, which creates a waist on the specimen

Fig. 24.3 Photograph of a fresh specimen after a conventional APE, with the typical waist at the level of the puborectal muscle

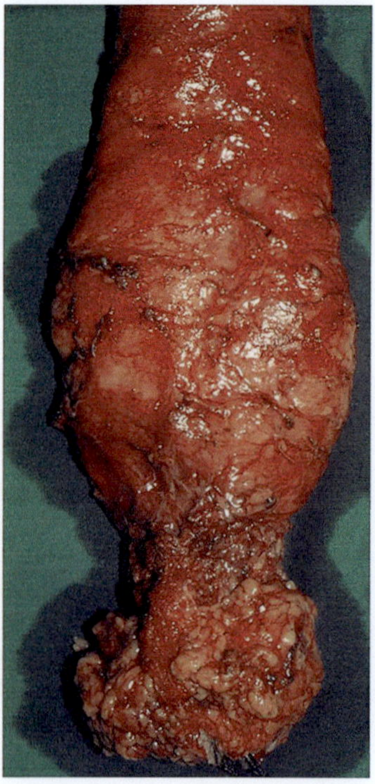

and also that perforation is a significant risk factor for adverse outcomes regarding local control and survival [16]. In addition, a publication based on the Dutch TME trial reported that tumor involvement of the CRM was an independent risk factor, both for local recurrence and survival, in patients undergoing APE [17]. Thus, the differences in oncological outcomes between the conventional type of APE and AR may to a substantial part be explained by the increased risk of tumor-involved margins and inadvertent bowel perforations, as both these factors are significantly related to local control and survival.

With the development of TME, leading to substantially improved results after AR, many surgeons have advocated low or ultralow anterior resection, even for tumors of the lower rectum. It has also been shown that these procedures are feasible and oncologically safe, provided that the tumor can be removed with a clear distal and circumferential margin. In dedicated and highly specialized centers, adopting intersphincteric AR for appropriate cases, the overall APE rate may be below 15% [18].

Although LAR and intersphincteric AR may be suitable for many patients with low rectal cancer, a substantial proportion of patients have advanced tumors where a restorative procedure is impossible and an APE necessary. Local tumor staging with MRI is crucial to detect low advanced tumors, growing close to or into the distal mesorectal fascia, the levator muscle, or the external sphincter (Fig. 24.4). In view of the fact that the results after conventional APE have been suboptimal, it is important to improve APE in order to reduce the rate of inadvertent bowel perforations and tumor-involved margins and to obtain better oncological outcomes. The extralevator APE (ELAPE) was described in order to reduce rates of perforation and involved CRM in such low, advanced tumors.

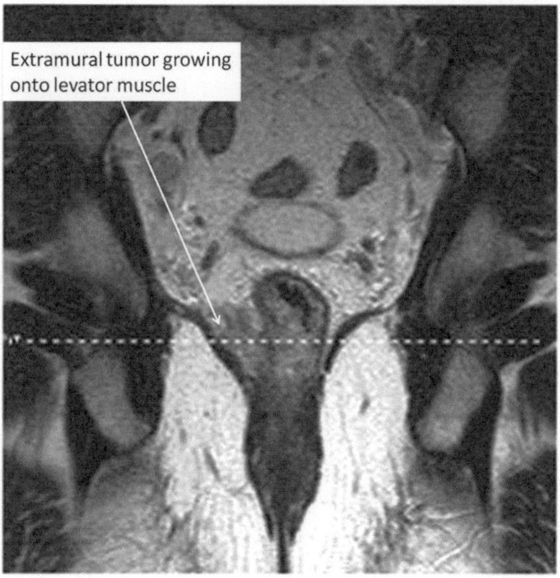

Fig. 24.4 Pelvic MRI showing a low, advanced rectal cancer with extramural tumor growth onto the levator muscle on the right side

The Concept of ELAPE

One obvious problem associated with the conventional type of APE is the lack of standardization and a clear definition of the details of the perineal part of this procedure [19]. Although the abdominal part of the operation follows the standard TME principles, there has been no obvious agreement on the surgical details of the perineal part of the operation. This probably explains the significant variability in the observed rates of tumor-involved margins, bowel perforations, local recurrence, and survival [20]. Due to this variability and the suboptimal results after APE, there has been a call for a different concept and a more standardized approach to APE [21].

The main purpose of ELAPE is to improve treatment results in low advanced tumors by reducing the risk of inadvertent bowel perforation and CRM involvement. This can be accomplished because the levator muscles are excised en bloc with the mesorectum, to protect the most distal part of the bowel and thereby avoiding "the waist" on the specimen. Since the levator muscles should not be separated from the mesorectum, the pelvic dissection during the abdominal part of an ELAPE differs from an AR or a conventional APE.

The Pelvic Dissection in ELAPE

In both AR and conventional APE, the dissection continues down to the pelvic floor and the puborectalis muscle, and the mesorectum is mobilized off the levator muscles. In ELAPE it is crucial not to take the mobilization of the mesorectum as far down as the pelvic floor. Instead, the dissection should proceed only down to the sacrococcygeal junction dorsally, just beyond the inferior hypogastric plexus anterolaterally, and the anterior dissection should stop just below the seminal vesicles in men or the cervix uteri in women. By terminating the mobilization at this level, the mesorectum is still attached to the levator muscles of the pelvic floor, which is a crucial feature of ELAPE.

The Perineal Dissection in ELAPE

The perineal part of ELAPE can be performed with the patient either in the supine or in the prone, jack-knife position. The prone position is often preferable, due to the excellent exposure of the operative field. Some surgeons prefer the supine position, mainly to avoid the time-consuming process of turning the patient with subsequent preparation and dressing of the perineal area.

Irrespective of the position, the perineal phase starts with closure of the anus to avoid any spillage of feces or mucus which may contain tumor cells. In ELAPE, less skin and ischioanal fat are excised as compared with Miles original description of the APE procedure. After incision of the skin, the external sphincter is identified, and the dissection is continued outside the sphincter up to the levator muscles on both sides. The levator muscles are then followed up to the pelvic sidewall (obturator internus muscle).

Once the external sphincter and levator muscles are exposed around the circumference, the pelvis is entered, either just below the tip of the coccyx or through the sacrococcygeal junction. At this stage it is important to identify the mesorectum in order not to injure the mesorectal fascia. The pelvic floor, i.e., the levator muscle, is now divided, and the division continues onto the prostate or vagina. The specimen is now still attached to the anterior aspect of the levator muscles and to the prostate or posterior wall of the vagina.

The dissection in the anterior plane during the perineal phase of ELAPE is the most difficult, and potentially most dangerous, part of the procedure because of the close relationship between the anterior rectal wall and the prostate or posterior vaginal wall. In addition, the neurovascular bundles derived from the inferior hypogastric plexus run anterolaterally on each side of the prostate or vagina and close to the rectum and can easily be damaged if they are not recognized at this stage of the operation (Fig. 24.5). The dissection along the anterior and lateral aspects of the lower rectum must therefore be performed meticulously and with great care. If the dissection is performed close to the rectal wall, there is a risk of inadvertent perforation or tumor-involved margin, and if the dissection is carried out too laterally or too anteriorly, there is a risk of damage to the neurovascular bundles or to the prostate or vagina. In anteriorly located tumors, it may be necessary to include the posterior vaginal wall or a slice of the posterior prostate with the specimen and sometimes even to sacrifice the neurovascular bundle on one side, to be able to achieve a negative CRM. However, this extension of the procedure should ideally be planned in advance, based on the preoperative MRI staging and digital examination, so that the surgeon is prepared for it and so that the patient is well informed about the consequences, which may be impairment of bladder and/or sexual function.

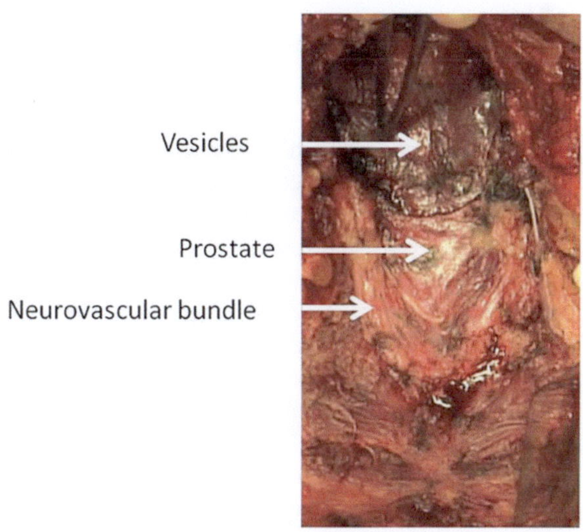

Fig. 24.5 Neurovascular bundles along the prostate after ELAPE (patient in prone position)

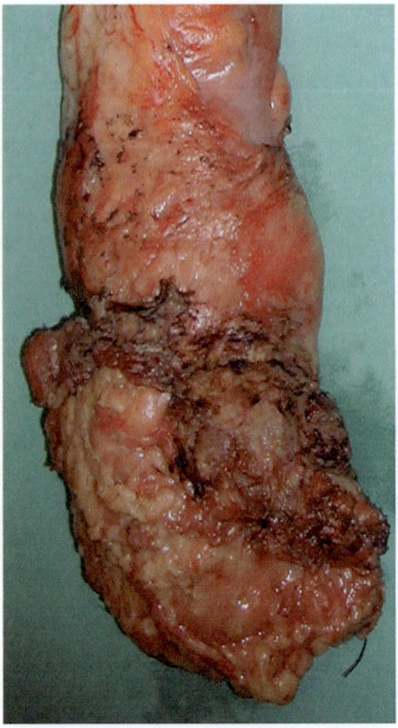

Fig. 24.6 Photograph of a fresh specimen after ELAPE. The specimen has no waist because the levator muscle is attached to the mesorectum

When the perineal dissection is carried out as described, the excised specimen is "cylindrical," usually without a waist, due to the fact that the levator muscle is still attached to the mesorectum, forming a cuff around the rectal muscle tube (Fig. 24.6).

Low Advanced Rectal Cancer: APE or ELAPE?

A description of the "extended abdominoperineal resection" or ELAPE was published in 2007, and since then, increasing numbers of surgeons have used the technique [22]. In 2010, West et al. published a comparative study on 176 extralevator APE procedures from 11 European colorectal surgeons with 124 standard excisions from one UK center and found that ELAPE removed more tissue from outside the smooth muscle layer and was associated with less CRM involvement and intraoperative perforations than standard surgery [23]. Stelzner et al. performed a literature search to identify articles reporting on APE after the introduction of TME and compared outcomes in 1097 patients after ELAPE with 4147 patients after conventional APE. They found significant risk reduction in the rates of inadvertent bowel perforation (4.1 vs. 10.4%), CRM involvement (9.6 vs. 15.4%), and the rate of local recurrence (6.6% vs. 11.9%) and concluded that "extended techniques of APE result in superior oncologic outcome as compared to standard techniques" [24].

Despite seemingly encouraging results after ELAPE, there have been disputes on the necessity of changing from the conventional type of APE to a more extensive ELAPE procedure. There has only been one small randomized trial comparing the two methods. The results from that study favored ELAPE [25]. Some other studies have reported similar or inferior results after ELAPE than after APE, but the conclusions have often been flawed because the ELAPE groups included lower and more advanced tumors than the APE groups [26, 27]. In a multicenter propensity score-matched analysis of conventional versus extended abdominoperineal excision for low rectal cancer from Spain, it was concluded that ELAPE does not improve rates of CRM involvement, intraoperative tumor perforation, local recurrence, or mortality [28]. The problem with this study was that matching was done for the quality of the specimen and that there was a very high proportion of excluded patients in the APE group compared to the ELAPE group—69 versus 3%.

In 2012, the Mayo group reported results from 655 consecutive patients with rectal cancer treated with curative intent, using surgery alone. All 246 patients having an APE were operated in the Lloyd-Davies position. The local recurrence rate at 5 years was 5.5% and not significantly different from the local recurrence rate after AR. Also, disease-free survival was similar after APE and AR. It was concluded that "commitment to a standardized wide resection should be the current approach to APR" [29]. However, when this paper is read in more detail, the operative technique for APE is described as follows: "the widest part of the perineal dissection was carried to the ischial tuberosities bilaterally and then extended upwards to incorporate a majority of the pelvic floor, joining the anterior dissection from the pelvic side without coning in." Thus, it is obvious that the authors' standard approach to APE is in fact ELAPE, performed in the supine position.

If the extent of excision of the levator muscle is not defined by the surgeon, the risk of misclassification is probably high, and with conventional APE, the surgical technique has probably varied considerably, which likely explains the reported significant differences in local control and survival. It is important to realize that the external sphincter is integrally related to the levator muscle and therefore removal of the external sphincter is, by definition, the initial part of an ELAPE. All that really is at issue is thus the extent of levator removal, which has often not been clarified in reports on results after conventional APE. Therefore, it is futile to compare ELAPE and conventional APE unless the exact extent of levator removal has been defined. When this is done, it may be evident that "standard APE" is in fact a more or less extensive ELAPE.

Summary

Although treatment results in rectal cancer have improved significantly during the recent two decades, local control and survival after APE have not improved to the same degree as that seen after AR. The reason is an increased risk of inadvertent bowel perforations and tumor-involved margins after APE as compared to AR. The conventional APE has not been a standardized procedure, and oncological outcomes have varied considerably between different institutions and different reports. All patients with rectal cancer should have a preoperative MRI of the pelvis for local staging of the tumor. In low advanced tumors, threatening or infiltrating the mesorectal fascia, levator, or external sphincter, a standard APE is not adequate. ELAPE, based on well-defined anatomical structures, was developed to treat such tumors. The key objective is to remove an intact specimen without perforation and with resection margins free from tumor cells, which obviously leads to improved local control and survival.

References

1. Miles WE. A method of performing abdomino-perineal excision for carcinoma of the rectum and of the terminal portion of the pelvic colon. Lancet. 1908;2:1812–3.
2. Collins DC. End-results of the Miles' combined abdominoperineal resection versus the segmental anterior resection. A 25-year postoperative follow-up in 301 patients. Am J Proctol. 1963;14:258–61.
3. Fick TE, Baeten CG, von Meyenfeldt MF, Obertop H. Recurrence and survival after abdominoperineal and low anterior resection for rectal cancer without adjunctive therapy. Eur J Surg Oncol. 1960;16:105–8.
4. Groves RA, Harrison RC. Carcinoma of the rectum and lower sigmoid colon: abdominoperineal or anterior resection? Can J Surg. 1962;5:393–403.
5. Slanetz CA, Herter FP, Grinnell RS. Anterior resection versus abdominoperineal resection for cancer of the rectum and rectosigmoid: an analysis of 524 cases. Am J Surg. 1972;123:110–7.
6. Vandertoll DJ, Beahrs OH. Carcinoma of the rectum and low sigmoid; evaluation of anterior resection in 1766 favourable lesions. Arch Surg. 1965;90:793–8.
7. Schmitz RL, Nelson PA, Martin GB, Boghossian HM. Synchronous (two-team) abdominoperineal resection of the rectum. AMA Arch Surg. 1958;77(4):492–7.
8. Påhlman L, Glimelius B. Local recurrences after surgical treatment for rectal carcinoma. Acta Chir Scand. 1984;150:331–5.
9. Heald RJ, Husband EM, Ryall RD. The mesorectum in rectal cancer surgery--the clue to pelvic recurrence? Br J Surg. 1982;69(10):613–6.
10. MacFarlane JK, Ryall RDH, Heald RJ. Mesorectal excision for rectal cancer. Lancet. 1993; 341:457–60.
11. Martling AL, Holm T, Rutqvist LE, Moran BJ, Heald RJ, Cedemark B. Effect of a surgical training programme on outcome of rectal cancer in the County of Stockholm. Stockholm Colorectal Cancer Study Group, Basingstoke Bowel Cancer Research Project. Lancet. 2000;356(9224):93–6.
12. Wibe A, Syse A, Andersen E, Tretli S, Myrvold HE, Soreide O. Oncological outcomes after total mesorectal excision for cure for cancer of the lower rectum: anterior vs. abdominoperineal resection. Dis Colon Rectum. 2004;47(1):48–58.
13. Marr R, Birbeck K, Garvican J, Macklin CP, Tiffin NJ, Parsons WJ, et al. The modern abdominoperineal excision: the next challenge after total mesorectal excision. Ann Surg. 2005; 242(1):74–82.
14. den Dulk M, Putter H, Collette L, Marijnen CA, Folkesson J, Bosset JF, et al. The abdominoperineal resection itself is associated with an adverse outcome: the European experience based on a pooled analysis of five European randomised clinical trials on rectal cancer. Eur J Cancer. 2009;45:1175.
15. Nagtegaal ID, van de Velde CJ, Marijnen CA, van Krieken JH, Quirke P. Low rectal cancer: a call for a change of approach in abdominoperineal resection. J Clin Oncol. 2005;23(36):9257–64.
16. Eriksen MT, Wibe A, Syse A, Haffner J, Wiig JN. Inadvertent perforation during rectal cancer resection in Norway. Br J Surg. 2004;91(2):210–6.

17. den Dulk M, Marijnen CA, Putter H, Rutten HJ, Beets GL, Wiggers T, et al. Risk factors for adverse outcome in patients with rectal cancer treated with an abdominoperineal resection in the total mesorectal excision trial. Ann Surg. 2007;246(1):83–90.
18. Chau A, Maggiori L, Debove C, Kanso F, Hennequin C, Panis Y. Toward the end of abdominoperineal resection for rectal cancer? An 8-year experience in 189 consecutive patients with low rectal cancer. Ann Surg. 2014;260(5):801–5. discussion 5–6
19. Moore TJ, Moran BJ. Precision surgery, precision terminology: the origins and meaning of ELAPE. Color Dis. 2012;14(10):1173–4.
20. Birbeck KF, Macklin CP, Tiffin NJ, Parsons W, Dixon MF, Mapstone NP, et al. Rates of circumferential resection margin involvement vary between surgeons and predict outcomes in rectal cancer surgery. Ann Surg. 2002;235(4):449–57.
21. Radcliffe A. Can the results of anorectal (abdominoperineal) resection be improved: are circumferential resection margins too often positive? Color Dis. 2006;8(3):160–7.
22. Holm T, Ljung A, Haggmark T, Jurell G, Lagergren J. Extended abdominoperineal resection with gluteus maximus flap reconstruction of the pelvic floor for rectal cancer. Br J Surg. 2007;94(2):232–8.
23. West NP, Anderin C, Smith KJ, Holm T, Quirke P. Multicentre experience with extralevator abdominoperineal excision for low rectal cancer. Br J Surg. 2010;97(4):588–99.
24. Stelzner S, Koehler C, Stelzer J, Sims A, Witzigmann H. Extended abdominoperineal excision vs. standard abdominoperineal excision in rectal cancer--a systematic overview. Int J Color Dis. 2011;26(10):1227–40.
25. Han JG, Wang ZJ, Wei GH, Gao ZG, Yang Y, Zhao BC. Randomized clinical trial of conventional versus cylindrical abdominoperineal resection for locally advanced lower rectal cancer. Am J Surg. 2012;204(3):274–82.
26. Klein M, Fischer A, Rosenberg J, Gogenur I, Danish Colorectal Cancer Group. Extralevatory abdominoperineal excision (ELAPE) does not result in reduced rate of tumor perforation or rate of positive circumferential resection margin: a nationwide database study. Ann Surg. 2015;261(5):933–8.
27. Prytz M, Angenete E, Ekelund J, Haglind E. Extralevator abdominoperineal excision (ELAPE) for rectal cancer--short-term results from the Swedish Colorectal Cancer Registry. Selective use of ELAPE warranted. Int J Color Dis. 2014;29(8):981–7.
28. Ortiz H, Ciga MA, Armendariz P, Kreisler E, Codina-Cazador A, Gomez-Barbadillo J, et al. Multicentre propensity score-matched analysis of conventional versus extended abdominoperineal excision for low rectal cancer. Br J Surg. 2014;101(7):874–82.
29. Mathis KL, Larson DW, Dozois EJ, Cima RR, Huebner M, Haddock MG, et al. Outcomes following surgery without radiotherapy for rectal cancer. Br J Surg. 2012;99(1):137–43.

Transanal TME: Why Go Bottom-Up!

25

Marta Penna and Roel Hompes

Rectal cancer surgery is one of the most difficult operations faced by colorectal surgeons. Whilst aiming to obtain a good oncological resection with complete total mesorectal excision (TME), the surgeon must also ensure that the surrounding structures, with the complex network of pelvic nerves and blood vessels, are also protected. Numerous studies and trials on laparoscopic and open 'top-down' approaches to TME surgery have highlighted how certain patient and tumour-related features can create a hostile pelvic environment that compromises adequate visualisation and accurate dissection [1–5]. Such risk factors include obese men with a narrow pelvis and low fixed bulky tumours. The 'bottom-up' or transanal approach was pioneered to overcome these difficult features by providing a new viewpoint of the dissection plane that is not restricted by a small pelvic diameter and avoids excessive manipulation of the specimen.

Transanal total mesorectal excisions (taTME) was inspired and developed by amalgamating various minimally invasive and transanal approaches, in particular, transanal endoscopic microsurgery (TEM) [6], transanal transabdominal approach (TATA) [7], natural orifice transluminal endoscopic surgery (NOTES) [8, 9] and transanal minimally invasive surgery (TAMIS) [10]. taTME has been further adapted for procedures other than anterior resections, including abdominoperineal excisions [11] and completion proctectomies [12, 13], as well as for benign disease. There is varying opinion amongst surgeons experienced in taTME on the indication and patient selection for this approach. Surgeons with taTME experience at the

M. Penna
Department of Colorectal Surgery, Oxford University Hospital, Oxford, UK
e-mail: m.penna@doctors.org.uk

R. Hompes (✉)
Department of GI and Oncologic Surgery, Academic Medical Center Amsterdam, Amsterdam, The Netherlands
e-mail: r.hompes@amc.uva.nl

C.M. Schlachta, P. Sylla (eds.), *Current Common Dilemmas in Colorectal Surgery*,
https://doi.org/10.1007/978-3-319-70117-2_25

Table 25.1 Patient selection criteria, indications and contraindications for transanal total mesorectal excision (taTME) established at the International taTME conference by surgeons experienced in taTME [14]

Indications and patient selection	
Disease	– Both benign and malignant
Patient characteristics	– Male gender – Narrow and/or deep pelvis – Visceral obesity and/or BMI >30 kg/m^2 – Prostatic hypertrophy
Tumour characteristics	– Rectal cancer <12 cm from anal verge, including very low cancers – Tumour diameter >4 cm – Distorted tissue planes following neoadjuvant radiotherapy – Impalpable, low primary tumour requiring accurate placement of the distal resection margin
Benign disease that may benefit from taTME	– Inflammatory bowel disease requiring proctectomy – Rectal strictures – Complex fistulae – Faecal incontinence – Familial adenomatous polyposis – Radiation proctitis – Need to remove the orphaned rectum following colectomy or permanent colonic diversion
Strategic conversion	– Failure to proceed during abdominal approach to TME
Contraindications	
Tumour characteristics	– T4 tumours – Obstructing rectal tumours
Presentation	– Emergency presentation

international taTME conference in 2014 provided a consensus statement with recommended criteria for patient selection [14] (outlined in Table 25.1).

The taTME pioneers and early adopters have published their individual operative technique and modifications along with post-operative morbidity, oncological and functional outcomes, which are summarised below.

The Technical Steps

The critical steps of taTME were initially developed and established following extensive preliminary work on animal models [15, 16] and human cadavers [9, 17], prior to the first live case reported in 2010 by Sylla et al. [18]. Although a purely transanal operation has been described [19], the most commonly adopted approach involves an abdominal (open, laparoscopic or robotic) and perineal phase, which can be performed synchronously by two teams or consecutively by one team [20, 21]. Once the preferred transanal access channel or platform is secured in place, the procedure can broadly be broken down into five key steps (Fig. 25.1): (1) distal purse string placement, (2) full-thickness rectotomy, (3) TME dissection, (4) specimen extraction and (5) anastomosis.

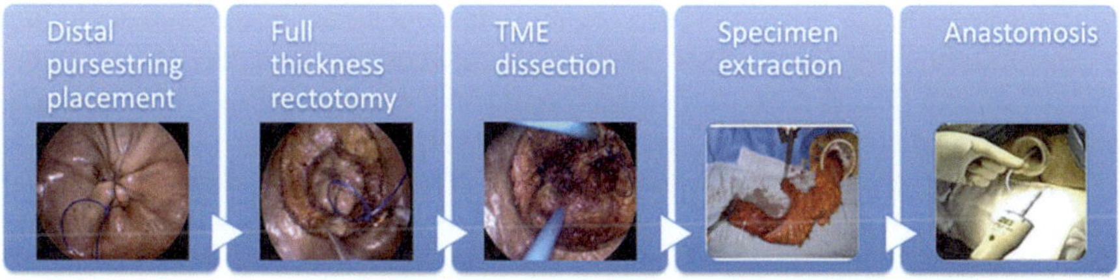

Fig. 25.1 Key operative steps to transanal total mesorectal excision

A circumferential distal purse string is placed at the start of the operation ensuring an adequate distal margin. The purse string must provide a tight seal to fully occlude the lumen throughout the operation, thus avoiding colonic insufflation and pelvic contamination by faecal spillage. In case the distal margin of the tumour is within 2 cm from the puborectal sling, another approach will be required: a mucosectomy and partial or complete intersphincteric dissection.

A full-thickness rectotomy is performed next by dissecting in a circle at the extremities of the radial folds formed by the purse string. The pneumopelvis created by the insufflation system through the transanal platform can be increased from an initial pressure of 8–10 mmHg to 10–15 mmHg, which will provide optimal distension as well as 'pneumo-dissection' to open up the plane. Dissection along the mesorectal 'holy' plane, found between the parietal endopelvic fascia and mesorectal envelope, can then proceed, starting around 5 or 7 o'clock and then joining at the posterior midline through the fibrotic raphe. TME dissection should continue in a cylindrical manner, alternating between posterior, anterior, and lateral dissection whilst advancing up the pelvis. This proposed sequence of dissection helps to prevent veering too laterally into the pelvic sidewall and injuring the neurovascular bundles. Likewise, the steep sacral angle must be acknowledged and followed in order to avoid creating defects in the mesorectum or even a rectal tube perforation by dissecting along a horizontal line from the anus. On the contrary, dissecting too posteriorly can lead to significant bleeding from presacral vessels. The most important structure anteriorly in males is the membranous urethra, which can be injured if dissecting too anteriorly or by inadvertently mobilising the prostate downwards.

To avoid unstabilising the pneumoperitoneum and draining fluid obscuring the perineal team's view, connection between the abdominal and transanal teams should occur once the anterior and posterior dissections are almost complete. The two teams will be able to work together, guiding each other to dissect along the correct remaining planes. The fully mobilised rectal specimen can be extracted either transanally or transabdominally. Transanal extraction should not be attempted with very bulky tumours due to the risk of specimen rupture or if too much tension is placed on the colonic mesentery.

A handsewn coloanal or stapled colorectal anastomosis can be formed with the open distal stump. Four anastomotic techniques (one handsewn and three stapled) have been described with suggestions as to which technique to use depending on the length of the anal/rectal stump and thickness of the tissues [22]. Whichever method is performed, the key principles for a reliable anastomosis are unchanged, including a tension-free, well-vascularised anastomosis. According to a recent systematic review, splenic flexure mobilisation was completed in approximately 90% of cases, whilst 98% had a defunctioning stoma formed [21].

More advances and modifications to the taTME technique are continuously being proposed, which, together with the creation of new bespoke equipment, are likely to lead to further improvements in this field.

Morbidity and Mortality Results

Two recently published systematic reviews on taTME found that perioperative mortality and morbidity was generally well reported [20, 21]. Similis et al. [20] reported on 37 studies (9 case reports, 24 case series and 4 comparative studies) with a total of 510 participants in his review, whilst Arunachalam et al. [21] included the largest cohort of 140 patients by Lacy et al. [23] together with another 14 predominantly retrospective studies involving 449 patients. The overall procedure-associated morbidity was 34% with a 30-day mortality rate of <1%, with results comparable to those reported for laparoscopic TME [4, 5]. The mean operative time ranged from 143 to 450 min, with 12 (2.3%) conversions to open surgery reported [20]. The causes for conversion were posterior fixity of the tumour, intra-abdominal adhesions after previous laparotomy, a bulky high tumour, technical difficulties in obese patients and a urethral injury. Three intra-operative urethral injuries were reported, two of which were sutured transanally with no further consequences [24, 25]. It is important to acknowledge risks associated with specific procedures, such as the initially unexpected urethral injury in taTME as well as the risk of rectal perforation, bladder/ureteric injury, prostatic bleeding, injury to neurovascular bundles and vaginal perforation. Effective training and awareness of features suggesting that the incorrect plane has been entered are vital in minimising such risks.

The reoperation rate was between 3.7 and 9.1% with an anastomotic leak rate of 6.1–9.1% [24, 25]. Unplanned return to the operating room occurred due to presacral abscesses requiring drainage, small bowel obstruction, anastomotic leaks and ischemic colon. The mean length of hospital stay reported by the included studies ranged from 4.3 to 16.6 days.

The international taTME registry collaborative has recently published the largest cohort to date including 720 taTME cases [26]. The majority of patients were male (68%) with a mean age of 62.4 years and BMI of 26.5 kg/m^2. The median tumour height from anorectal junction on MRI was 3 cm, and 57% received neoadjuvant therapy. The overall morbidity and mortality rates at 30 days were 33% and 0.5%, respectively. Reassuringly, the anastomotic leak rate was 5.4% (32 cases); however, five intra-operative urethral injuries occurred. These registry cases included the experience of the pioneers and early adopters of taTME; together they encourage all surgeons who wish to adopt this technique to receive appropriate training and education. Table 25.2 summarises key post-operative and histological outcomes reported in the largest cohorts of patients published so far.

Table 25.2 Comparative clinicopathological outcomes for series describing over 50 taTME cases of rectal cancer

	Lacy et al. [23]	Veltcamp Helbach et al. [48]	Tuech et al. [30]	Burke et al. [49]
Number of patients	140	80	56	50
Study period	October 2011–November 2014	June 2012–September 2014	February 2010–June 2012	March 2012–July 2015
Patient and tumour characteristics				
Gender, M:F	89:51	48:32	41:15	30:20
Age, mean ± SD or median (range), years	65.5 ± 12.7	66.5 (42–86)	65 (39–83)	56.5 (50–65)
Body mass index, mean ± SD or median (range), kg/m^2	25.2 ± 3.9	27.5(19.5–40)	27 (20–42)	26.0 (22.7–31.2)
Tumour height on MRI, mean ± SD or median (range), cm	From AV, 7.6 ± 3.6	From dentate line, 5.3 (1–10)	From AV, 4.0 (0–5.0)	From AV, 4.4 (3.0–5.5)
Pre-operative T stage, *n* (%) T1–2 T3 T4	29 (20.7) 90 (64.3) 11 (7.9)	All T2 or T3	10 (17.9) 44 (78.5) 2 (3.6)	7 (14) 35 (70) 8 (16)
Received neoadjuvant therapy, *n* (%)	94 (67.1)	65 (81.3)	47 (84)	43 (86)
Clinical outcomes				
Total operative time, median (range), minutes	166 (60–360)	204 (91–447)	270 (150–495)	267 (227–331)
Conversions, *n* (%)	0	–	3 (7.3)	1 (2.2)
Overall morbidity at 30 days, %	34	39	26	36
Overall mortality at 30 days, *n* (%)	0	1 (1.2)	0	0
Anastomotic leak, %	12 (8.6)	–	3 (5.4)	3 (6)
Unplanned re-operations, %	12 (8.6)	9 (11.3)	–	6 (12)
Length of hospital stay, median (range), days	6 (3–39)	8 (3–41)	10 (6–21)	4.5 (4–8)
Histological outcomes				
Positive CRM, *n* (%)	9 (6.4)	2 (2.5)[a]	3 (5.4)	2 (4)
Positive DRM, *n* (%)	0	0	0	1 (2)

(continued)

Table 25.2 (continued)

	Lacy et al. [23]	Veltcamp Helbach et al. [48]	Tuech et al. [30]	Burke et al. [49]
TME quality, *n* (%) Complete Nearly complete Incomplete	136 (97.1) 3 (2.1) 1 (0.7)	71 (88.7) 7 (8.8) 2 (2.5)	47 (84) 9 (16) 0	36 (72) 13 (26) 1 (2)
Number of lymph nodes, mean ± SD or median (range)	14.7 ± 6.8	14 (6–30)	12 (7–29)	18 (12–24)
Recurrence rate, *n* (%)	Median 15 months	Mean 21 months	Median 29 months	Median 15 months
Local	1 (0.8)	2 (2.5)	1 (1.7)	2 (4)
Distant	8 (6.1)	–	–	7 (15)
Both local and distant	2 (1.5)	–	–	–

AV anal verge, *CRM* circumferential resection margin
[a]Positive CRM defined as tumour present <2 mm instead of <1 mm

Oncological Outcomes

The aim of an oncological resection for rectal cancer is to obtain a good-quality intact TME specimen, as described by Quirke et al. [27], as well as negative circumferential (CRM) and distal resection margins (DRM). One of the pioneers of taTME, Professor Antonio Lacy, recently published his initial 140 cases and achieved a complete TME specimen in over 97% of cases with a positive CRM of 6.4% and early recurrence rate of <3% over a mean follow-up period of 15 months [23]. In the systematic review by Similis et al. [20] that included 510 patients, the mesorectum was described as complete or nearly complete in 88% and 6%, respectively, whilst the CRM was negative in 95% and DRM negative in 99.7%. The international registry data [26] included 634 cancer cases and also showed promising results with low CRM positivity and good-quality TME specimens in 2.4% and 96%, respectively. Further analysis by multivariate logistic regression identified three factors that significantly increased the risk of obtaining poor histological features (R1, rectal perforation and poor TME quality): (1) low tumour height of <2 cm from anorectal junction, (2) positive CRM on staging MRI and (3) more extensive posterior pelvic dissection performed abdominally. Direct visualisation of the tumour prior to placing the distal purse string at the start of the taTME procedure explains the low rates of positive DRM. Better visualisation of the anatomy and hence more accurate dissection are likely to be the main reasons for obtaining such reassuring CRM rates and good-quality TME specimens, especially when the majority of cases included were overweight male patients with T3 tumours. Such results compare favourably to those reported for open and laparoscopic TME, with an overall positive CRM rate of 16% and 10% in the CLASSIC [4] and COLOR II [5] trials, respectively. Even the two most recent randomised controlled trials (RCTs) comparing laparoscopic to open surgery for rectal cancer, ACOSOG Z6051 [28] and ALaCaRT [29], could not demonstrate non-inferiority of laparoscopic TME over open TME for histopathological outcomes and morbidity. The positive CRM rate for laparoscopic versus open TME surgery in these trials was 7–12.1% vs. 3–7.7%, respectively.

Tuech et al. [30] published recurrence rates and survival for one of the longest follow-up periods, with a median of 29 (18–52) months, reporting an overall survival rate of 96.4%, disease-free survival rate of 94.2% and local recurrence rate of 1.7%. Metastatic disease was diagnosed after surgery in 2 out of 52 patients (3.8%). Further studies on long-term oncological outcomes are pending.

Quality of Life and Functional Outcomes

Injury to the pelvic hypogastric or sacral splanchnic nerves is a recognised complication of rectal resection and can lead to urinary and sexual dysfunction [31, 32]. The incidences of urinary and sexual dysfunction after laparoscopic or open TME have been reported to be 0–26% and 11–38%, respectively [33–35]. One of the most common complications found in Similis et al.'s review was urinary retention and transient urinary dysfunction following taTME at a rate of 5% [20]. Sylla et al. demonstrated with urodynamic testing the presence of minimal detrusor activity secondary to parasympathetic nerve injury on their two cases of urinary dysfunction [36].

Four studies collected postoperative Wexner scores for bowel function over a follow-up period ranging from 3 to 12 months and found a mean score of 4.3 (good function) [30, 37–39]. More detailed and longer-term functional outcomes and quality of life questionnaires are still pending.

Evidence so far suggests that taTME may provide a better view for more accurate dissection of the 'holy plane', which subsequently protects the autonomic pelvic nerves, and therefore potentially has a lower incidence of urinary and sexual dysfunction. However, longer-term results are still needed, and the effects of constant prolonged anal dilatation by both rigid and flexible transanal platforms remain to be explored.

Future of taTME

As the interest and evidence for taTME continue to grow, so does the number of surgeons wishing to learn this new technique. It is therefore vitally important to ensure that adequate training is available with a system that fully supports surgeons and allows a strong network of communication. The need to create a structured educational curriculum for taTME was acknowledged and proposed at the first international taTME educational group meeting in the United Kingdom in October 2015 [40]. The educational group aims to broaden the knowledge in this field by sharing experiences amongst surgeons and facilitating international research collaborations. An interactive online website (www.tatme.com) has been launched by the International taTME Educational Collaborative and provides valuable training material, up-to-date literature, access to the taTME registry and information on upcoming taTME workshops [41].

The true benefits and risks of taTME now need to be confirmed in randomised controlled trials. The first to be initiated in Europe include the national multicentre study in France called ETAP-GRECCAR 11 [42] and the international RCT COLOR III [43]. Results from these studies will not be available for at least 3–5 years but will be eagerly awaited. During this time, however, taTME is likely to undergo further modifications. Early studies have already shown promising results with the application of the robot to the transanal component [38, 44–46]. Furthermore, Atallah et al. demonstrated the feasibility of using intra-operative CT-guided navigation for the first case of frameless stereotactic navigation in transanal rectal surgery [47]. The expanding field of surgical innovation and development is likely to introduce even more specialised equipment and adjuncts to the 'standard' taTME technique, making this a truly exciting journey to follow and be part of.

In conclusion, the strive to obtain better oncological resections with less functional compromise has led to the fascinating evolution of rectal cancer surgery. taTME resulted from the combination of various minimally invasive approaches and detailed preliminary animal and cadaveric work. Results from large cohort studies and comparative studies so far are promising, although they do highlight the importance of adequate training and experience in the new technique in order to avoid unforeseen complications, namely, urethral injury. Results from the recently started European RCTs will be eagerly awaited, as well as the latest innovative advances in technology and innovation.

Disclosures None

Consent Written informed patient consent for the use of anonymised images in research has been obtained.

References

1. Targarona EM, Balague C, Pernas JC, Martinez C, Berindoague R, Gich I, et al. Can we predict immediate outcome after laparoscopic rectal surgery? Multivariate analysis of clinical, anatomic, and pathologic features after 3-dimensional reconstruction of the pelvic anatomy. Ann Surg. 2008;247(4):642–9.
2. SJ O, Shin JY. Risk factors of circumferential resection margin involvement in the patients with extraperitoneal rectal cancer. J Korean Surg Soc. 2012;82(3):165–71.
3. Cecil TD, Taffinder N, Gudgeon AM. A personal view on laparoscopic rectal cancer surgery. Color Dis. 2006;8:30–2.
4. Jayne DG, Guillou PJ, Thorpe H, Quirke P, Copeland J, Smith AM, et al. Randomized trial of laparoscopic-assisted resection of colorectal carcinoma: 3-year results of the UK MRC CLASICC trial Group. J Clin Oncol. 2007;25:3061–8.

5. van der Pas MHGM, Haglind E, Cuesta MA, Furst A, Lacy AM, Hop WC, et al. Laparoscopic versus open surgery for rectal cancer (COLOR II): short-term outcomes of a randomized, phase 3 trial. Lancet Oncol. 2013;14:210–8.
6. Buess G, Theiss R, Hutterer F, Pichlmaier H, Pelz C, Holfeld T, et al. Transanal endoscopic surgery of the rectum: testing a new method in animal experiments. Leber Magen Darm. 1983;13:73–7.
7. Marks JH, Frenkel JL, D'Andrea AP, Greenleaf CE. Maximizing rectal cancer results: TEM and TATA techniques to expand sphincter preservation. Surg Oncol Clin N Am. 2011;20:501–20.
8. Rattner D, Kalloo A. ASGE/SAGES Working Group on natural orifice transluminal endoscopic surgery. Surg Endosc. 2006;20:329–33.
9. Whiteford MH, Denk PM, Swanstrom LL. Feasibility of radical sigmoid colectomy performed as natural orifice transluminal endoscopy surgery (NOTES) using transanal endoscopic microsurgery. Surg Endosc. 2007;21:1870–4.
10. Atallah S, Albert M, Larach S. Transanal minimally invasive surgery: a giant leap forward. Surg Endosc. 2010;24:2200–5.
11. Buchs NC, Kraus R, Mortensen NJ, Cunningham C, George B, Jones O, et al. Endoscopically assisted extralevator abdominoperineal excision. Color Dis. 2015;17(12):O277–80.
12. Liyanage C, Ramwell A, Harris GJ, Levy BF, Simson JN. Transanal endoscopic microsurgery: a new technique for completion proctectomy. Color Dis. 2013;15(9):e542–7.
13. de Buck van Overstraeten A, Wolthuis AM, D'Hoore A. Transanal completion proctectomy after total colectomy and ileal pouch-anal anastomosis for ulcerative colitis: a modified single stapled technique. Color Dis. 2016;18(4):O141–4.
14. Motson RW, Whiteford MH, Hompes R, Albert M, Miles WF, Expert Group. Current status of trans-anal total mesorectal excision (TaTME) following the Second International Consensus Conference. Color Dis. 2016;18(1):13–18
15. Sylla P, Willingham FF, Sohn DK, Gee D, Brugge WR, Rattner DW. NOTES rectosigmoid resection using transanal endoscopic microsurgery (TEM) with transgastric endoscopic assistance: a pilot study in swine. J Gastrointest Surg. 2008;12:1717–23.
16. Trunzo JA, Delaney CP. Natural orifice proctectomy using a transanal endoscopic microsurgical technique in a porcine model. Surg Innov. 2010;17:48–52.
17. Sylla P, Kim M, Dursun A, et al. NOTES rectosigmoid resection using transanal endoscopic microsurgery (TEM): experience in human cadavers. Dis Colon Rectum. 2010;53:640.
18. Sylla P, Rattner DW, Delgado S, Lacy AM. NOTES transanal rectal cancer resection using transanal endoscopic microsurgery and laparoscopic assistance. Surg Endosc. 2010;24:1205–10.
19. Leroy J, Barry BD, Melani A, Mutter D, Marescaux J. No-scar transanal total mesorectal excision: the last step to pure NOTES for colorectal surgery. JAMA Surg. 2013;148:226–30.
20. Similis C, Hompes R, Penna M, Rasheed S, Tekkis PPA. systematic review of transanal total mesorectal excision: is this the future of rectal cancer surgery? Color Dis. 2015;18:19–36.
21. Arunachalam L, O'Grady H, Hunter IA, Killeen S. A systematic review of outcomes after transanal mesorectal resection for rectal cancer. Dis Colon Rectum. 2016;59:340–50.
22. Penna M, Knol KK, Tuynman JB, Tekkis PP, Mortensen NJ, Hompes R. Four anastomotic techniques following transanal total mesorectal excision (TaTME). Tech Coloproctol. 2016;20(3): 185–91.
23. Lacy AM, Tasende MM, Delgado S, Fernandez-Hevia M, Jimenez M, De Lacy B, et al. Transanal total mesorectal excision for rectal cancer: outcomes after 140 patients. J Am Coll Surg. 2015;221(2):415–23.
24. Rouanet P, Mourregot A, Azar CC, Carrere S, Gutowski M, Quenet F, et al. Transanal endoscopic proctectomy: an innovative procedure for difficult resection of rectal tumors in men with narrow pelvis. Dis Colon Rectum. 2013;56:408–15.
25. Schirnhofer J, Brunner E, Mittermair C, et al. Technical issues in transanal minimal invasive surgery: total mesorectal excision (TAMIS-TME). Eur Surg. 2014;46:S58.
26. Penna M, Hompes R, Arnold S, TaTME Registry Collaborative, et al. Transanal total mesorectal excision international registry results of the first 720 cases. Ann Surg. 2016;266(1):111–7. https://doi.org/10.1097/SLA.0000000000001948.

27. Quirke P, Durdey P, Dixon MF, Williams NS. Local recurrence of rectal adenocarcinoma due to inadequate surgical resection. Histopathological study of lateral tumor spread and surgical excision. Lancet. 1986;2(8514):996–9.
28. Fleshman J, Branda M, Sargent DJ, Am B, George V, Abbas M, et al. Effect of laparoscopic-assisted resection vs open resection of stage II or III rectal cancer on pathologic outcomes: the ACOSOG Z6051 randomized clinical trial. JAMA. 2015;314(13):1346–55.
29. Stevenson AR, Solomon MJ, Lumley JW, Hewett P, Clouston AD, Gebski VJ, et al. Effect of laparoscopic-assisted resection vs open resection on pathological outcomes in rectal cancer: the ALaCaRT randomized clinical trial. JAMA. 2015;314(13):1356–63.
30. Tuech JJ, Karoui M, Lelong B, De Chaisemartin C, Bridoux V, Manceau G, et al. A step toward NOTES total mesorectal excision for rectal cancer: endoscopic transanal proctectomy. Ann Surg. 2015;261:228–33.
31. Kim NK, Aahn TW, Park JK, Lee KY, Lee WH, Sohn SK, et al. Assessment of sexual and voiding function after total mesorectal excision with pelvic autonomic nerve preservation in males with rectal cancer. Dis Colon Rectum. 2002;45:1178–85.
32. Morino M, Parini U, Allaix ME, Monasterolo G, Brachet Contul R, Garrone C. Male sexual and urinary function after laparoscopic total mesorectal excision. Surg Endosc. 2009;23:1233–40.
33. Maurer CA. Urinary and sexual function after total mesorectal excision. Recent Results Cancer Res. 2005;165:196–204.
34. Pocard M, Zinzindohoue F, Haab F, Caplin S, Parc R, Tiret E. A prospective study of sexual and urinary function before and after total mesorectal excision with autonomic nerve preservation for rectal cancer. Surgery. 2002;131:368–72.
35. Quah HM, Jayne DG, Eu KW, Seow-Choen F. Bladder and sexual dysfunction following laparoscopically assisted and conventional open mesorectal resection for cancer. Br J Surg. 2002;89:1551–6.
36. Sylla P, Bordeianou LG, Berger D, Han KS, Lauwers GY, Sahani DV, et al. A pilot study of natural orifice transanal endoscopic total mesorectal excision with laparoscopic assistance for rectal cancer. Surg Endosc. 2013;27:3396–405.
37. Dumont F, Goéré D, Honoré C, Elias D. Transanal endoscopic total mesorectal excision combined with single-port laparoscopy. Dis Colon Rectum. 2012;55:996–1001.
38. Gómez Ruiz M, Parra IM, Palazuelos CM, Martin JA, Fernandez CC, Diego CC, et al. Robotic-assisted laparoscopic transanal total mesorectal excision for rectal cancer: a prospective pilot study. Dis Colon Rectum. 2015;58:145–53.
39. Elmore U, Fumagalli Romario U, Vignali A, Sosa MF, Angiolini MR, Rosati R. Laparoscopic anterior resection with transanal total mesorectal excision for rectal cancer: preliminary experience and impact on postoperative bowel function. J Laparoendosc Adv Surg Tech A. 2015; 25:364–9.
40. Penna M, Hompes R, Mackenzie H, Carter F, Francis NK. First international training and assessment consensus workshop on transanal total mesorectal excision (taTME). Tech Coloproctol. 2016;20(6):343–52. https://doi.org/10.1007/s10151-016-1454-2.
41. International taTME Educational Collaborative website, available at www.tatme.com. Accessed 20 Aug 2016.
42. ClinicalTrials.gov website. Evaluate efficacy, morbidity and functional outcome of endoscopic transanal proctectomy vs standard transabdominal laparoscopic proctectomy for rectal cancer (ETAP). https://clinicaltrials.gov/ct2/show/NCT02584985. Accessed 26 Aug 2016.
43. Deijen CL, Velthuis S, Tsai A, Mavroveli S, de Lange-Klerk ES, Sietses C, et al. COLOR III: a multicentre randomized clinical trial comparing transanal TME versus laparoscopic TME for mid and low rectal cancer. Surg Endosc. 2015;30(8):3210–5. https://doi.org/10.1007/s00464-015-4615-x.
44. Atallah S, Nassif G, Polavarapu H, deBeche-Adams T, Ouyang J, Albert M, Larach S. Robotic-assisted transanal surgery for total mesorectal excision (RATS-TME): a description of a novel surgical approach with video demonstration. Tech Coloproctol. 2013;17:441–7.

45. Gomez Ruiz M, Palazuelos CM, Martin Parra JI, Alonso Martin J, Cagigas Fernandez C, del Castillo Diego J, et al. New technique of transanal proctectomy with completely robotic total mesorectal excision for rectal cancer. Cir Esp. 2014;92:356–61.
46. Verheijen PM, Consten EC, Broeders IA. Robotic transanal total mesorectal excision for rectal cancer: experience with a first case. Int J Med Robot. 2014;10:423–6.
47. Atallah S, Nassif G, Larach S. Stereotactic nagivation for TAMIS-TME: opening the gateway to frameless, image-guided abdominal and pelvic surgery. Surg Endosc. 2015;29:207–11.
48. Veltcamp Helback M, Deijen CL, Velthius S, Bonjer HJ, Tuynman JB, Sietses C. Transanal total mesorectal excision for rectal carcinoma: short-term outcomes and experience after 80 cases. Surg Endosc. 2016;30(2):464–70.
49. Burke JP, Martin-Perez B, Khan A. Transanal total mesorectal excision for rectal cancer: early outcomes in 50 consecutive patients. Color Dis. 2016;18(6):570–7.

Part VIII

Sphincter-Preserving Strategies for Low Rectal Cancer

Management of Low Rectal Cancer After Complete Clinical Response

26

Angelita Habr-Gama, Guilherme Pagin São Julião, Cecilia Beatriz Rossi, Bruna Borba Vailati, and Rodrigo Oliva Perez

Introduction

Rectal cancer management has become increasingly complex over the last few decades [1]. The widespread use of neoadjuvant therapies has introduced a new variable, tumor response, which may dramatically change the ultimate surgical decision from radical surgery to local excision, transanal endoscopic microsurgery, or even no surgery at all for the management of these patients.

Assessing Tumor Response

The rationale for assessing tumor response after neoadjuvant therapy is to define final treatment strategy based upon the current status of the tumor, that is, after therapy. Following neoadjuvant therapy, tumors present significant changes in size, depth, and proximity to the mesorectal fascia. Even if total mesorectal excision (TME) will be the definitive treatment strategy, it may be considerably useful to know ahead of time what challenges are expected during surgical resection.

In up to 42% of patients undergoing neoadjuvant chemoradiotherapy (nCRT), however, complete tumor regression may develop [2]. The problem is that most of the times radical surgery is required to appropriately confirm the presence of complete pathological response (cPR). In an effort to spare patients from potentially unnecessary surgery, colorectal surgeons have attempted to assess tumor response in order to estimate pathological response by clinical, endoscopic, and radiological means. In this setting, the term complete clinical response (cCR) has been used for

A. Habr-Gama • G.P. São Julião • C.B. Rossi • B.B. Vailati • R.O. Perez (✉)
Department of Surgery, Angelita and Joaquim Gama Institute, São Paulo, Brazil
e-mail: gamange@uol.com.br; guilhermepc91@gmail.com; ceciliarossi_86@hotmail.com; brunabvailati@gmail.com; rodrigo.operez@gmail.com

C.M. Schlachta, P. Sylla (eds.), *Current Common Dilemmas in Colorectal Surgery*,
https://doi.org/10.1007/978-3-319-70117-2_26

patients with no clinical evidence of residual cancer after nCRT therapy. However, the features of a cCR may be quite subjective and dependent on surgeon's experience, different diagnostic tools, and treatment-related factors. Attempts to standardize the definition of a cCR are already available, particularly with the use of endoscopic and radiological imaging [3]. Still, clinical assessment remains highly subjective and surgeon-dependent.

It has been suggested that patients with cCR (*using very stringent criteria*) could be offered no immediate radical surgery. Instead, a strict surveillance program, also known as the "watch and wait" (WW) strategy, with frequent visits to the colorectal surgeon and the use of multiple staging modalities, could provide safe follow-up. Initial studies trying to estimate the accuracy of clinical assessment in predicting pCR were disappointing [4]. However, more recent studies have shown that clinical assessment can accurately detect pathological response when stringent criteria are used [5]. In a recent retrospective study, surgeons were asked to indicate the presence of pCR based on photographs of resected specimens without any information on radiological imaging or digital rectal examination (DRE). Curiously, negative and positive predictive values were ≥90% using these stringent criteria. On one hand, this means that using these criteria would be considerably safe to offer no immediate surgery to these patients [5, 6]. On the other hand, the low overall specificity of these features in identifying a pCR will inevitably lead to a significant proportion of patients that still undergo radical surgery. In fact, recent reports suggest that the majority of patients that develop pCR still harbor incomplete clinical response at the time of assessment of response [7, 8] (Fig. 26.1). Altogether, these data suggest that there is significant room for improvement to allow a more substantial proportion of patients to avoid unnecessary radical surgery after developing pCR [7].

Intervals between CRT completion and assessment of response may also be relevant. Studies suggest that longer intervals are associated with higher pCR rates [9–11]. The only randomized study comparing two different intervals between CRT completion and surgery demonstrated that patients undergoing a 6-week interval developed

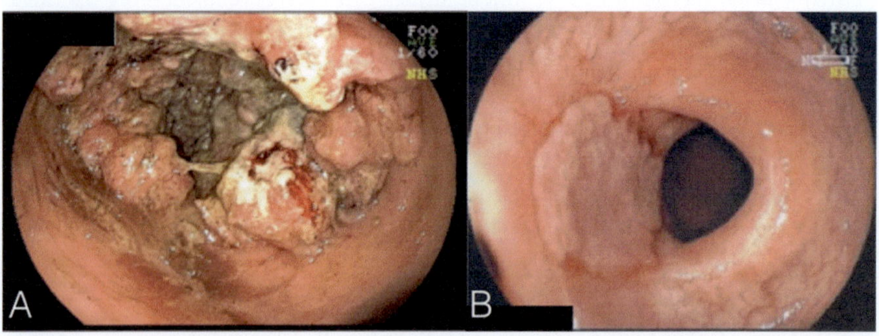

Fig. 26.1 (**a**) Endoscopic view of rectal tumor before neoadjuvant treatment. (**b**) Endoscopic view of the same patient 10 weeks after neoadjuvant treatment showing residual ulcer, considered incomplete clinical response based on stringent criteria used to define complete response. This patient did not undergo surgery and is sustaining a complete response after 30 months of follow up

more significant tumor regression when compared to a 2-week interval. Retrospective data has further suggested that intervals longer than 6 weeks could be associated with even higher rates of tumor regression. In fact, several small series reported on higher rates of pCR after 7 weeks of CRT. Another study suggested that pCR rates would only plateau after 12 weeks from CRT completion [9, 10, 12, 13]. These findings led to the prospective non-randomized study using CRT and consolidation chemotherapy (delivered after CRT completion). In this study, patients were enrolled in different treatment regimens with progressively longer intervals from CRT completion (8, 12, 16, and 20 weeks). During these intervals, patients would receive additional cycles of consolidation chemotherapy (0, 2, 4, and 6, respectively). The use of longer intervals and additional cycles of FOLFOX was independently associated with the development of a pCR (18%, 25%, 30%, and 38%, respectively; $p = 0.003$) [14].

There are ongoing randomized studies to address these issues that will provide us further information on the ideal interval between CRT and assessment of response, in an effort to maximize the chances of a patient developing a complete response [12]. There is a chance, however, that intervals will need to be tailored or individualized for each patient, as tumors may respond differently as a function of time since treatment [15]. It has been our practice to assess tumor response at least 8 weeks from CRT completion. As said, longer intervals (up to 12 weeks) have been used for the majority of patients unless there is worsening of symptoms or radiological evidence of disease progression. Even though this is rarely seen, it is not impossible.

Response assessment always begins with characterization of symptoms. Symptomatic patients rarely have complete tumor regression, even though this feature has very low specificity. DRE is perhaps one of the most relevant tools in tumor response assessment. There is currently no single diagnostic tool that can possibly replace the information given by DRE. Very frequently, irregularities of the rectal wall are better felt than seen and should be considered as highly suspicious for residual cancer. In the presence of rectal wall irregularities, mass ulceration, or stenosis, patients are recommended standard radical resection. In terms of DRE, a cCR is the absence of any irregularity of the rectal wall. The area can be thickened and firm, but to be considered a cCR, the surface has to be regular and smooth [3].

Endoscopic assessment is also very important. Whitening of the mucosa and telangiectasia are usually seen in patients with a cCR (Fig. 26.2). The presence of any ulceration or mucosal irregularity missed on DRE should prompt additional investigations and usually rule out a cCR. During flexible or rigid proctoscopy, biopsies are frequently considered for assessment of response.Forceps biopsies rarely add clinically relevant information if there is clinical evidence (DRE and endoscopic) of a cCR [16]. On the other hand, in the presence of clinical evidence of residual cancer (incomplete response), endoscopic biopsies are also rarely useful, except for convincing patients there is residual disease there. Even in the presence of negative endoscopic biopsies, patients with incomplete clinical response should not be offered a nonoperative approach [16]. Considering the poor results with forceps endoscopic biopsies, a novel strategy using incisional biopsies in an ex vivo model has been attempted. In the presence of an incomplete pathological response, incisional biopsies were able to detect only 55%. As such, incisional biopsy is

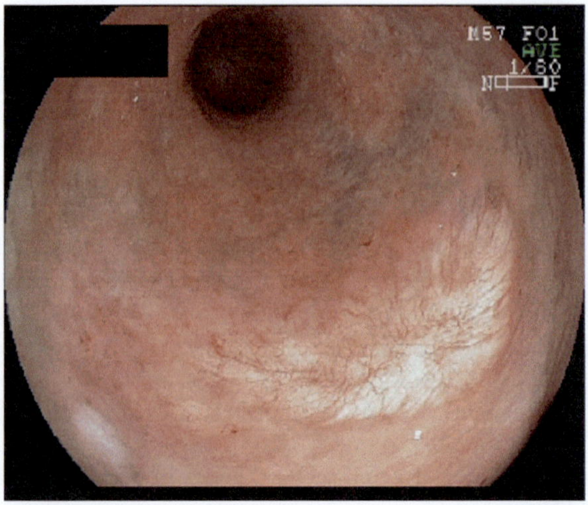

Fig. 26.2 Endoscopic view of rectal cancer that developed cCR after neoadjuvant chemoradiation, showing whitening of the mucosa and telangiectasia

certainly not suitable as a stand-alone method to deem patients fit for WW [17]. The potential utility of incisional biopsy may be restricted in its ability to identify patients with residual disease that may otherwise have been considered for a WW approach. It is likely that the reason for the poor sensitivity for residual disease using incisional biopsy was due to the fragmented and scattered distribution of some residual tumors [18].

Local Excision of the Tumor Site

A full-thickness excision of a residual lesion following nCRT may be an interesting alternative in patients with incomplete clinical response. However, the use of TEM for resection of a scar in the setting of a cCR may not the best treatment alternative [19]. Resection of a scar in a patient with a cCR would provide pathological confirmation of a complete response (pCR). However, this may be the sole benefit of this approach in the setting of a cCR [19].

In this setting, TEM may also have significant disadvantages including perioperative morbidity and functional consequences. Although many studies have demonstrated the significantly lower morbidity rates after local excision when compared to radical surgery, perioperative complications after TEM in the setting of neoadjuvant chemoradiation are much higher [20, 21]. The most frequent complication associated with this procedure after CRT is wound dehiscence. Frequently, wound separations lead to considerable rectal pain and need for readmission for pain control [21].

In addition, patients undergoing TEM after CRT may also develop significant functional consequences in terms of fecal continence. The comparison of anorectal function between patients undergoing neoadjuvant CRT and nonoperative management or TEM resulted in superior outcomes for patients managed nonoperatively.

Full-thickness transanal local excision using TEM for residual cancers in patients with near-complete response to neoadjuvant CRT resulted in significant decreases in anal resting and pressures, rectal capacity, and sensitivity. Moreover, these differences translated into significant worsening of fecal continence and quality-of-life scores in the TEM group. In fact, patients managed by CRT developing a cCR managed nonoperatively had normal anorectal function nearly 3 years after CRT completion [22].

Therefore, when deciding between local excision and observation alone for the management of patients with cCR following neoadjuvant CRT, these issues need to be taken into account: First, both strategies have been considered to be organ-sparing alternatives, but function preservation may be truly only achieved with non-operative management. Second, the benefits of TEM either for diagnostic or therapeutic purposes become significantly restricted to highly selected patients that can potentially avoid a major operation but will still face a significantly morbid and painful procedure.

Special Consideration: Residual Adenoma

A considerable number of patients with complete regression of the primary cancer after CRT may still harbor residual adenomas at the site of the primary rectal cancer. These lesions usually harbor high-grade dysplasia adenomatous tissue and may be more resistant to CRT than we expected. They seem to represent areas of the primary cancer that ultimately did not respond to CRT as their invasive counterpart. Residual adenomas should not be considered as cCR or pCR even though there is no residual invasive cancer. Despite their inability to invade and disseminate, these lesions require some type of surgical or endoscopic resection as progression to invasive adenocarcinoma is likely to occur. In this setting, full-thickness excision of these lesions provides appropriate management of the adenoma in addition to accurate assessment of primary cancer response to CRT within the rectal wall and should be the preferred initial treatment [23].

Radiological Imaging

Radiological assessment of response is of paramount importance to appropriately select patients for an alternative treatment strategy such as the WW approach following a cCR. As a matter of fact, the developments in radiological imaging, including both PET/CT and MR, have been quite significant. Proper magnetic resonance imaging (MRI) with the use of diffusion-weighted techniques is now used routinely for the assessment of response in these patients. Currently, we would only consider a true complete responder: (1) a patient showing low-signal intensity area replacing the area of the previous tumor or (2) a patient with no detectable abnormalities in standard MR associated with no evidence of disease on clinical and endoscopic examination (Fig. 26.3). A recent publication has reported three different patterns of

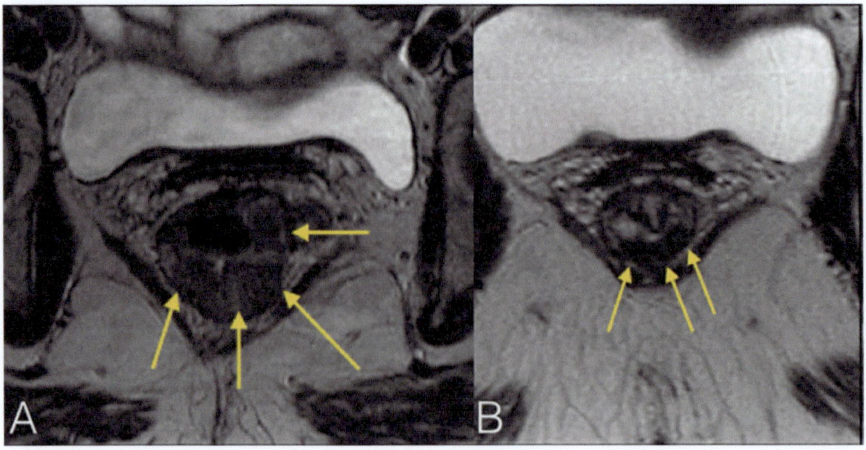

Fig. 26.3 Axial high-resolution T2WI magnetic resonance (MR) imaging (**a**) showing pretreatment rectal tumor—yellow arrow. (**b**) MR imaging from the same patient after neoadjuvant treatment showing complete radiological response, as low-signal intensity

low-signal intensity that are compatible with a cCR: minimal fibrosis, transmural fibrosis, and irregular fibrosis [24]. Others have attempted to estimate tumor regression grades (as described for pathological assessment) [25] by standard MRI [26]. In addition, diffusion-weighted MR series may provide evidence of absence of restriction to diffusion to fulfill the criteria for a radiological complete response [27]. In our previously reported experiences with this WW treatment strategy, MR imaging was not available to a significant proportion of patients [28]. Therefore, there is a hope that incorporation of these findings for the selection of patients with cCR will significantly impact the outcomes of the WW strategy. The presence of mixed signal intensity within the area of the previous cancer should raise a suspicion of an incomplete clinical response. In addition to the assessment of the rectal wall, the mesorectum is also at risk for the presence of residual cancer despite complete primary regression (ypT0N1). Therefore, MRI should also provide the colorectal surgeon with information regarding possible mesorectal (or even lateral node) involvement regardless of primary tumor response.

Molecular imaging may also play a role in the assessment of tumor response. PET/CT imaging offers information on tumor metabolism in addition to standard radiological anatomical features. In this setting, PET/CT has been used for the assessment of tumor response to neoadjuvant chemoradiation therapy [29, 30]. In addition to the visual identification of FDG uptake within the area of the rectal wall harboring the tumor or within the mesorectum, PET/CT allows the estimation of the metabolism profile [15]. Even though we have used PET/CT to distinguish between complete and incomplete responses in the setting of a prospective study with acceptable overall accuracy (85%), its ability for the detection of a cCR (or its negative predictive value) was rather disappointing (<80%). More recent data, incorporating variations in tumor volume and metabolism together (total lesion glycolysis variation) using PET/CT imaging has resulted in improved detection of complete responders with a negative predictive value of >90%. Therefore, the use of this imaging modality in the setting of precise metabolic tumor volume estimation prior to and following nCRT is a promising tool in the assessment of tumor response to be validated in future studies [31].

Follow-Up

When a nonoperative strategy for cCR in rectal cancer is considered, a relatively intensive follow-up is certainly required. Patients should be encouraged to adhere to this strict follow-up program in order to allow early recognition of any local or systemic recurrence and therefore increasing the chance of a successful salvage treatment. After initial assessment of response confirming a cCR, visits should be performed every 1–2 months during the first year, every 3 months during the second year, and every 6 months thereafter. DRE, proctoscopy, and CEA level determination are recommended for all visits. Timing for radiological assessment during follow-up has not yet been standardized. Routine MRI for the assessment of the rectal wall, mesorectum, and pelvic nodes every 6 months for the first 2 years and yearly thereafter has been our practice.

Outcomes

Patients managed nonoperatively under the WW strategy after a cCR following neoadjuvant chemoradiation were originally reported to have similar long-term oncological outcomes to patients with pCR after radical surgery [32]. Additional retrospective studies have been consistently reported by other groups showing similar oncological outcomes between these subgroups of patients [33–39]. These findings further support the idea that patients with a cCR may be spared from the surgical morbidity and mortality of radical surgery with no oncological compromise [40]. In addition, functional outcomes of patients managed nonoperatively appear to be better not only to radical surgery but also to other organ-preserving strategies (transanal local excision) [22, 33].

Local recurrences after this treatment strategy are still a concern and may develop at any time during follow-up. The majority of local recurrences appears to develop within the first 12 months of follow-up and may represent limitations in the precise identification of microscopic residual disease among "apparent" complete clinical responders. For these reasons, these "early recurrences" developing within the initial 12 months of follow-up have been called "early regrowths" instead [41]. Still, close and strict follow-up may allow early detection of regrowths leading to identical oncological outcomes to patients with incomplete clinical response immediately after 8–12 weeks from CRT completion [42]. In addition, local recurrences (late and early regrowths) are usually amenable to salvage therapies, often allowing sphincter preservation and associated with excellent long-term local disease control [41].

Considering that the rate of complete clinical or pathological response was historically <30% of patients across most of the studies, one could assume that this treatment strategy could benefit a rather limited proportion of patients with rectal cancer. However, the observation of increased rates of complete response (clinical or pathological) using regimens with consolidation chemotherapy and with the inclusion of earlier stages of disease (cT2N0 otherwise candidates for ultra-low resections or APRs) may result in nearly 50% that ultimately avoid surgical resection [14, 43]. This has been further confirmed in a prospective trial including patients with T2 and T3 rectal cancer managed by CRT and an additional endorectal high-dose brachytherapy boost (total 65Gy) that showed a 58% cCR rate at 2 years of follow-up without surgical resection [34].

A recent study using a propensity score matched cohort analysis comparing WW and radical surgery has been designed to demonstrate the non-inferiority of the WW approach. Curiously, however, the comparison between groups demonstrated a slight superiority of the nonoperative management of these patients in terms of survival and a clear benefit in colostomy-free survival even when accounting for the development of local recurrences [39, 44].

Patients with a complete clinical or pathological response to CRT are still at risk for developing systemic recurrences. In a pooled analysis of patients undergoing neoadjuvant CRT followed by radical surgery and pCR, 5-year distant metastases-free survival was 88.8% (11.2% systemic recurrence rate) even though nearly 40% of these patients did receive adjuvant systemic chemotherapy [45]. In contrast, the systemic recurrence rate among patients with cCR managed nonoperatively without routine adjuvant chemotherapy has been reported to be 14% [41].

References

1. Kosinski L, Habr-Gama A, Ludwig K, Perez R. Shifting concepts in rectal cancer management: a review of contemporary primary rectal cancer treatment strategies. CA Cancer J Clin. 2012;62(3):173–202.
2. Sanghera P, Wong DW, McConkey CC, Geh JI, Hartley A. Chemoradiotherapy for rectal cancer: an updated analysis of factors affecting pathological response. Clin Oncol. 2008;20(2):176–83.
3. Habr-Gama A, Perez RO, Wynn G, Marks J, Kessler H, Gama-Rodrigues J. Complete clinical response after neoadjuvant chemoradiation therapy for distal rectal cancer: characterization of clinical and endoscopic findings for standardization. Dis Colon Rectum. 2010;53(12):1692–8.
4. Hiotis SP, Weber SM, Cohen AM, Minsky BD, Paty PB, Guillem JG, et al. Assessing the predictive value of clinical complete response to neoadjuvant therapy for rectal cancer: an analysis of 488 patients. J Am Coll Surg. 2002;194(2):131–5. Discussion 5–6.
5. Smith FM, Chang KH, Sheahan K, Hyland J, O'Connell PR, Winter DC. The surgical significance of residual mucosal abnormalities in rectal cancer following neoadjuvant chemoradiotherapy. Br J Surg. 2012;99(7):993–1001.
6. Habr-Gama A, Perez RO. The surgical significance of residual mucosal abnormalities in rectal cancer following neoadjuvant chemoradiotherapy. Br J Surg. 2012;99(11):1601. Author reply 2.
7. Smith FM, Wiland H, Mace A, Pai RK, Kalady MF. Clinical criteria underestimate complete pathological response in rectal cancer treated with neoadjuvant chemoradiotherapy. Dis Colon Rectum. 2014;57(3):311–5.

8. Nahas SC, Rizkallah Nahas CS, Sparapan Marques CF, Ribeiro U Jr, Cotti GC, Imperiale AR, et al. Pathologic complete response in rectal cancer: can we detect it? Lessons learned from a proposed randomized trial of watch-and-wait treatment of rectal cancer. Dis Colon Rectum. 2016;59(4):255–63.
9. Kalady MF, de Campos-Lobato LF, Stocchi L, Geisler DP, Dietz D, Lavery IC, et al. Predictive factors of pathologic complete response after neoadjuvant chemoradiation for rectal cancer. Ann Surg. 2009;250(4):582–9.
10. Tulchinsky H, Shmueli E, Figer A, Klausner JM, Rabau M. An interval >7 weeks between neoadjuvant therapy and surgery improves pathologic complete response and disease-free survival in patients with locally advanced rectal cancer. Ann Surg Oncol. 2008;15(10):2661–7.
11. Francois Y, Nemoz CJ, Baulieux J, Vignal J, Grandjean JP, Partensky C, et al. Influence of the interval between preoperative radiation therapy and surgery on downstaging and on the rate of sphincter-sparing surgery for rectal cancer: the Lyon R90-01 randomized trial. J Clin Oncol. 1999;17(8):2396.
12. Evans J, Tait D, Swift I, Pennert K, Tekkis P, Wotherspoon A, et al. Timing of surgery following preoperative therapy in rectal cancer: the need for a prospective randomized trial? Dis Colon Rectum. 2011;54(10):1251–9.
13. Wolthuis AM, Penninckx F, Haustermans K, De Hertogh G, Fieuws S, Van Cutsem E, et al. Impact of interval between neoadjuvant chemoradiotherapy and TME for locally advanced rectal cancer on pathologic response and oncologic outcome. Ann Surg Oncol. 2012;19(9):2833–41.
14. Garcia-Aguilar J, Chow OS, Smith DD, Marcet JE, Cataldo PA, Varma MG, et al. Effect of adding mFOLFOX6 after neoadjuvant chemoradiation in locally advanced rectal cancer: a multicentre, phase 2 trial. Lancet Oncol. 2015;16(8):957–66.
15. Perez RO, Habr-Gama A, Sao Juliao GP, Gama-Rodrigues J, Sousa AH Jr, Campos FG, et al. Optimal timing for assessment of tumor response to neoadjuvant chemoradiation in patients with rectal cancer: do all patients benefit from waiting longer than 6 weeks? Int J Radiat Oncol Biol Phys. 2012;84(5):1159–65.
16. Perez RO, Habr-Gama A, Pereira GV, Lynn PB, Alves PA, Proscurshim I, et al. Role of biopsies in patients with residual rectal cancer following neoadjuvant chemoradiation after downsizing: can they rule out persisting cancer? Color Dis. 2012;14(6):714–20.
17. Smith FM, Wiland H, Mace A, Pai RK, Kalady MF. Assessment of a novel, full-thickness incisional biopsy model to restage rectal tumours after neoadjuvant chemoradiotherapy: results of an ex vivo pilot study. Tech Coloproctol. 2015;19(3):159–64.
18. Perez RO, Habr-Gama A, Smith FM, Kosinski L, Sao Juliao GP, Grzona E, et al. Fragmented pattern of tumor regression and lateral intramural spread may influence margin appropriateness after TEM for rectal cancer following neoadjuvant CRT. J Surg Oncol. 2014;109(8):853–8.
19. Habr-Gama A, Sao Juliao GP, Perez RO. Pitfalls of transanal endoscopic microsurgery for rectal cancer following neoadjuvant chemoradiation therapy. Minim Invasive Ther Allied Technol. 2014;23(2):63–9.
20. Marks JH, Valsdottir EB, DeNittis A, Yarandi SS, Newman DA, Nweze I, et al. Transanal endoscopic microsurgery for the treatment of rectal cancer: comparison of wound complication rates with and without neoadjuvant radiation therapy. Surg Endosc. 2009;23(5):1081–7.
21. Perez RO, Habr-Gama A, Sao Juliao GP, Proscurshim I, Scanavini Neto A, Gama-Rodrigues J. Transanal endoscopic microsurgery for residual rectal cancer after neoadjuvant chemoradiation therapy is associated with significant immediate pain and hospital readmission rates. Dis Colon Rectum. 2011;54(5):545–51.
22. Habr-Gama A, Lynn PB, Jorge JMN, São Julião GP, Proscurshim I, Gama Rodrigues J, et al. Impact of organ-preserving strategies on anorectal function in patients with distal rectal cancer following neoadjuvant chemoradiation. Dis Colon Rectum. 2016;59(4):264–9.
23. Habr-Gama A, Vianna MR, Sao Juliao GP, Rawet V, Gama-Rodrigues J, Proscurshim I, et al. Management of adenomas within the area of rectal cancer that develop complete pathological response. Int J Color Dis. 2015;30(9):1285–7.

24. Lambregts DM, Maas M, Bakers FC, Cappendijk VC, Lammering G, Beets GL, et al. Long-term follow-up features on rectal MRI during a wait-and-see approach after a clinical complete response in patients with rectal cancer treated with chemoradiotherapy. Dis Colon Rectum. 2011;54(12):1521–8.
25. Restivo A, Zorcolo L, Cocco IM, Manunza R, Margiani C, Marongiu L, et al. Elevated CEA levels and low distance of the tumor from the anal verge are predictors of incomplete response to chemoradiation in patients with rectal cancer. Ann Surg Oncol. 2013;20(3):864–71.
26. Patel UB, Taylor F, Blomqvist L, George C, Evans H, Tekkis P, et al. Magnetic resonance imaging-detected tumor response for locally advanced rectal cancer predicts survival outcomes: MERCURY experience. J Clin Oncol. 2011;29(28):3753–60.
27. Lambregts DM, Vandecaveye V, Barbaro B, Bakers FC, Lambrecht M, Maas M, et al. Diffusion-weighted MRI for selection of complete responders after chemoradiation for locally advanced rectal cancer: a multicenter study. Ann Surg Oncol. 2011;18(8):2224–31.
28. Habr-Gama A, Perez RO, Nadalin W, Nahas SC, Ribeiro U Jr, Silva ESAH Jr, et al. Long-term results of preoperative chemoradiation for distal rectal cancer correlation between final stage and survival. J Gastrointest Surg. 2005;9(1):90–9; discussion 9–101.
29. Perez RO, Habr-Gama A, Gama-Rodrigues J, Proscurshim I, Juliao GP, Lynn P, et al. Accuracy of positron emission tomography/computed tomography and clinical assessment in the detection of complete rectal tumor regression after neoadjuvant chemoradiation: long-term results of a prospective trial (National Clinical Trial 00254683). Cancer. 2012;118(14):3501–11.
30. Kristiansen C, Loft A, Berthelsen AK, Graff J, Lindebjerg J, Bisgaard C, et al. PET/CT and histopathologic response to preoperative chemoradiation therapy in locally advanced rectal cancer. Dis Colon Rectum. 2008;51(1):21–5.
31. Dos Anjos DA, Habr-Gama A, Vailati BB, Rossi CB, Coturel AE, Perez RO, et al. ^{18}F-FDG uptake by rectal cancer is similar in mucinous and nonmucinous histological subtypes. Ann Nucl Med. 2016;30:513–7.
32. Habr-Gama A, Perez RO, Nadalin W, Sabbaga J, Ribeiro U Jr, Silva e Sousa AH Jr, et al. Operative versus nonoperative treatment for stage 0 distal rectal cancer following chemoradiation therapy: long-term results. Ann Surg. 2004;240(4):711–7. Discussion 7–8.
33. Maas M, Beets-Tan RG, Lambregts DM, Lammering G, Nelemans PJ, Engelen SM, et al. Wait-and-see policy for clinical complete responders after chemoradiation for rectal cancer. J Clin Oncol. 2011;29(35):4633–40.
34. Appelt AL, Ploen J, Harling H, Jensen FS, Jensen LH, Jorgensen JC, et al. High-dose chemoradiotherapy and watchful waiting for distal rectal cancer: a prospective observational study. Lancet Oncol. 2015;16(8):919–27.
35. Vaccaro CA, Yazyi FJ, Ojra Quintana G, Santino JP, Sardi ME, Beder D, et al. Locally advanced rectal cancer: Preliminary results of rectal preservation after neoadjuvant chemoradiotherapy. Cir Esp. 2016;94(5):274–9.
36. Smith RK, Fry RD, Mahmoud NN, Paulson EC. Surveillance after neoadjuvant therapy in advanced rectal cancer with complete clinical response can have comparable outcomes to total mesorectal excision. Int J Color Dis. 2015;30(6):769–74.
37. Dalton RS, Velineni R, Osborne ME, Thomas R, Harries S, Gee AS, et al. A single-centre experience of chemoradiotherapy for rectal cancer: is there potential for nonoperative management? Color Dis. 2012;14(5):567–71.
38. Araujo RO, Valadao M, Borges D, Linhares E, de Jesus JP, Ferreira CG, et al. Nonoperative management of rectal cancer after chemoradiation opposed to resection after complete clinical response. A comparative study. Eur J Surg Oncol. 2015;41(11):1456–63.
39. Renehan AG, Malcomson L, Emsley R, Gollins S, Maw A, Myint AS, et al. Watch-and-wait approach versus surgical resection after chemoradiotherapy for patients with rectal cancer (the OnCoRe project): a propensity-score matched cohort analysis. Lancet Oncol. 2015;17(2):174–83. https://doi.org/10.1016/S1470-2045(15)00467-2.
40. Smith FM, Rao C, Oliva Perez R, Bujko K, Athanasiou T, Habr-Gama A, et al. Avoiding radical surgery improves early survival in elderly patients with rectal cancer, demonstrating

complete clinical response after neoadjuvant therapy: results of a decision-analytic model. Dis Colon Rectum. 2015;58(2):159–71.
41. Habr-Gama A, Gama-Rodrigues J, Sao Juliao GP, Proscurshim I, Sabbagh C, Lynn PB, et al. Local recurrence after complete clinical response and watch and wait in rectal cancer after neoadjuvant chemoradiation: impact of salvage therapy on local disease control. Int J Radiat Oncol Biol Phys. 2014;88(4):822–8.
42. Habr-Gama A, Perez RO, Proscurshim I, Nunes Dos Santos RM, Kiss D, Gama-Rodrigues J, et al. Interval between surgery and neoadjuvant chemoradiation therapy for distal rectal cancer: does delayed surgery have an impact on outcome? Int J Radiat Oncol Biol Phys. 2008;71(4):1181–8.
43. Habr-Gama A, Sabbaga J, Gama-Rodrigues J, Sao Juliao GP, Proscurshim I, Bailao Aguilar P, et al. Watch and wait approach following extended neoadjuvant chemoradiation for distal rectal cancer: are we getting closer to anal cancer management? Dis Colon Rectum. 2013;56(10):1109–17.
44. Perez RO. Complete clinical response in rectal cancer: a turning tide. Lancet Oncol. 2016;17(2):125–6.
45. Maas M, Nelemans PJ, Valentini V, Das P, Rodel C, Kuo LJ, et al. Long-term outcome in patients with a pathological complete response after chemoradiation for rectal cancer: a pooled analysis of individual patient data. Lancet Oncol. 2010;11(9):835–44.

Optimizing Function for Very Low Rectal Tumors: Intersphincteric Resection or APR?

27

Srikanth Parsi, Jean Salem, and John H. Marks

Introduction

Rectal cancer is a challenging entity posing technical problems of operating in the confines of the bony pelvis with proximity to the anal sphincter.

Traditionally rectal cancer was managed by abdominoperineal resection (APR) which was first described by Miles in 1908 [1]. APR was the only surgical option until Dixon performed anterior resection for upper rectal carcinoma in 1948. It took a while for surgeons to adopt the technique of anterior resection as an alternative to APR as it was associated with significant morbidity from anastomotic leak and mortality. In 1986, Heald described total mesorectal excision (TME) which dramatically improved local recurrence rate for rectal carcinoma [2]. The introduction of surgical staples in 1980s allowed ultralow anterior resection for mid-rectal tumors.

However, for low rectal cancers, APR remained the only surgical option until the transanal abdominal transanal (TATA) proctectomy and transanal endoscopic microsurgery (TEM) options emerged in the 1980s [3]. These techniques evolved with the introduction of chemoradiation in the management of rectal carcinoma which revolutionized sphincter-preserving surgery (SPS) for low rectal tumors. As part of a long-standing rectal cancer management program, we were the first to perform full-thickness local excision (FTLE) after preoperative radiation therapy in 1984 [4].

SPS in the lower pelvis has deterred surgeons because of the challenge of obtaining adequate distal and circumferential margins as well as the difficulty in performing a low anastomosis. This is due to the confines of the bony pelvis as well as the tapering

S. Parsi • J. Salem • J.H. Marks (✉)
Marks Colorectal Surgical Associates, Lankenau Institute for Medical Research, Wynnewood, PA, USA

Division of Colorectal Surgery, Lankenau Medical Center, Wynnewood, PA 19096, USA
e-mail: parsis@mlhs.org; salemj@mlhs.org; marksj@mlhs.org

C.M. Schlachta, P. Sylla (eds.), *Current Common Dilemmas in Colorectal Surgery*,
https://doi.org/10.1007/978-3-319-70117-2_27

of the mesorectum. Historically, resections in this area have been prone to local recurrence (LR) and have posed significant incontinence and poor quality of life.

To address these issues, Gerard Marks in 1984 described the transanal abdominal transanal proctectomy (TATA) with descending coloanal anastomosis for low rectal tumors following high-dose preoperative radiation [5]. The main advantage of TATA is avoidance of a permanent colostomy with preservation of the anal sphincter as this obviates the need for placement of a stapler from above. In the last few years, a modification of TATA emerged in the form of taTME (bottom-up TATA) using single-port laparoscopy to extend the dissection from below. This has even been extended to natural orifice transluminal endoscopic surgery (NOTES) where the entire procedure including splenic flexure mobilization is performed transanally [6].

Treatment Strategies for Low Rectal Cancer

Management of low rectal cancer involves a multidisciplinary team and is based on TNM staging of the disease. As part of our multidisciplinary rectal cancer management program, we offer neoadjuvant chemoradiation therapy for all tumors in the distal third of the rectum and unfavorable cancers at all levels of the rectum (i.e., ≥T3 or N+). The hallmark to extending sphincter preservation and optimizing the benefit of the downstaging effect of chemoradiation is that final decisions regarding surgical treatment are made after completion of the neoadjuvant therapy. TEM can be offered for tumors <4 cm in size, <40% of circumference, mobile, and which have regressed to within the rectal wall (≤T2).

For >T2 low rectal tumors, intersphincteric resection (ISR) should be considered along with APR. Sphincter-preserving surgery (SPS) is offered for all patients, except those whose cancer remains fixed at or below the 3 cm level.

Our standard practice is to wait 8–12 weeks and reassess clinically to decide upon the final surgical plan.

APR Vs Sphincter-Preserving Surgery

Neoadjuvant chemoradiotherapy has led to an increase in the rate of SPS by downstaging the tumor and, coupled with improved surgical technique, a decrease in the locoregional recurrence [7].

In choosing the right procedure in surgical treatment of low rectal carcinoma, one has to take into account several important factors. Patient baseline sphincter function is of course important as are tumor size and involvement of sphincter complex, response to neoadjuvant chemoradiation, level of surgeon's experience in intersphincteric surgery, and lastly patient preference after discussing pros and cons of each procedure. However, it must be emphasized that final decisions regarding sphincter preservation should be held until the 8–12-week interval to maximize the benefit of chemoradiation.

Despite this, APR rates in the literature remain as high as 32–67% [8]. We advocate that all cancers of the distal 3 cm of the rectum that are not fixed 8–12 weeks after neoadjuvant chemoradiotherapy are managed either by taTME, laparoscopic TATA, ultralow LAR, or TEM.

Preoperative Planning

Preoperative work-up includes complete blood count, metabolic profile, coagulation profile, liver function test, and baseline carcinoembryonic antigen (CEA). Digital rectal examination (DRE) along with flexible sigmoidoscopy and biopsy is performed in the office during the initial visit. Colonoscopy to rule-out synchronous lesions is performed if not done recently. Tumors are evaluated for extent of invasion by computed tomography (CT), magnetic resonance imaging (MRI), or endorectal ultrasound.

Metastatic disease is evaluated with a CT of the abdomen, pelvis, and chest. Positron-emission tomography CT is not routinely performed unless CT or MRI is equivocal for metastasis.

Patients who undergo neoadjuvant chemoradiation are initially evaluated by DRE and flexible endoscopy. Size, fixity, position, degree of ulceration, shape, clinical T stage, and level in the rectum relative to the anorectal ring are noted originally and at 8–10 weeks post-radiation therapy. At 8–12 weeks after completion of chemoradiation, final assessment is performed to determine whether ISR or APR is indicated [9]. All patients with adequate sphincter function, except those cancers that remained fixed on examination after completion of their neoadjuvant chemoradiation, undergo sphincter-preserving surgery. The TATA is utilized for patients whose cancer resides in the distal 3cm of the rectum.

Every patient undergoing an APR is seen by an ostomy specialist for ostomy teaching. A very high level of preoperative education and expectation from either surgery are discussed in detail prior to surgery.

TATA Procedure

This operation is offered to patients with non-fixed cancers in the distal 3 cm of the rectum. Patients are positioned in extreme lithotomy position with Yellofins® Stirrups (Allen Medical Systems, Acton, MA) for adequate perianal exposure (Fig. 27.1). It is therefore essential that patients are secured firmly to the operating table. Preoperative antibiotic is given along with alvimopan for faster gastrointestinal recovery in the postoperative period. The abdomen and anus are prepped with povidone-iodine and drapes secured to the anus with 2-0 nylon suture. We use lighted suction device that is very helpful during the procedure (VitalVue™, Medtronic Minimally Invasive Therapies, New Haven, CT).

To start, the perineum is injected with lidocaine and epinephrine for hemostasis and to facilitate dissection.

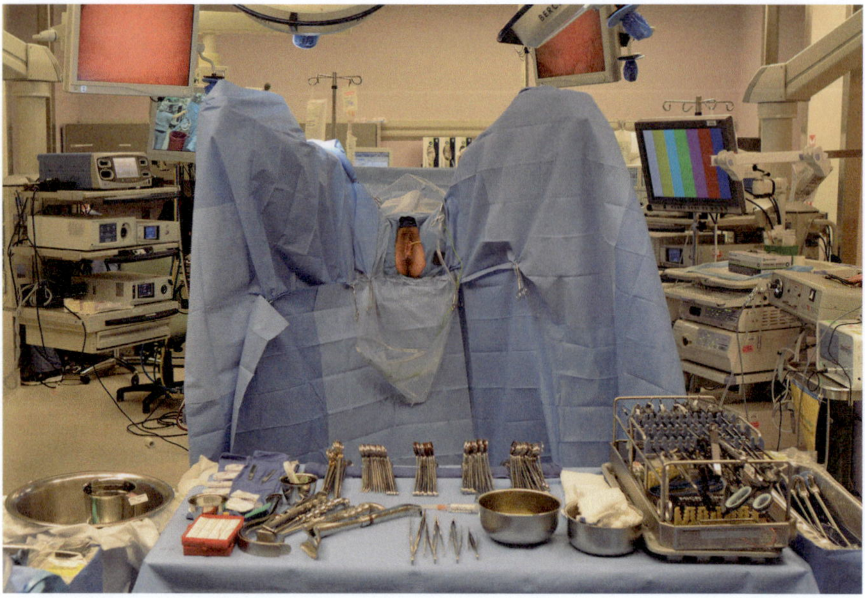

Fig. 27.1 Patient positioning and operating room setup

Allis-Adair clamps are used to evert the anal canal and to identify the dentate line (Fig. 27.2). The hallmark of the TATA is starting the operation transanally by performing a full-thickness circumferential incision at or just above the dentate line, followed by an intersphincteric dissection (Fig. 27.3). The dissection is carried out in the intersphincteric plane between the puborectalis and the internal sphincter circumferentially (Fig. 27.4). The TATA is classically performed by making an incision at the dentate line, therefore excising the upper half of the internal sphincter, while preserving the external sphincter, puborectalis, and levator ani. When the tumor invades the upper anal canal, at times a complete resection of the internal sphincter is carried out, but the functional outcome is likely impaired in this situation. The rectum is mobilized transanally to the level of the cervix in female subjects and the seminal vesicles in male subjects. This allows for a known distal margin while sparing the external sphincter and the distal half of the internal sphincter muscles. The rectum is then oversewn in a watertight fashion followed by placement of a transanal access platform (GelPOINT Path, Applied Medical, Rancho Santa Margarita, CA) and a flexible-tip Olympus videoscope (Fig. 27.5). Driving the camera is a significant challenge because of the infrequent use of flexible-tip cameras and the constant need to avoid collision with the surgeon instruments in a narrow working space. We continue the dissection with the help of a LigaSure™ (Medtronic Minimally Invasive Therapies, New Haven, CT) bipolar energy device, transanally as proximal as possible, including opening the peritoneal cavity, mobilization of the left colon and the splenic flexure, and ligation of the inferior mesenteric artery and vein, when possible.

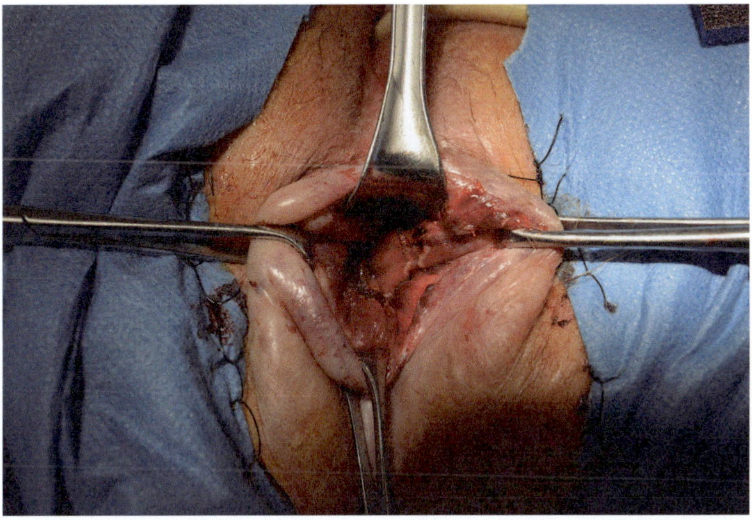

Fig. 27.2 Allis-Adair clamps are used to evert the anal canal and identify the dentate line. Dissection is started by doing a full-thickness circumferential incision at the dentate line

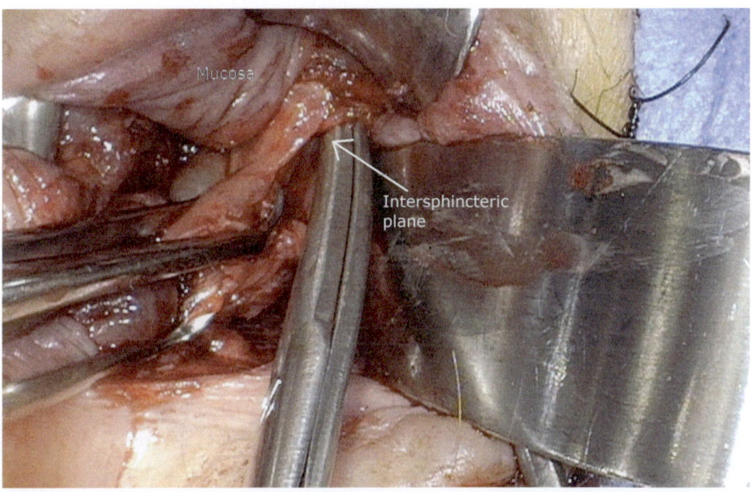

Fig. 27.3 Intersphincteric dissection carried circumferentially

The abdominal dissection is completed by open, laparoscopic, or robotic techniques. In our early experience, the abdominal portion was completed in an open fashion. Over the last decade, we began using minimally invasive transanal and transabdominal platforms for the completion of the dissection. The abdominal portion is completed laparoscopically either with a single-port or multiport technique. The rectum and sigmoid colon are then delivered transanally and transected at the sigmoid-colic junction (Fig. 27.6). A hand-sewn coloanal anastomosis is performed

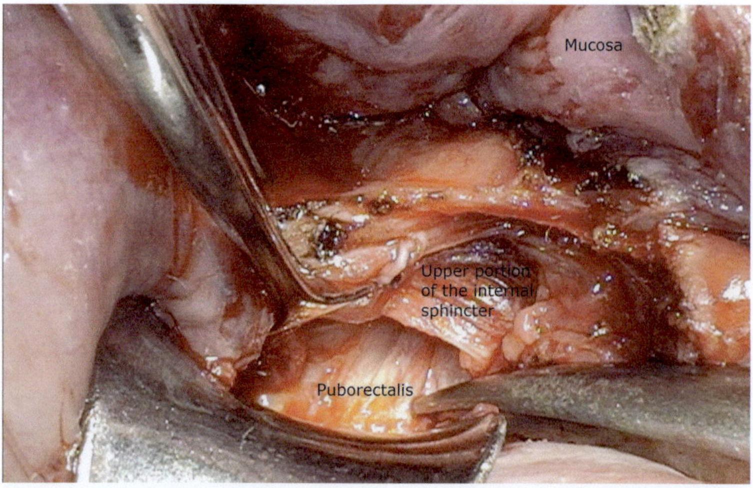

Fig. 27.4 Intersphincteric dissection landmarks: dissection carried out in the intersphincteric plane between the puborectalis and the internal sphincter. The upper portion of the internal sphincter is resected en bloc with the rectal specimen

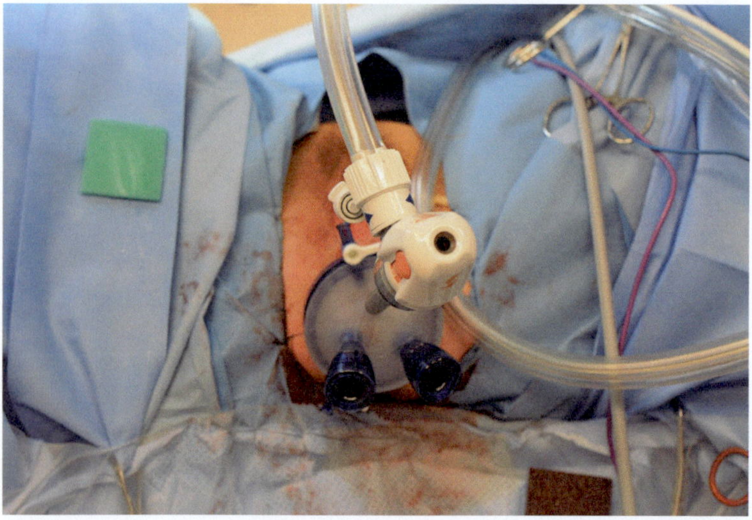

Fig. 27.5 Placement of a transanal access platform

transanally with 0 Vicryl sutures (Ethicon. Cincinnati, OH). Different options of anastomosis exist: straight coloanal, colonic J-pouch-anal, side-to-end anastomosis. A temporary diverting stoma is made to protect the coloanal anastomosis. In case of SILS abdominal approach, we use the same site for the diverting ileostomy in the right lower abdomen [10].

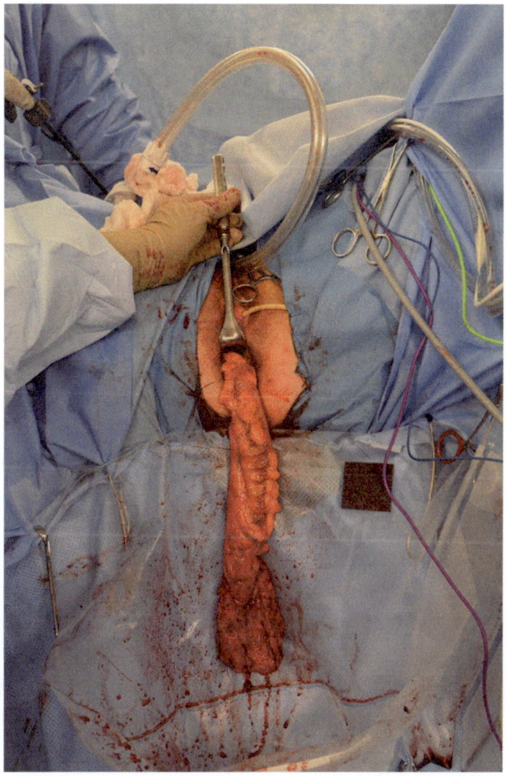

Fig. 27.6 Delivery of the specimen transanally

Complications

Early complications pertaining to TATA include anastomotic dehiscence/leak (5–48%), pelvic abscess (0–9%), intra-abdominal bleeding (0–3.8%), small bowel obstruction (0–16%), and internal hernia [11, 12]. Delayed complications include anastomotic stricture (2% to 16%) and neorectal prolapse (0.8–3.7%) [12].

Postoperative Management

Postoperatively, intravenous doxycycline is provided while the patient is hospitalized; this is continued orally for 10 days after discharge for all patients. Our postoperative pain regime includes IV ketorolac and intramuscular meperidine. Very rarely, patients need patient-controlled analgesia (PCA). A clear liquid diet is initiated immediately postoperatively. Patients are assessed at follow-up at 2 weeks after surgery, every 3 months for the first 2 years, every 4 months for the next 2 years, every 6 months for the fifth year, and yearly thereafter.

Clinical and digital examinations are performed at each postoperative visit. Flexible sigmoidoscopy is performed at 6-month intervals for the first 2 years. Full colonoscopy is performed at 1 year followed by every 3 years. CEA is measured at each visit, and CT of the abdomen and pelvis is performed at 6 months, 1 year, and then annually. PET scan is performed selectively if recurrence is suspected.

Results

Between 1984 and 2015, we have performed 373 TATA procedures. The mean tumor level from the anorectal ring was 1.7 cm. About 97.7% of patients received neoadjuvant radiation with a mean dose of 5405 cGy. Seventy-seven percent of patients received concurrent chemotherapy with infusional 5FU or capecitabine. Mean time from completion of neoadjuvant therapy was 11 weeks.

The TME was initiated transanally in all cases with the abdominal portion completed in an open fashion in 48% (n = 180) and laparoscopic approach in 52% (n = 193) of cases. Of patients who underwent laparoscopic surgery, the abdominal portion was carried out by multiport access in 147 patients, SILS in 34 patients, and robotic access in 13 patients. In 38 patients, the transanal TME dissection was continued further using a single-port platform into the peritoneal cavity as in the taTME fashion. A hand-sewn coloanal anastomosis was performed via a colonic J-pouch, side-to-end , or straight coloanal anastomosis depending on the length of the remaining colon. A temporary diverting loop stoma was made in all patients. Overall mean blood loss was 550 mL and incidence of transfusion was 12.6%. Mean length of stay was 6.2 days.

In regard to complications, there was one perioperative mortality due to myocardial infarction (0.3%).

The overall morbidity rate was 25.7%. Early morbidity was 13.4% with 4 anastomotic dehiscences, 3 pelvic abscesses, and 3 small bowel obstructions. Reoperation was performed in two patients, one for internal hernia and the other for intra-abdominal bleeding. Delayed morbidity rate was 12.3% with 10 pelvic abscesses, 10 anastomotic strictures, and 10 patients with neorectal prolapse.

Overall 25.3% had complete pathological response. Tumor's final pathological stages were as follows: 9.6% were ypT1, 33.1% ypT2, 31.7% ypT3, and 0.34% ypT4. About 4.8% had positive circumferential resection margin of <1 mm.

Mean follow-up was 65.7 months. The overall 5-year survival was 90% (KM5YAS) and was better in patients who underwent a laparoscopic abdominal completion of transanally initiated TME rather than open abdominal approach (93 vs 87%, $p = 0.03$). Overall local recurrence rate was 7.4%. LR was also less in laparoscopic group when compared to open group (4.3 vs 10.85%, $p = 0.02$).

Distance metastasis was observed in 19.5%. Only four patients required salvage APR.

Functional Outcomes: ISR Vs APR

Surgical resection represents the mainstay treatment of rectal cancer. However, for patients with very low rectal cancer, this usually entails removing the anal sphincter and committing the patient to a permanent colostomy. Although APR offers the chance of cure, it is correlated with a worse quality of life (QoL) and an increased prevalence of depression because of the permanent colostomy [12].

Around one-quarter of stoma patients experience clinically significant psychological symptoms postoperatively. The most common symptoms are those of an anxiety disorder and major depressive episode. Twenty-nine percent of the patients improve psychologically after surgery, 23% deteriorate, and 48% of patients experience no change in psychological symptoms [13].

Studies suggest that patients with a stoma have also a poorer QoL than those without a stoma, and although many patients accept a colostomy without issue, many patients consider life with a permanent colostomy to be unacceptable [14, 15]. Stoma patients seem to report similar concerns. These can be broadly categorized into concerns about changed body image and attractiveness, noise, odor, and leakage. To tackle these psychological and QoL issues, we were the first to describe the TATA proctosigmoidectomy, a sphincter-preserving surgery designed to simultaneously cure the rectal cancer and avoid a permanent colostomy [16]. Although this approach has been well described, for a variety of reasons, its adoption in the surgical community has been limited. A major concern voiced has been, ironically, concerns over the QoL of patients in terms of continence and functional status. Indeed, a common refrain from many surgeons reluctant to the approach of expanded sphincter preservation has been either "The patient would be better off with a colostomy" or "Why give the patient a perineal colostomy?".

To address these concerns, we have recently published our data on QoL after TATA [17]. It is one of the largest studies in the literature with 90 patients included, and it adds significantly to the understanding of QoL of patients in the United States after ISR and TATA. Patients were surveyed using the FIQLS, EORTC QLQ-C30, CR38, and the Marks Metric for Effect of Continence on QoL. We concluded that patient's QoL was not significantly different after surgery. However, in subgroup analysis, we found that patients with more proximal tumors had better lifestyle and physical and emotional scores and that older patients performed better on multiple levels; this is perhaps related to the fact that older patients coped better and had more realistic expectations than younger ones [8]. When we compared our results with those published in the literature for APR using standardized questionnaires, patients who underwent TATA scored better in all of the functional scales, including general QoL, physical, role, emotional, cognitive, and social [17].

Konanz et al. compared the QoL of patients after low anterior resection, ISR, and APR using the EORTC QLQ-C30, CR38, and the Wexner score [18]. They found that global QoL was comparable between the groups. However, physical and sexual functions were significantly better after ISR compared with APR, but diarrhea and constipation were higher after ISR [18].

All the published studies address the issues of QoL and functional outcomes based on established scales.

However, none of them clearly asked the patients if they were satisfied with their surgery or whether they would prefer a permanent colostomy. We addressed this issue in our study by asking the patients if they would have preferred having a colostomy rather than TATA. One-hundred percent of the patients preferred their current level of function over a permanent colostomy, and more than 90% of the patients responded that they never would have preferred to have a colostomy. This measurement reflects that patients have a high level of subjective satisfaction with sphincter-sparing surgery [17].

Furthermore, it has been demonstrated that psychological morbidity among patients who have undergone SPS is lower than that experienced by patients after APR [19]. When compared to non-stoma patients, stoma patients have higher levels of psychologic distress and more restrictions in their level of social and sexual functioning [20].

Although it is clear that patients after rectal surgery will never have the same bowel function that they enjoyed before developing rectal cancer, data support that they develop a new normal, which, although not perfect, is one that they are very pleased with and prefer over having a permanent colostomy [18]. However, patient selection is very important. A large number of the patients included in our QoL study came to be treated specifically because they refused to accept a permanent colostomy. This patient selection effect on the QoL and their satisfaction with the outcome cannot be overstated, because this is clearly a very motivated population of patients with rectal cancer.

Conclusion

Cancer of the distal third of rectum presents the greatest challenge for colorectal surgeons. As of yet, the best surgical approach is still unclear. The two main goals of any rectal cancer surgery are oncological outcomes and quality of life. SPR should be offered when feasible following high-dose chemoradiation in a properly motivated patient with good sphincter function. APR is recommended in patients with poor sphincter function and whose cancer is fixed to sphincter complex despite neoadjuvant therapy.

Further standardization of technique and multicenter prospective randomized studies to define the best surgical approach for distal rectal cancer are needed. Future direction of complete transanal approach by single-port robotic platform is under investigations.

Acknowledgement This work was supported by the Harry Mirabile Colorectal Center fund of the Marks Colorectal Surgical Foundation.

References

1. Miles WE. Discussion on the treatment of carcinoma of the rectum. Proc R Soc Med. 1924;17:79.
2. Heald RJ, et al. The mesorectum in rectal cancer surgery-the clue to pelvic recurrence? Br J Surg. 1982;69:613–61.
3. Buess G, Theiss R, Gunther M, Hutterer F, Hepp M, Pichlmaier H. Endoscopic operative procedure for the removal of rectalpolyps. Coloproctology. 1984;84:254–61.
4. Marks G, Mohiuddin M, Masoni L, Pecchioli L. High-dose preoperative radiation and full-thickness local excision. Dis Colon Rectum. 1990;33(9):735–9.
5. Marks GJ, Marks JH, Mohiuddin M, Bradley L. Radical Sphincter-preservation surgery with coloanal anastomosis following high dose external irradiation for the very low lying rectal cancer. Recent Results Cancer Res. 1998;146:161–74.
6. Marks JH, Lopez-Acevedo N, Krishnan B, Johnson MN, Montenegro GA, Marks GJ. True NOTES TME resection with splenic flexure release, high ligation of IMA, and side-to-end hand-sewn coloanal anastomosis. Surg Endosc. 2016;30(10):4626–31.
7. Sauer R, Liersch T, Merkel S, et al. Preoperative versus postoperative chemoradiotherapy for locally advanced rectal cancer: results of the German CAO/ARO/AIO-94 randomized phase III trial after a median follow-up of 11 years. J Clin Oncol. 2012;30:1926.
8. Wibe A, Syse A, Andersen E, Tretli S, Myrvold HE, Soreide O. Oncologic outcomes after total mesorectal excision forcure of cancer of the lower rectum: anterior vs abdominoperineal resection. Dis Colon Rectum. 2004;47:48–58.
9. Marks JH, Nassif G, Schoonyoung H, DeNittis A, Zeger E, Mohiuddin M, Marks GJ. Sphincter-sparing surgery for adenocarcinoma of the distal 3 cm of the true rectum: results after neoadjuvant therapy and minimally invasive radical surgery or local excision. Surg Endosc. 2013;27:4469–77.
10. Marks JH, Valsdottir EB. Total mesorectal excision with coloanal anastomosis: laparoscopic technique. In: Mulholland M, editor. Operative techniques in surgery, vol. 2. Exeter: Lippincott Williams & Wilkins; 2015. p. 1177–89.
11. Tiret E, Poupardin B, McNamara D, Dehni N, Parc R. Ultralow anterior resection with intersphincteric dissection-what is the limit of safe sphincter preservation? Color Dis. 2003;5:454–7.
12. Cipe G, Muslumanoglu M, Yardimci E, Memmi N, Aysan E. Intersphincteric resection and coloanal anastomosis in treatment of distal rectal cancer. Int J Surg Oncol. 2012;2012:581258.
13. White CA, Hunt JC. Psychological factors in postoperative adjustment to stoma surgery. Ann R Coll Surg Engl. 1997;79:3–7.
14. Thomas C, Madden F, Jehu D. Psychological morbidity in the first three months following stoma surgery. J Psychosom Res. 1984;28:251–7.
15. Wilson TR, Alexander DJ. Clinical and non-clinical factors influencing postoperative health-related quality of life in patients with colorectal cancer. Br J Surg. 2008;95:1408–15.
16. Engel J, Kerr J, Schlesinger-Raab A, Eckel R, Sauer H, Holzel D. Quality of life in rectal cancer patients: a four-year prospective study. Ann Surg. 2003;238:203–13.
17. Marks G, Mohiuddin M, Goldstein SD. Sphincter preservation for cancer of the distal rectum using high dose preoperative radiation. Int J Radiat Oncol Biol Phys. 1988;15:1065–8.
18. Marks JH, Salem JF, Valsdottir EB, Yarandi SS, Marks GJ. Quality of life and functional outcome after transanal abdominal transanal proctectomy for low rectal cancer. Dis Colon Rectum. 2017;60(3):258–65.
19. Konanz J, Herrle F, Weiss C, Post S, Kienle P. Quality of life of patients after low anterior, intersphincteric and abdominoperineal resection for rectal cancer – a matched-pair analysis. Int J Color Dis. 2013;28:679–88.
20. Sprangers MAG, et al. Quality of life in colorectal cancer. Stoma vs nonstoma patients. Dis Colon Rectum. 1995;38(4):361–9.

Optimal Coloanal Reconstruction: J-pouch, Straight, Stapled, and Hand Sewn

28

Andrea M. Petrucci and Steven D. Wexner

Introduction

Coloanal anastomosis (CAA) is technically challenging given its distal location within the limited confines of the pelvis. Different coloanal anastomotic techniques including straight, colonic J-pouch, coloplasty, end-to-side (ETS), and other creative techniques including cecorectal anastomosis have all been described and challenged in the literature. In addition, these anastomoses can be performed trans-abdominally or trans-perineally, using either a hand-sewn or a stapled technique. They are undertaken for both benign and malignant diseases [1]. One concern following surgery is the possibility of impaired bowel function from the loss of the rectal reservoir [2]. Regardless, the goal is to provide patients with intestinal continuity with acceptable function, while preserving anal sphincter anatomy and physiology.

Construction of a coloanal anastomosis must follow basic anastomotic principles that will allow healing and minimize complications. These steps include ensuring that the anastomosis is well vascularized and is tension-free. In order to meet these goals, regardless of the type of anastomosis performed, the splenic flexure is mobilized in order to gain length, and the inferior mesenteric artery and vein are both ligated at their respective origins to allow for the proximal colon to reach the deep pelvis, thereby eliminating any tension. Another important consideration is the patient's sphincter function. Sphincter-preserving surgery has allowed surgeons to provide patients with intestinal continuity; however, patients with poor sphincter function prior to surgery may not be ideal candidates and may suffer from poor quality of life secondary to poor continence. A good history and physical exam help to identify these patients. Furthermore, diagnostic tests such as a pelvic MRI, endoanal ultrasound, and manometric studies assess sphincter integrity and allow surgeons to

A.M. Petrucci • S.D. Wexner (✉)
Department of Colorectal Surgery, Cleveland Clinic Florida, Weston, FL, USA
e-mail: apetru1@gmail.com; wexners@ccf.org

C.M. Schlachta, P. Sylla (eds.), *Current Common Dilemmas in Colorectal Surgery*,
https://doi.org/10.1007/978-3-319-70117-2_28

select patients who would benefit from having sphincter-preserving surgery as opposed to having a permanent colostomy. Therefore a detailed discussion with the patient must be undertaken prior to surgery.

Overview of Sphincter-Preserving Coloanal Anastomotic Techniques

The original coloanal anastomosis described by Parks in 1982 included performing a mucosectomy and a hand-sewn coloanal anastomosis (HCAA) at the level of the dentate line [3]. Shortly thereafter in 1986, the colonic J-pouch (CJP) reconstruction was described by both Lazorthes et al. [4] and Parc et al. [5], who published their techniques during the same year. The CJP quickly became the preferred method for creating a new reservoir as the efferent limb provides no functional peristalsis and creates a pouch [6]. This design allows accommodation of more volume and acts as a neorectum, which results in better function when compared to a straight coloanal anastomosis (SCAA) [7]. After resecting the diseased colon, the proximal colon is either exteriorized through the abdomen or through the anus. Regardless, the CJP is created the same way, by using 6 cm of the distal ends of a well-mobilized descending colon, folded onto itself to create a J limb (Fig. 28.1) [8].

The antimesenteric borders are then stapled together using a 60 mm linear cutting stapler where each arm of the stapler is inserted through a common colotomy made at the apex of the pouch. Ensuring that the antimesenteric borders are re-approximated helps eliminate the incorporation of small vessels located near the

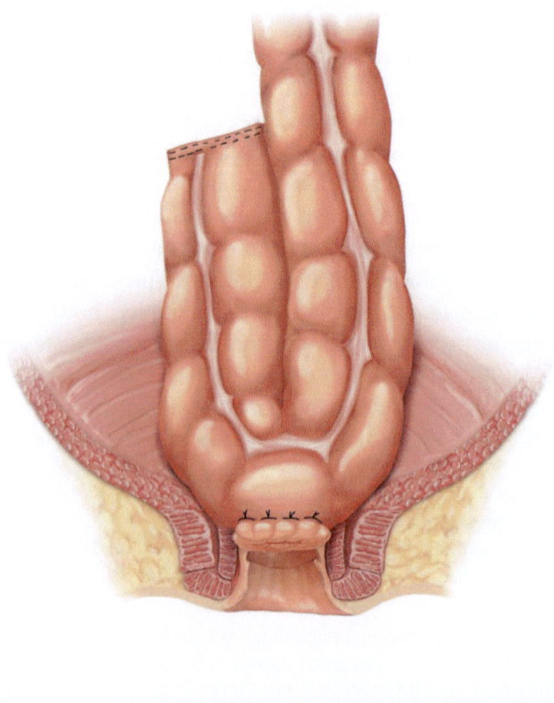

Fig. 28.1 The colonic J-pouch (CJP). With permission from [8]. © 2011 Wolters Kluwer Health, Inc

mesenteric side and decreases bleeding from the staple line. The afferent limb is secured to the efferent limb with 3.0 polydioxanone sutures. It may be desirable to suture the afferent limb to the efferent limb prior to firing the stapler, especially when the CJP is constructed through the transanal approach. Once the pouch is created, the colotomy is used as the proximal end and is anastomosed to the anus either using a stapled or hand-sewn approach. When using a stapled approach, a ≥ 2 cm cuff above the dentate line is preserved in order to accommodate the circular stapler, as opposed to a hand-sewn approach which can be undertaken at any level. A purse-string suture using a 0-polypropylene is placed around the proximal colotomy, and the anvil is inserted and secured by tying the purse string around the anvil shaft. A tight seal is necessary in order to avoid displacement of the anvil proximally into the J-pouch. The proximal limb is then returned into the abdominal cavity either through the abdominal incision or pushed into the pelvis through the perineal opening.

When using a trans-perineal approach, the distal end must also be purse-stringed with a 0-polypropylene suture. In this approach, the proximal colon containing the secured anvil is connected to the spike of the end-to-end anastomotic stapler. Only then is the stapler advanced into the anal canal and the distal purse string is secured and tied down around the trocar. Once secured, the stapler is closed and fired, and the anastomosis is created.

If using a transabdominal approach, the circular stapler is inserted into the stapled distal cuff with the spike piercing through the stapled rectum, preferably through the staple line. The anvil is mated to the stapler, which is then closed, and the stapler is fired, creating the CJP anastomosis.

This optimal CJP length was studied by Lazorthes et al. [9] in a prospective randomized controlled trial (RCT) wherein they compared a small (6 cm) versus a larger (10 cm) CJP. The authors showed that, despite no differences in frequency, urgency, and fecal incontinence at 2 years, 30% of the larger-pouch patients compared to 10% of the small-pouch group used laxatives or enemas for stool evacuation and constipation [9]. As a result, the authors determined that the "ideal" length of the CJP to avoid long-term evacuatory complications is 6–7 cm [1, 7, 9]. These findings were confirmed by Hida et al. who demonstrated that the enlargement and the horizontal inclination of the longitudinal axis of the CJP in patients with longer pouches (10 vs 5 cm) lead to evacuation difficulty [10, 11].

Alternatives to the CJP are the ETS anastomosis, also known as the "Baker" anastomosis (Fig. 28.2) [12], and anastomosis with transverse coloplasty (TC), originally described by Z'graggen in 2001 (Fig. 28.3) [13]. Both of these techniques can be considered if a CJP is not feasible. A study by Harris et al. [14] that assessed reasons for failure to construct a CJP found seven factors overall, which were divided into technical factors including a narrow pelvis, bulky anal sphincters, the need for mucosectomy, diverticulosis, insufficient colon length, or pregnancy and nontechnical factors including complex surgery or distant metastases.

The ETS anastomosis is created by inserting the anvil through the proximal opened end of the healthy colon, and the tip of the anvil is pierced through the colonic wall, roughly 3 cm from the colotomy edge. The colotomy is then stapled closed, and the stapled anastomosis is created using the circular stapler, leaving a small efferent limb that acts as the reservoir.

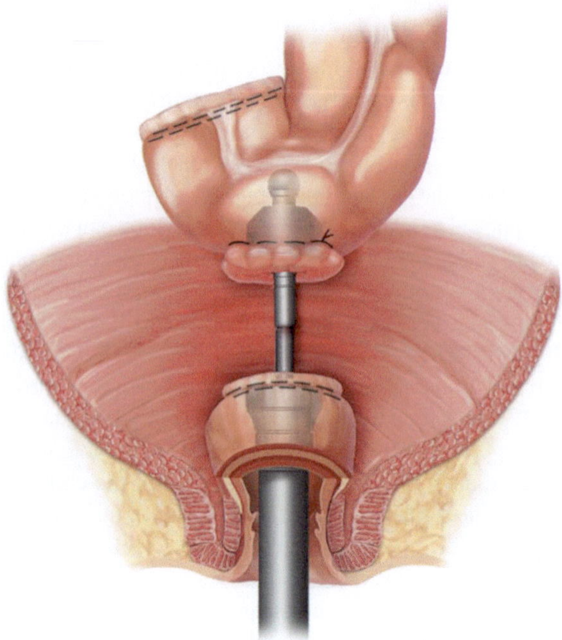

Fig. 28.2 The end-to-side "Baker" anastomosis (ETS). With permission from [8]. © 2011 Wolters Kluwer Health, Inc

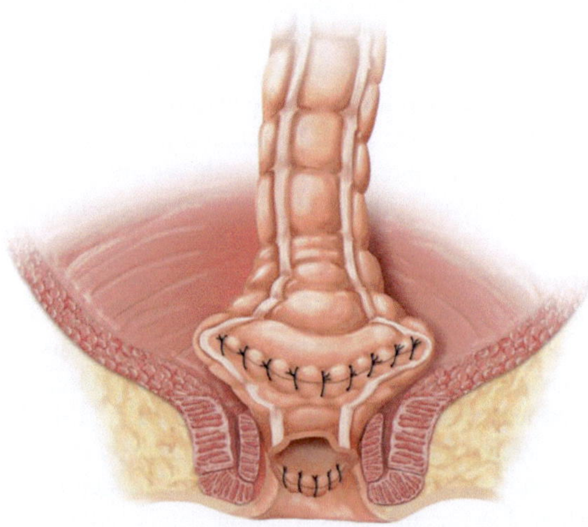

Fig. 28.3 The transverse coloplasty (TC). With permission from [8]. © 2011 Wolters Kluwer Health, Inc

Transverse coloplasty is performed prior to the CAA. Early studies showed that a TC is a feasible alternative to CJP [14, 15]. After securing the anvil around a purse string of the proximal colon, a neorectal reservoir is created by performing an 8–10 cm longitudinal colotomy in the distal colonic end of the proximal limb, with the most distal point located 2–4 cm from the anvil. The defect is closed in a transverse fashion, using a single layer of absorbable interrupted or running sutures [8,

16]. Unfortunately, due to the prohibitively high rate of sepsis mostly attributed to anastomotic leaks, this procedure has been largely abandoned [17].

The SCAA is still performed in situations when constructing a colonic reservoir is not feasible. The anastomosis is created in the standard fashion, either hand sewn (Fig. 28.4) or using a circular stapler (Fig. 28.5). Although not the preferred method

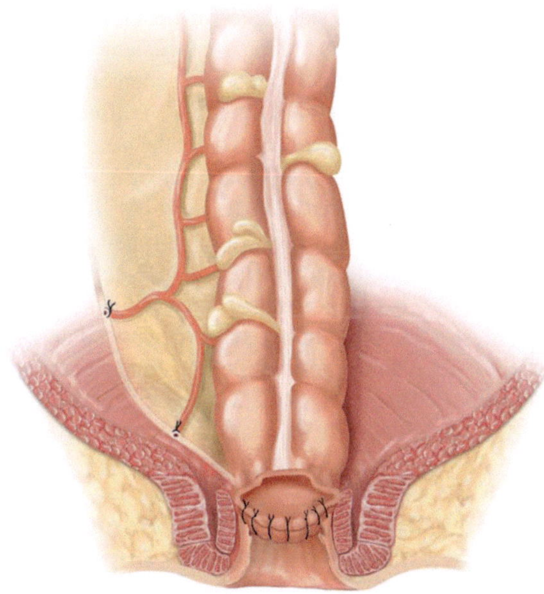

Fig. 28.4 The hand-sewn straight coloanal anastomosis. With permission from [8]. © 2011 Wolters Kluwer Health, Inc

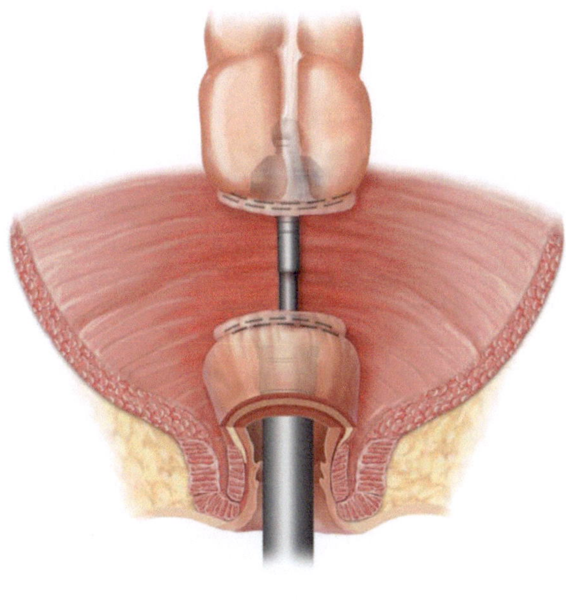

Fig. 28.5 The stapled straight coloanal anastomosis. With permission from Wexner SD, Fleshman JW, eds. Colon and Rectal Surgery: Abdominal Operations. © Wolters Kluwer Health, Inc., Philadelphia, 2011 [8]

for reconstruction for reasons described later, a SCAA may be the only available option in specific cases. Unfortunately, due to the loss of the rectal reservoir, many patients experience the *low anterior resection syndrome*, consisting of increased stool frequency, urgency, and fecal incontinence, which has a great impact on the patient's quality of life [7].

Another creative option for constructing a reservoir is the ileocecal interposition (ICI), also known as the "cecum pouch," which was introduced in 1994 by von Flüe and Harder as a new technique for pouch reconstruction following rectal surgery [18]. This technique of rectal replacement consists of creating an antiperistaltic cecoproctostomy that is rotated 180° counterclockwise to anastomose to the residual rectum or anal canal [18]. It can be used following subtotal colectomy after recurrent low anterior resection or in the case of metachronous rectal cancers [18].

A randomized controlled trial comparing ICI with CJP construction after TME for rectal cancer showed similar quality of life outcomes between both approaches at up to 5 years after surgery, although patients with ICI had higher frequency of defecation and more complications including bowel obstruction and stricture formation [19]. This procedure has been popularized by Sarli et al. from Perna, Italy. They showed that the antiperistaltic cecorectal anastomosis is safe and effective for patients with colonic inertia following total colectomy. The 10 female patients in the study reported an average of 2.2 bowel movements per day, with no major morbidity and good quality of life at 1 year following surgery [20].

Stapled Vs Hand-Sewn (Transabdominal Vs Transperineal) Coloanal Anastomosis and the Impact of Intersphincteric Resection

The use of staplers in the field of colorectal surgery has revolutionized how anastomoses are created. Ever since their introduction in 1979 by Ravitch and Steichen [21], stapled anastomoses have been found to have lower complications such as leaks and contribute to a shorter operative time [22]. The distal point of transection influences whether a stapled CAA is technically feasible. In certain cases of very low anastomoses, the hand-sewn technique is the only option. In the case of sphincter preservation surgery, the main concern is functional outcome as this will affect the patient's quality of life. The superiority of the hand-sewn or stapled approaches has been a topic of great debate for years. A prospective study in 2002 by Takase et al. [23] included 15 patients who underwent intersphincteric resection with hand-sewn CAA for rectal cancer over a 59-month period and compared these patients to 16 who underwent stapled CAA. Overall, patients with a hand-sewn coloanal anastomosis (HCAA) had impaired internal sphincter muscle function at 12 months, although overall evacuatory function in both groups was similar. In addition, oncologic outcome such as local recurrence was found in four patients in the HCAA group who went on to have a curative abdominal perineal resection (APR). Although tumor height was lower in the HCAA group, all patients had adequate distal resection margins [23]. A prospective randomized study by Laurent et al. [24] compared the stapled versus hand-sewn techniques specifically for CJP anastomoses in 37 patients undergoing restorative proctectomy with total mesorectal excision for rectal cancer. The authors found no difference in function and morbidity at 12 months between the groups; however, there was a decrease in operating time in the stapled group. Moreover, three patients in the HCAA group developed anastomotic stricture requiring dilation, but this was not statistically significant. The authors concluded that a stapled CJP anastomosis should be considered when technically feasible [24]. An earlier systematic review by Lustosa et al. [25] in 2002 comparing stapled versus hand-sewn colorectal anastomosis found insufficient evidence to state that one technique is superior to the other, regardless of the level of anastomosis. Ten years later, an updated systematic review comparing both types of colorectal anastomoses in 1233 patients was also not able to demonstrate superiority of one anastomotic technique over the other. However, the authors did find that stapled anastomosis had a higher incidence of anastomotic stricture when compared to HCAA, whereas the latter took longer to complete [26]. Nonetheless, this review classified the level of anastomosis as either above or below the peritoneal reflection and found no significant differences between both [26].

For patients with very low rectal cancer, an intersphincteric resection (ISR) is a method of sphincter preservation performed in an effort to achieve negative distal resection margins and has been shown to have acceptable oncologic outcomes [27]. In select patients who do not have tumor invasion of the external sphincter or levator muscles and have good sphincter function, it is feasible to perform either a partial (distal resection margin at the level of the dentate line) or a complete (distal resection margin at the intersphincteric groove) ISR with a hand-sewn coloanal anastomosis. The type of ISR is dictated by the level of the tumor in relation to the anorectal ring as described by Rullier et al. [28] where a partial ISR is appropriate for tumors located less than 1 cm from the sphincter complex (juxta-anal Type II) and a complete ISR for those with internal sphincter invasion (intra-anal Type III). The anastomotic leak rate following an ISR is quite variable ranging from 0.9 to 48% and thus should be performed by experienced surgeons [27]. An interesting study looked at complications and functional outcomes in patients undergoing laparoscopic ISR with a stapled CAA and retrospectively compared these patients to a group who had undergone hand-sewn CAA. None of these patients were diverted, and the median tumor distance from the dental line was 2.1 cm. The stapled CAA group had significantly lower rates of anastomotic leak and stricture formation compared to the hand-sewn group at the 24-month follow-up; functional outcomes, however, were surprisingly similar [29]. Despite these problems, some patients are willing to accept the complications over having a permanent colostomy.

Outcomes: Which Coloanal Anastomotic Technique is Best?

The technical decision regarding which anastomotic technique to employ is frequently made in the operating room while preparing for the anastomosis as many intraoperative factors including patient's body habitus, bowel vascularization, and anatomy play a significant role. Short- and long-term outcomes such as anastomotic leak, bowel function, and quality of life have been studied for each type of coloanal anastomotic technique. The most devastating complication besides recurrent carcinoma following a coloanal anastomosis is anastomotic leak. A recent study found anastomoses less than 10 cm from the anal verge to be an independent risk factor for anastomotic leak regardless whether the anastomosis was hand sewn or stapled [30]. The definition of an anastomosis ≤ 10 cm from the anal verge as being "high risk" has been included in many recent studies" [31–34]. The majority of patients who undergo coloanal anastomosis after restorative proctectomy for rectal cancer are proximally diverted as diversion has been shown to decrease the incidence of anastomotic leak requiring urgent or emergent surgery [35]. Anastomotic leaks are not only problematic in the immediate postoperative period but also lead to functional problems in the long term. Ashburn et al. [36, 37] looked at function following anastomotic leak in patients who had undergone proctectomy for rectal cancer and found that function was worse in those who had leaked; patients suffered more day- and nighttime bowel movements as well as worse control of solid stool and worse physical and metal scores.

Poor functional outcomes following restorative proctectomy have a significant impact on the patient's quality of life. It has been shown that poor preoperative function with high incontinence scores and low anastomoses (<5 cm) following proctectomy for rectal cancer predict persistent incontinence after a restorative procedure [36]. Moreover, oncologic outcomes may be worse following anastomotic leak [38].

CJP Vs SCAA

Many studies have compared CJP with the standard SCAA. In 1995, a small RCT that included 40 patients who underwent ultralow anterior resection (median distance from the anal verge of 3.25 cm) with either CJP ($n = 20$) or SCAA ($n = 20$) and diverting loop ileostomy found that anal function was significantly better with CJP. These patients experienced less frequency ($p < 0.05$), use of antidiarrheal medications ($p < 0.008$), and number of bowel movements per day ($p < 0.05$) at 12 months following ileostomy closure [39]. In addition, at the 12-month follow-up, all patients with CJP had return of normal continence after ileostomy reversal compared to only 70% of patients with a SCAA [39]. Hallböök et al. [40] randomized 100 patients with rectal cancer located within 12 cm from the anal verge to undergo either CJP or SCAA with or without a diverting loop ileostomy. Patients randomized to the CJP group were found to have a lower postoperative anastomotic leak rate (2% vs 15%, $p = 0.03$) as well as fewer bowel movements per 24 h, less nocturnal evacuations, urgency, and incontinence at 2 months and 1 year following surgery (after temporary stoma closure in applicable patients) [38]. Moreover, these patients rated their overall well-being significantly higher than patients who received a SCAA after 1 year [40]. In an early study, Joo et al. [1] assessed long-term functional and clinical outcomes between SCAA and CJP. They found patients with CJP had superior function compared to those with SCAA at up to 1 year after surgery;

following the 1-year mark, function appears to be similar between CJP and SCAA [1]. Another study by Hida et al. [41] compared functional outcomes between CJP and SCAA for low (5–8 cm from verge) and ultralow (4 cm from verge) anastomoses over a longer follow-up period of 5 years. The authors found that patients with CJP had less urgency, soiling, and nocturnal bowel movements. In addition, reservoir function was better in the CJP group for both low and ultralow anastomoses [41]. Surgical approach was also studied. Liang et al. [42] compared CJP to SCAA in 48 patients specifically undergoing laparoscopic-assisted surgery for rectal cancer. Because patients with CJP had improved postoperative bowel function, this leads to better short-term outcomes such as decreased disability after surgery and quicker return to partial activity ($p = 039$), full activity ($p < 0.001$), and work ($p < 0.001$) [42].

CJP Vs ETS

The CJP is one of many colonic reservoirs available for reconstruction of a neorectum, with the goal being to mitigate symptoms of poor anal function. A prospective randomized trial by Machado et al. [43] studied 100 patients and looked at functional and surgical outcomes of an ETS anastomosis compared to the CJP. Surgical outcomes such as anastomotic height, blood loss, length of procedure, length of stay, and mortality were similar. Functional outcomes were also similar between the two groups, except for the ability to evacuate the bowel in less than 15 min at 6 months after surgery, which favored the CJP group. The authors concluded that both reservoirs result in similar long-term outcomes, thus making them both acceptable options for reconstruction. A meta-analysis by Siddiqui et al. [44] looked at four randomized controlled trials including 273 patients comparing CJP and ETS anastomoses. The authors demonstrated that patients with CJP had less urgency at 6 months, but this difference was not significant by 24 months, as were the use of pads and enemas, stool frequency, and incomplete evacuation. In addition, pressure and volumetric outcomes as well as surgical outcomes were all similar between the groups, concluding that CJP or ETS anastomoses are acceptable and safe options after anterior resection for rectal cancer. A more recent randomized study by Doeksen et al. [45] looked at ETS anastomosis versus CJP in 107 patients and found functional outcomes to be better in the CJP group at up to 12 months after surgery. However, other outcomes including quality of life and complications were similar, concluding that ETS anastomosis is an acceptable alternative when CJP is not feasible.

CJP Vs Transverse Coloplasty

Transverse coloplasty has also been challenged against CJP reconstruction. Furst et al. [15] performed a RCT focusing specifically on technical feasibility, anal manometry findings, and stool frequency between the CJP and TC in patients with distal rectal cancer. Creating a TC was technically feasible in 100% of the patients, whereas CJP was possible in only 75%. The lack of feasibility to construct a CJP can be due to variation in the amount of mesenteric adipose tissue surrounding the colon a narrow pelvis, a short left colon, or diverticula in the left colon [15]. Stool frequency and manometric measurements were similar except that the TC group had higher neorectal sensitivity, concluding that TC is a safe and feasible alternative to CJP [15]. Ho et al. [17] compared CJP to TC in a RCT of 80 patients and followed them for up to 12 months after surgery. Transverse coloplasty resulted in significantly higher leak rates (15.9% vs 0%; $p = 0.01$) and higher overall complications (31.8% vs 9.1%; $p = 0.03$) with minimal differences in bowel function, confirming that CJP remains the favored option for coloanal reconstruction [17]. As previously noted in this chapter, high complication rates associated with TC have led to its abandonment.

Comparing All Types of Anastomoses

Several studies have compared the various types of anastomoses. In 2005, Remzi et al. [2] studied quality of life, functional outcomes, and complications among TC, SCAA, and CJP. They performed a retrospective review of all patients with benign and malignant diseases who underwent a low colorectal or coloanal anastomosis at or below 3 cm from the dentate line with or without a diverting loop ileostomy. They stratified each anastomotic technique into two groups: stapled or hand sewn. Overall, QOL was better in patients with CJP and TC. In addition, both of these anastomoses resulted in less nighttime bowel movements compared to the SCAA. Patients with TC also had less daytime bowel movements, stool clustering, and less use of antidiarrheal medications. Although overall complications were similar between each group, the authors noted a specifically higher anastomotic leak rate in patients who underwent a hand-sewn CJP compared to the hand-sewn TC anastomosis (44% vs 3.6%), which is unusually high. For patients who underwent either a stapled CJP or TC anastomosis, the anastomotic leak rate was 4.8% vs 5.8%, respectively. Transverse coloplasty was deemed a safe and feasible alternative to CJP [2]. Although the outcomes for TC seem favorable, a 2007 multicenter RCT that included 364 patients performed by the same group looked at the same outcomes, including long-term function (at 24 months) including urinary and sexual function, as well as bowel function [6]. Interestingly, the groups were divided based on whether a CJP construction was feasible: one subgroup consisted in transverse coloplasty (CP-1) or SCAA if CJP was not feasible, and the other group was transverse coloplasty (CP-2) or CJP if CJP was feasible. Overall, there were no significant differences among the four subgroups of patients. Of the 364 patients, 297 were evaluated for functional outcomes. There were no functional differences between the CP-1 and SCAA groups; however, patients with CJP had improved function (fewer bowel movements, less clustering, less use of pads, and a lower incontinence score) relative to the CP-2 group [6]. Quality of life and complications were similar among all four groups [6]. This study showed that when CJP is not feasible, transverse coloplasty was not superior to SCAA with regard to bowel function but remains a reconstructive option [6].

A meta-analysis by Heriot et al. [45] looked at complications and outcomes between CJP, SCAA, and TC after anterior resection measured at 6 months, 1 year, and 2 years after surgery. Results demonstrated no difference in complications, including anastomotic leak, wound infection, and postoperative mortality, between the different types of anastomoses. However, CJP proved to have less frequency of defecation and less urgency than the SCAA. When CJP was compared to TC, results were similar [46]. A 2008 systematic review by Brown et al. [47] assessed functional outcomes from 16 randomized controlled trials comparing different combinations of the four coloanal anastomotic techniques, namely, SCAA, CLP, side-to-end, and TC. Overall, CJP had superior functional outcomes that were most apparent in the first 18 months after surgery; following this period, it was difficult to show a significant benefit of one technique over the other as there was a paucity of studies that looked at long-term outcomes [47].

Conclusion

Coloanal anastomosis is a technically challenging procedure with high potential morbidity. Surgeons performing restorative proctectomy should combine clinical judgment and evidence-based results with respect to short- and long-term outcomes following coloanal anastomoses to determine which anastomosis is most appropriate for each patient. Transverse coloplasty is limited to historic interest. The CJP reconstruction remains the most favored option when technically feasible; however, when it cannot be constructed, an ETS anastomosis seems preferable to a SCAA.

References

1. Joo JS, Latulippe JF, Alabaz O, Weiss EG, Nogueras JJ, Wexner SD. Long-term functional evaluation of straight coloanal anastomosis and colonic J-pouch: is the functional superiority of colonic J-pouch sustained? Dis Colon Rectum. 1998;41(6):740–6.
2. Remzi FH, Fazio VW, Gorgun E, Zutshi M, Church JM, Lavery IC, et al. Quality of life, functional outcome, and complications of coloplasty pouch after low anterior resection. Dis Colon Rectum. 2005;48(4):735–43.
3. Parks AG, Percy JP. Resection and sutured colo-anal anastomosis for rectal carcinoma. Br J Surg. 1982;69(6):301–4.
4. Lazorthes F, Fages P, Chiotasso P, Lemozy J, Bloom E. Resection of the rectum with construction of a colonic reservoir and colo-anal anastomosis for carcinoma of the rectum. Br J Surg. 1986;73(2):136–8.
5. Parc R, Tiret E, Frileux P, Moszkowski E, Loygue J. Resection and colo-anal anastomosis with colonic reservoir for rectal carcinoma. Br J Surg. 1986;73(2):139–41.
6. Fazio VW, Zutshi M, Remzi FH, Parc Y, Ruppert R, Furst A, et al. A randomized multicenter trial to compare long-term functional outcome, quality of life, and complications of surgical procedures for low rectal cancers. Ann Surg. 2007;246(3):481–8. Discussion 8–90.
7. de la Fuente SG, Mantyh CR. Reconstruction techniques after proctectomy: what's the best? Clin Colon Rectal Surg. 2007;20(3):221–30.
8. Wexner SD, Fleshman JW, editors. Colon and rectal surgery: abdominal operations. Philadelphia: Wolters Kluwer; 2011.

9. Lazorthes F, Gamagami R, Chiotasso P, Istvan G, Muhammad S. Prospective, randomized study comparing clinical results between small and large colonic J-pouch following coloanal anastomosis. Dis Colon Rectum. 1997;40(12):1409–13.
10. Hida J, Yasutomi M, Maruyama T, Tokoro T, Uchida T, Wakano T, et al. Horizontal inclination of the longitudinal axis of the colonic J-pouch: defining causes of evacuation difficulty. Dis Colon Rectum. 1999;42(12):1560–8.
11. Hida J, Yasutomi M, Maruyama T, Tokoro T, Wakano T, Uchida T. Enlargement of colonic pouch after proctectomy and coloanal anastomosis: potential cause for evacuation difficulty. Dis Colon Rectum. 1999;42(9):1181–8.
12. Baker JW. Low end to side rectosigmoidal anastomosis; description of technic. Arch Surg. 1950;61(1):143–57.
13. Z'Graggen K, Maurer CA, Birrer S, Giachino D, Kern B, Buchler MW. A new surgical concept for rectal replacement after low anterior resection: the transverse coloplasty pouch. Ann Surg. 2001;234(6):780–5. Discussion 5–7.
14. Harris GJ, Lavery IJ, Fazio VW. Reasons for failure to construct the colonic J-pouch. What can be done to improve the size of the neorectal reservoir should it occur? Dis Colon Rectum. 2002;45(10):1304–8.
15. Furst A, Suttner S, Agha A, Beham A, Jauch KW. Colonic J-pouch vs. coloplasty following resection of distal rectal cancer: early results of a prospective, randomized, pilot study. Dis Colon Rectum. 2003;46(9):1161–6.
16. Z'Graggen K, Maurer CA, Buchler MW. Transverse coloplasty pouch. A novel neorectal reservoir. Dig Surg. 1999;16(5):363–6.
17. Ho YH, Brown S, Heah SM, Tsang C, Seow-Choen F, KW E, et al. Comparison of J-pouch and coloplasty pouch for low rectal cancers: a randomized, controlled trial investigating functional results and comparative anastomotic leak rates. Ann Surg. 2002;236(1):49–55.
18. von Flue M, Harder F. New technique for pouch-anal reconstruction after total mesorectal excision. Dis Colon Rectum. 1994;37(11):1160–2.
19. Rink AD, Haaf F, Knupper N, Vestweber KH. Prospective randomised trial comparing ileocaecal interposition and colon-J-pouch as rectal replacement after total mesorectal excision. Int J Color Dis. 2007;22(2):153–60.
20. Sarli L, Costi R, Sarli D, Roncoroni L. Pilot study of subtotal colectomy with antiperistaltic cecoproctostomy for the treatment of chronic slow-transit constipation. Dis Colon Rectum. 2001;44(10):1514–20.
21. Ravitch MM, Steichen FM. A stapling instrument for end-to-end inverting anastomoses in the gastrointestinal tract. Ann Surg. 1979;189(6):791–7.
22. Korolija D. The current evidence on stapled versus hand-sewn anastomoses in the digestive tract. Minim Invasive Ther Allied Technol. 2008;17(3):151–4.
23. Takase Y, Oya M, Komatsu J. Clinical and functional comparison between stapled colonic J-pouch low rectal anastomosis and hand-sewn colonic J-pouch anal anastomosis for very low rectal cancer. Surg Today. 2002;32(4):315–21.
24. Laurent A, Parc Y, McNamara D, Parc R, Tiret E. Colonic J-pouch-anal anastomosis for rectal cancer: a prospective, randomized study comparing handsewn vs. stapled anastomosis. Dis Colon Rectum. 2005;48(4):729–34.
25. Lustosa SA, Matos D, Atallah AN, Castro AA. Stapled versus handsewn methods for colorectal anastomosis surgery: a systematic review of randomized controlled trials. Sao Paulo Med J. 2002;120(5):132–6.
26. Neutzling CB, Lustosa SA, Proenca IM, da Silva EM, Matos D. Stapled versus handsewn methods for colorectal anastomosis surgery. Cochrane Database Syst Rev. 2012;2:CD003144.
27. Martin ST, Heneghan HM, Winter DC. Systematic review of outcomes after intersphincteric resection for low rectal cancer. Br J Surg. 2012;99(5):603–12.
28. Rullier E, Denost Q, Vendrely V, Rullier A, Laurent C. Low rectal cancer: classification and standardization of surgery. Dis Colon Rectum. 2013;56:560–7.
29. Cong JC, Chen CS, Ma MX, Xia ZX, Liu DS, Zhang FY. Laparoscopic intersphincteric resection for low rectal cancer: comparison of stapled and manual coloanal anastomosis. Color Dis. 2014;16(5):353–8.

30. Trencheva K, Morrissey KP, Wells M, Mancuso CA, Lee SW, Sonoda T, et al. Identifying important predictors for anastomotic leak after colon and rectal resection: prospective study on 616 patients. Ann Surg. 2013;257(1):108–13.
31. Senagore A, Lane FR, Lee E, Wexner S, Dujovny N, Sklow B, et al. Bioabsorbable staple line reinforcement in restorative proctectomy and anterior resection: a randomized study. Dis Colon Rectum. 2014;57(3):324–30. https://doi.org/10.1097/DCR.0000000000000065.
32. Jafari, MD, Wexner SD, Martz JE, McLemore EC, Margolin DA, Sherwinter DA, et al. Perfusion assessment in laparoscopic left-sided/anterior resection (PILLAR II): a multi-institutional study. J Am Coll Surg. 2015;220(1):82–92 e1.
33. A Study Assessing Perfusion Outcomes With PINPOINT® Near Infrared Fluorescence Imaging in Low Anterior Resection (PILLAR III). Clinical trial identifier NCT02205307. Study terminated. Available from https://clinicaltrials.gov/ct2/show/NCT02205307.
34. LifeSeal™ Pilot Study in Subjects Undergoing Circular Stapled Anastomosis Created Within 10 cm of the Anal Verge. Clinical trial identifier NCT02046278. Available from https://clinicaltrials.gov/ct2/show/NCT02046278.
35. Montedori A, Cirocchi R, Farinella E, Sciannameo F, Abraha I. Covering ileo- or colostomy in anterior resection for rectal carcinoma. Cochrane Database Syst Rev. 2010;5:CD006878.
36. Ashburn JH, Stocchi L, Kiran RP, Dietz DW, Remzi FH. Consequences of anastomotic leak after restorative proctectomy for cancer: effect on long-term function and quality of life. Dis Colon Rectum. 2013;56(3):275–80.
37. Lee TG, Kang SB, Heo SC, Jeong SY, Park KJ. Risk factors for persistent anal incontinence after restorative proctectomy in rectal cancer patients with anal incontinence: prospective cohort study. World J Surg. 2011;35(8):1918–24.
38. Kim IY, Kim BR, Kim YW. The impact of anastomotic leakage on oncologic outcomes and the receipt and timing of adjuvant chemotherapy after colorectal cancer surgery. Int J Surg. 2015;22:3–9.
39. Seow-Choen F, Goh HS. Prospective randomized trial comparing J colonic pouch-anal anastomosis and straight coloanal reconstruction. Br J Surg. 1995;82(5):608–10.
40. Hallbook O, Pahlman L, Krog M, Wexner SD, Sjodahl R. Randomized comparison of straight and colonic J-pouch anastomosis after low anterior resection. Ann Surg. 1996;224(1):58–65.
41. Hida J, Yoshifuji T, Tokoro T, Inoue K, Matsuzaki T, Okuno K, et al. Comparison of long-term functional results of colonic J-pouch and straight anastomosis after low anterior resection for rectal cancer: a five-year follow-up. Dis Colon Rectum. 2004;47(10):1578–85.
42. Liang JT, Lai HS, Lee PH, Huang KC. Comparison of functional and surgical outcomes of laparoscopic-assisted colonic J-pouch versus straight reconstruction after total mesorectal excision for lower rectal cancer. Ann Surg Oncol. 2007;14(7):1972–9.
43. Machado M, Nygren J, Goldman S, Ljungqvist O. Similar outcome after colonic pouch and side-to-end anastomosis in low anterior resection for rectal cancer: a prospective randomized trial. Ann Surg. 2003;238(2):214–20.
44. Siddiqui MR, Sajid MS, Woods WG, Cheek E, Baig MK. A meta-analysis comparing side to end with colonic J-pouch formation after anterior resection for rectal cancer. Tech Coloproctol. 2010;14(2):113–23.
45. Doeksen A, Bakx R, Vincent A, van Tets WF, Sprangers MA, Gerhards MF, et al. J-pouch vs side-to-end coloanal anastomosis after preoperative radiotherapy and total mesorectal excision for rectal cancer: a multicentre randomized trial. Color Dis. 2012;14(6):705–13.
46. Heriot AG, Tekkis PP, Constantinides V, Paraskevas P, Nicholls RJ, Darzi A, et al. Meta-analysis of colonic reservoirs versus straight coloanal anastomosis after anterior resection. Br J Surg. 2006;93(1):19–32.
47. Brown CJ, Fenech DS, McLeod RS. Reconstructive techniques after rectal resection for rectal cancer. Cochrane Database Syst Rev. 2008;2:CD006040.

Part IX

Optimizing TME Outcomes

Short-Course Vs Long-Course Radiotherapy: Pros and Cons

29

Nicolas D. Prionas, Albert C. Koong, and Daniel T. Chang

Background

It has long been recognized that surgical resection of rectal cancer suffers from local-regional failures in the pelvis due to the lack of a barrier to spread, the rich lymphatic tissue in the pelvis, and the difficulty of achieving wide surgical margins in a narrow pelvic cavity. As such, the addition of radiotherapy has been a mainstay of treatment for decades, given either preoperatively or postoperatively. There are several important advantages of preoperative radiotherapy over postoperative radiotherapy: (1) better tissue perfusion and oxygenation due to the intact blood supply, (2) decreased dose of radiation due to better oxygenation, (3) reduced size of treatment fields due to lack of surgical disruption, (4) sterilization of margins allowing for an R0 resection, (5) determination of pathologic response, which can provide important prognostic information, and (6) potential downstaging of the tumor allowing for organ preservation. The primary purpose of neoadjuvant radiation for rectal cancer is to reduce the risk of pelvic failure by sterilizing both the lymphatic tissue within the mesorectum and pelvis as well as the circumferential resection margin. An additional benefit is organ preservation by downsizing tumors in the lower and mid-rectum to facilitate low-anterior resection and avoid abdominoperineal resection.

Currently, the standard of care for locally advanced rectal cancer (T3–4 and/or node positive), as outlined by the National Comprehensive Cancer Network Guidelines, includes neoadjuvant radiotherapy followed by surgical resection and adjuvant chemotherapy [1]. Recommended radiotherapy schedules include either

N.D. Prionas • D.T. Chang (✉)
Department of Radiation Oncology, Stanford Cancer Institute, Stanford, CA, USA
e-mail: nprionas@stanford.edu; dtchang@stanford.edu

A.C. Koong
Department of Radiation Oncology, MD Anderson Cancer Center, Houston, TX, USA
e-mail: akoong@stanford.edu

C.M. Schlachta, P. Sylla (eds.), *Current Common Dilemmas in Colorectal Surgery*,
https://doi.org/10.1007/978-3-319-70117-2_29

long-course (LC) radiation (45–50.4 Gy in 25–28 fractions) with concurrent 5-fluorouracil (5-FU) or short-course (SC) radiotherapy alone (25 Gy in 5 fractions). To understand why these alternative regimens exist, it is important to review the historical contexts of each regimen.

Historical Perspective

Given the problem of local failure following surgical resection and prior to establishing systemic therapy as a standard, investigators in Europe, primarily in Scandinavia, the Netherlands, and the United Kingdom, chose a SC regimen of preoperative radiotherapy alone. This schedule was convenient and less expensive, and many randomized trials demonstrated its efficacy with reduced local failures (Table 29.1). There have been 12 modern randomized trials of SC preoperative radiotherapy, all of which used low to moderate doses of radiation. Most showed a decrease in local recurrence, though only five reached statistical significance [2–4]. Two meta-analyses showed decreased local recurrence with SC radiotherapy [5]. The Swedish Rectal Cancer Trial was the only trial to show an improvement in overall survival [6], though like many others, it was conducted prior to the total mesorectal excision (TME) era. In the Dutch CKVO trial, 1805 eligible patients with resectable rectal cancer were randomized to preoperative SC radiotherapy, delivering 25 Gy in 5 fractions, followed by TME, versus TME alone. Preoperative radiotherapy halved the rate of local recurrence at 5 years (6% vs 12%). Overall survival at 2 years was 82% in both groups [7].

However, in the United States, initial combined modality approaches involved postoperative radiotherapy, as established in multiple clinical trials [8–11] and included in a 1990 NIH consensus statement which standardized this approach [12]. These trials showed that in the postoperative setting, LC chemoradiation could be safely tolerated and had improved local and systemic control at a time before multi-agent systemic chemotherapy was developed.

Preoperative chemoradiation then became the standard of care following the German Rectal Trial, which compared preoperative chemoradiotherapy delivering 50.4 Gy with concurrent 5-FU followed by TME to postoperative chemoradiotherapy delivering 55.8 Gy with concurrent 5-FU in 797 patients with locally advanced rectal cancer. Preoperative chemoradiation improved local failure (6% vs 13%, $p = 0.006$), grade 3 or 4 acute toxicity (27% vs 40%, $p = 0.001$), late toxicity (14% vs 24%, $p = 0.01$), and sphincter preservation (39% vs 19%, $0 = 0.004$) [13]. An updated report showed the 10-year cumulative incidence of local relapse was still improved in the preoperative arm (7.1% vs 10.1%, $p = 0.048$) [14].

With two acceptable regimens, however, questions remain about whether they are equivalent in terms of outcomes and toxicity as well as which clinical scenarios are better suited for one over the other. The purpose of this chapter is to discuss the differences and similarities between SC and LC radiotherapy in terms of clinical outcomes, toxicity profiles, impact on subsequent surgical resection, and future directions.

Table 29.1 Selected short-course radiotherapy trials prior to and after the standardization of total mesorectal excision

Trial	Design	*N*	Local failure		Disease-free survival		Overall survival	
Pre-TME era								
Swedish Rectal Cancer Trial (2005) [6, 26]	5 Gy × 5 fx + surgery	583	9% (13 years)	$p < 0.001$	72% (13 years)	$p = 0.04$	38% (13 years)	$p = 0.008$
	Surgery	585	26% (13 years)		62% (13 years)		30% (13 years)	
SCCSG I (1990) [2]	5 Gy × 5 fx + surgery	424	11%	$p < 0.01$	68%[a] (5 years)	$p < 0.01$	45%[a] (5 years)	p = NS
	Surgery	425	25%		60%[a] (5 years)		43%[a] (5 years)	
SCCSG II (1996) [27]	5 Gy × 5 fx + surgery	272	10% (4.2 years)	$p < 0.01$	74%	$p = 0.02$		
	Surgery	285	21% (4.2 years)		65%			
NRCG (1994) [28]	5 Gy × 5 fx + surgery	143	12.8% (8 years)	$p = 0.0001$			26%[a] (8 years)	$p = 0.21$
	Surgery	141	36.5% (8 years)				18%[a] (8 years)	
TME era								
Dutch CKVO (2011) [7, 29]	5 Gy × 5 fx + TME	897	5% (10 years)	$p < 0.0001$			48% (10 years)	$p = 0.86$
	TME	908	11% (10 years)				49% (10 years)	
MRC CR07 (2009) [30]	5 Gy × 5 fx + TME vs	674	4.4% (3 years)	$p < 0.0001$	77.5% (3 years)	$p = 0.013$	80.3% (3 years)	$p = 0.40$
	TME + 1.8 Gy × 25 fx	676	10.6% (3 years)		71.5% (3 years)		78.6% (3 years)	

fx fractions, *TME* total mesorectal excision, *NS* not significant
[a]Estimated from published Kaplan-Meier curve

Principles of Radiotherapy/Hypofractionation

Fractionated radiation has long been the mainstay of radiotherapy due to concerns of normal tissue tolerance with large daily doses of radiation. The efficacy of conventionally fractionated radiotherapy is radiobiologically predicated on the principles of repair of sublethal cell damage, redistribution of cells within the cell cycle, repopulation of cells, and reoxygenation. In other words, dividing a total dose into multiple fractions spares normal tissues because of repair of sublethal damage between fractions and repopulation of cells, if given sufficient time. Furthermore, the opportunity for reoxygenation and redistribution of cells into radiosensitive phases of the cell cycle increases the efficacy of cancer cell kill.

On the other hand, it has been classically demonstrated that delivering a given total dose over fewer fractions, or hypofractionating, has a higher biological effectiveness but leads to increased late normal tissue injury, which is determined primarily by fraction size. In other words, the larger the dose per fraction, the higher the risk of damage to normal organs. Therefore, SC radiotherapy is based on the principles of delivering an effective dose in a shortened timeframe, but it is associated with the potential for higher normal tissue toxicity compared with conventionally fractionated LC radiotherapy.

Criticisms of Short Course Vs Long Course

There are three main criticisms of SC radiotherapy followed by immediate surgery. First, 25 Gy in 5 fractions is not thought to be as biologically effective as 50.4 Gy in 28 fractions based on classic radiobiologic principles, leading to the concern of inferior disease outcomes. Secondly, the standard schedule, 25 Gy in 5 fractions followed by surgery 1 week later, does not allow adequate time for tumor downstaging, which negates the benefit of margin sterilization for tumors involving or approaching the mesorectal fascia, and the potential for organ preservation for tumors in the lower rectum. Finally, the larger doses per fraction may have a higher rate of late toxicity. Long-term follow-up data after 5.1 years from the Dutch CKVO trial which used SC radiation showed higher rates of fecal incontinence (62% vs 38%, $p < 0.001$), pad wearing (56% vs 33%, $p < 0.001$), anal blood loss (11% vs 3%, $p = 0.004$), and mucus loss (27% vs 15%, $p = 0.005$) in the radiation group compared to the surgery alone group [15].

There are criticisms of LC chemoradiation as well. It is conventionally given with 5-FU followed by surgical resection 1–2 months after completion, which delays the administration of multi-agent systemic therapy to address micrometastatic disease for at least 3–4 months. There are increased costs and patient inconvenience of a 5.5-week course of treatment with higher potential of acute radiation toxicity as compared to a 1-week schedule. Finally, the concurrent use of 5-FU requires additional costs and resources and has potential added toxicity.

Short-Course Vs Long-Course Direct Comparison

Recent trials have directly compared SC radiation and LC chemoradiation (Table 29.2). In the first, the Polish Colorectal Study Group compared SC radiotherapy followed by surgery after 7 days to LC chemoradiation (50.4 Gy with bolus 5-FU and leucovorin with surgery after 4–6 weeks) in 312 patients and demonstrated a nonsignificant difference in local recurrence rates (9% vs 14% in favor of SC, $p = 0.170$). There was no significant difference in the rate of distant metastases between SC and LC therapies (31.4% vs 34.6%, $p = 0.540$). SC radiotherapy had a lower pathologic complete response (pCR) rate compared to LC (1% vs 16%) and a higher rate of circumferential radial margin (CRM) positivity (4% vs 13% $p = 0.017$) (Table 29.3). Furthermore, tumor shrinkage and pCR did not translate into a difference in sphincter preservation rate (61% with SC and 58% with LC, $p = 0.57$). No difference in overall survival at 4 years (67% vs 66%, $p = 0.960$) and disease-free survival (58% vs 55%, $p = 0.820$) was seen between SC and LC therapy. SC had lower acute toxicity (3% vs 18%, $p < 0.001$) but similar severe late toxicity (10% vs 7%, $p = 0.360$) compared to LC [16].

The Trans-Tasman Radiation Oncology Group (TROG 01.04) randomized 326 patients with T3 N0–2 rectal cancer to SC radiotherapy vs LC chemoradiotherapy showing similar local recurrence rates at 3 years (7.5% with SC vs 4.4% with LC, $p = 0.24$). For distal tumors (<5 cm from anal verge), local recurrence was non-significantly higher with SC (6 of 48 SC patients vs 1 of 31 LC patients, $p = 0.21$). Also, no difference in distant recurrence rates at 5 years was noted between SC (27%) and LC (30%, $p = 0.92$) [17]. Pathologic downstaging was more common after LC than SC (28% vs 45%, $p = 0.002$) as was pCR (1% vs 15%). However, no difference in APR rates (79% vs 77%, $p = 0.87$) and sphincter preservation (63% vs 69%, $p = 0.22$) was noted. Overall survival between groups was no different between SC and LC (74% vs 70%, $p = 0.62$). Late grade 3–4 toxicities were similar as well (5.8% vs 8.2%, $p = 0.53$). This trial also reported on quality of life within 12 months of treatment, showing no overall difference in health-related quality of life between the two arms [18].

In addition, the Stockholm III trial randomized 385 patients to: 1) SC radiotherapy with surgery within 1 week (SC), 2) SC radiotherapy with surgery delayed 4-8 weeks later (SC-delay), or 3) LC radiotherapy (50 Gy in 25 fractions) alone with surgery 4-8 weeks later. The cumulative incidence of local recurrence was 2%, 3%, and 5% in the SC, SC-delay, and LC patients, respectively, which was not statistically significant. The recurrence free survival and OS were similar in all 3 arms. [19]

The consistent results of these three studies strongly suggest the equivalency of SC vs LC radiation. However, longer-term follow-up is needed to determine disease outcomes beyond 5 years. It is unclear why the improved response with LC chemoradiation did not lead to a higher rate of sphincter preservation. One reason may be the reluctance of surgeons to alter their initial surgical plan despite a good clinical response.

Table 29.2 Head-to-head randomized trials comparing short-course and long-course neoadjuvant radiotherapy

Trial	Design	*N*	Local failure		Overall survival		Acute toxicity		Late toxicity (%)	
TROG 01.04 (2012) [17]	5 Gy × 5 fx + early TME	163	7.5% (5 years)	$p = 0.24$	74 (5 years)	$p = 0.62$	NR		5.8	$p = 0.53$
	1.8 Gy × 28 fx + chemo + TME	163	4.4% (5 years)		70% (5 years)		NR		8.2	
Polish I (2006) [16]	5 Gy × 5 fx + early TME	155	9% (4 years)	$p = 0.17$	67% (4 years)	$p = 0.96$	3.2%	$p < 0.001$	10.1	$p = 0.36$
	1.8 Gy × 28 fx + chemo + TME	157	14% (4 years)		66% (4 years)		18.2%		7.1	
Polish II (2016) [24]	5 Gy × 5 fx + chemo + TME	271	22% (3 years)	$p = 0.82$	73% (3 years)	$p = 0.046$	46% (Gr 2+) 24% (Gr3+)	$p = 0.006$	8	$p = 0.54$
	1.8 Gy × 28 fx + chemo + TME	270	21% (3 years)		65% (3 years)		60% (gr 2+) 24% (Gr3+)		6	

fx fractions, *TME* total mesorectal excision, *NR* not reported

Table 29.3 Pathologic complete response rates of short-course and long-course neoadjuvant radiotherapy

Trial	Design	*N*	Pathologic complete response (%)	
Trials with immediate surgery after short-course radiation				
TROG 01.04 (2012) [17]	5 Gy × 5 fx + early TME	163	1[a]	$p < 0.001$
	1.8 Gy × 28 fx + chemo + TME	163	15[a]	
Polish I (2006) [16]	5 Gy × 5 fx + early TME	155	0.7	NR
	1.8 Gy × 28 fx + chemo + TME	157	16.1	
Trials with delayed surgery after short-course radiation				
Polish II (2016) [24]	5 Gy × 5 fx + chemo + TME	271	16	$p = 0.17$
	1.8 Gy × 28 fx + chemo + TME	270	12	
Kaunas (2011) [22]	5 Gy × 5 fx + delayed TME	37	2.7	$p = 0.03$
	2 Gy × 25 fx + chemo + TME	46	13.1	
Stockholm III (2010) [20, 21]	5 Gy × 5 fx + TME	118	0.8	NR
	5 Gy × 5 fx + delayed TME	120	12.5	
	2 Gy × 25 fx + TME	65	5	

fx fractions, *TME* total mesorectal excision, *NR* not reported
[a]pathologic T0 rates

Alternative Approaches

Because the short interval between SC radiation and surgery does not allow time for tumor downsizing, one method to address this shortcoming is to delay the interval between radiation and surgery, which was tested in the Stockholm III Trial SC delayed surgery improved pCR rates (12.5% vs 0.5%) [20]. Postoperative complication rates were similar across the three arms (46.6, 40.0, and 32% respectively, $p = 0.164$). In the SC radiotherapy arm, postoperative complications were significantly more common 11–17 days after the initiation of radiotherapy as compared to <11 or >17 days after initiating treatment (38.7, 64.9, 33.3%, $p = 0.036$). APR rates (30, 33, 20%, $p = 0.381$) and postoperative death rates were similar across groups (0.8, 0.8, 2%, $p = 0.999$) [21]. The rate of radiation toxicity requiring hospitalization was higher in SC-delay patients vs. the SC patients (7% vs. <1%). However, the overall complication rate and surgical complication rate was lower for SC-delay patients (41% and 28%) vs. the SC patients (53% and 36%) [19].

In a much smaller trial by the Kaunas University of Medicine, 83 patients with stage II–III rectal adenocarcinoma were randomized to SC radiotherapy (25 Gy in 5 fractions) or LC chemoradiotherapy with surgery performed 6 weeks later. LC chemoradiation offered higher pCR rates (2.7% vs 13.1%, $p = 0.03$) and smaller tumors (33.1 vs 25.5 mm, $p = 0.009$). However, there was no impact on R0 resection rate (86.5% vs 91.3%, $p = 0.734$), sphincter preservation (70.3% vs 69.6%, $p = 0.342$), and postoperative complication rates (40.5% vs 26.1%, $p = 0.221$) [22].

Another approach is to give chemotherapy following SC radiation to address systemic disease earlier and to consolidate the effect of radiation. This strategy has been used by investigators at Washington University who gave 25 Gy in 5 fractions followed by four cycles of FOLFOX chemotherapy and then radical resection in 76 patients. The pCR rate was 25%, and 68% of patients were pathologically N0, despite only 22% staged initially as N0. At 3 years, the local control was 95% [23].

The Polish II trial prospectively evaluated SC radiotherapy (25 Gy in 5 fractions) followed by consolidation chemotherapy (FOLFOX4 for three cycles) vs LC chemoradiotherapy (50.4 Gy in 28 fractions with bolus 5-FU, leucovorin, and oxaliplatin), with surgery at 12 weeks in both arms, in patients with unresectable cT3–4 rectal cancer. Postoperative complication rates were similar between arms (29% vs 25%) as was the need for reoperation (14% vs 11%) and surgery-related death (0% vs 2%, $p = 0.18$). There was no difference in local recurrence at 3 years (22% vs 21%, $p = 0.82$) or distant failure at 3 years (30% vs 27%, $p = 0.25$) and no differences in pCR rates (16% vs 12%, $p = 0.17$) and R0 resection rates (77% vs 71%, $p = 0.07$), trending in favor of SC radiotherapy. While no difference in disease-free survival (53% vs 52%, $p = 0.85$) was seen, this trial was notable for showing an overall survival benefit at 3 years with SC therapy (73% vs 65%, $p = 0.046$). The SC arm had fewer dose reductions (0% vs 8%, $p < 0.001$) and fewer prolongations of treatment (0% vs 5%, $p < 0.001$) compared with LC. The rate of preoperative treatment acute toxicity was lower with SC radiotherapy ($p = 0.006$), with grade 3–4 toxicities of 21% vs 23%. There were also fewer acute toxic deaths with SC therapy (1% vs 3%, $p = 0.0006$) with all deaths occurring during chemotherapy. Similarly, late grade 3–4 (8% vs 5%, $p = 0.54$) and grade 5 (0.5% vs 1%) toxicities were no different [24].

Taken together, these data suggest that altering the SC regimen by delaying surgery does in fact allow time for tumor downsizing and improves pathologic response rates, thus dispelling two major criticisms of SC radiation. However, longer-term follow-up is needed to determine local control and survival. The addition of chemotherapy between radiation and surgery offers an intriguing new paradigm that serves to achieve the best of both worlds, allowing time for tumor downsizing and addressing systemic disease early in the treatment course. The RAPIDO trial, currently underway, is designed very similarly to the Polish II trial, randomizing patients to LC chemoradiation with oral 5-fluorouracil (capecitabine) vs SC 5 Gy × 5 and 6 cycles of capecitabine and oxaliplatin [25]; the results will further determine the efficacy of this approach.

Summary/Patient Selection

In summary, head-to-head data with early follow-up shows no difference in local failure or survival between SC radiotherapy and LC chemoradiotherapy. Pathologic downstaging and pCR rates are higher with long-course radiotherapy but without an apparent improvement in sphincter preservation rates or difference in postoperative complications. Acute toxicity is worse with LC radiotherapy, but there is no significant difference in late toxicity. Based on the available literature, both regimens can be considered acceptable standards of care for patients with locally advanced rectal cancer.

There may be situations where SC preoperative radiotherapy with immediate surgery may be ideal. For example, oligometastatic disease with few liver metastases may be a scenario in which addressing the primary as rapidly as possible may help control the few distant lesions before disease progression. On the other hand, LC chemoradiotherapy has a clear benefit in terms of pathologic downstaging and pCR rates prior to surgery. As such, patients who require tumor shrinkage in preparation for optimal surgery, such as in patients with larger tumors with threatened circumferential resection margins, might benefit more from this approach. However, as more data emerges regarding delaying surgery or regarding the addition of systemic chemotherapy immediately following SC radiation, the use of SC will likely expand.

References

1. Network NCC. NCCN clinical practive guidelines in oncology (NCCN Guidelines): rectal cancer (Version 2.2016) [July 17, 2016]. Available from: https://www.nccn.org/professionals/physician_gls/pdf/rectal.pdf.
2. Preoperative short-term radiation therapy in operable rectal carcinoma. A prospective randomized trial. Stockholm Rectal Cancer Study Group. Cancer. 1990;66(1):49–55.
3. Cedermark B, Johansson H, Rutqvist LE, Wilking N. The Stockholm I trial of preoperative short term radiotherapy in operable rectal carcinoma. A prospective randomized trial. Stockholm Colorectal Cancer Study Group. Cancer. 1995;75(9):2269–75.
4. Frykholm GJ, Glimelius B, Pahlman L. Preoperative or postoperative irradiation in adenocarcinoma of the rectum: final treatment results of a randomized trial and an evaluation of late secondary effects. Dis Colon Rectum. 1993;36(6):564–72.
5. Camma C, Giunta M, Fiorica F, Pagliaro L, Craxi A, Cottone M. Preoperative radiotherapy for resectable rectal cancer: a meta-analysis. JAMA. 2000;284(8):1008–15.
6. Improved survival with preoperative radiotherapy in resectable rectal cancer. Swedish Rectal Cancer Trial. N Engl J Med. 1997;336(14):980–7.
7. Kapiteijn E, Marijnen CA, Nagtegaal ID, Putter H, Steup WH, Wiggers T, et al. Preoperative radiotherapy combined with total mesorectal excision for resectable rectal cancer. N Engl J Med. 2001;345(9):638–46.
8. Prolongation of the disease-free interval in surgically treated rectal carcinoma. Gastrointestinal Tumor Study Group. N Engl J Med. 1985;312(23):1465–72.
9. Krook JE, Moertel CG, Gunderson LL, Wieand HS, Collins RT, Beart RW, et al. Effective surgical adjuvant therapy for high-risk rectal carcinoma. N Engl J Med. 1991;324(11):709–15.
10. Fisher B, Wolmark N, Rockette H, Redmond C, Deutsch M, Wickerham DL, et al. Postoperative adjuvant chemotherapy or radiation therapy for rectal cancer: results from NSABP protocol R-01. J Natl Cancer Inst. 1988;80(1):21–9.
11. Wolmark N, Wieand HS, Hyams DM, Colangelo L, Dimitrov NV, Romond EH, et al. Randomized trial of postoperative adjuvant chemotherapy with or without radiotherapy for carcinoma of the rectum: National Surgical Adjuvant Breast and Bowel Project Protocol R-02. J Natl Cancer Inst. 2000;92(5):388–96.

12. Adjuvant therapy for patients with colon and rectum cancer. NIH Consens Statement. 1990; 8(4):1–25.
13. Sauer R, Becker H, Hohenberger W, Rodel C, Wittekind C, Fietkau R, et al. Preoperative versus postoperative chemoradiotherapy for rectal cancer. N Engl J Med. 2004;351(17):1731–40.
14. Sauer R, Liersch T, Merkel S, Fietkau R, Hohenberger W, Hess C, et al. Preoperative versus postoperative chemoradiotherapy for locally advanced rectal cancer: results of the German CAO/ARO/AIO-94 randomized phase III trial after a median follow-up of 11 years. J Clin Oncol. 2012;30(16):1926–33.
15. Peeters KC, van de Velde CJ, Leer JW, Martijn H, Junggeburt JM, Kranenbarg EK, et al. Late side effects of short-course preoperative radiotherapy combined with total mesorectal excision for rectal cancer: increased bowel dysfunction in irradiated patients—a Dutch colorectal cancer group study. J Clin Oncol. 2005;23(25):6199–206.
16. Bujko K, Nowacki MP, Nasierowska-Guttmejer A, Michalski W, Bebenek M, Kryj M. Long-term results of a randomized trial comparing preoperative short-course radiotherapy with preoperative conventionally fractionated chemoradiation for rectal cancer. Br J Surg. 2006;93(10):1215–23.
17. Ngan SY, Burmeister B, Fisher RJ, Solomon M, Goldstein D, Joseph D, et al. Randomized trial of short-course radiotherapy versus long-course chemoradiation comparing rates of local recurrence in patients with T3 rectal cancer: Trans-Tasman Radiation Oncology Group trial 01.04. J Clin Oncol. 2012;30(31):3827–33.
18. McLachlan SA, Fisher RJ, Zalcberg J, Solomon M, Burmeister B, Goldstein D, et al. The impact on health-related quality of life in the first 12 months: a randomised comparison of preoperative short-course radiation versus long-course chemoradiation for T3 rectal cancer (Trans-Tasman Radiation Oncology Group Trial 01.04). Eur J Cancer. 2016;55:15–26.
19. Erlandsson, J., et al., Optimal fractionation of preoperative radiotherapy and timing to surgery for rectal cancer (Stockholm III): a multicentre, randomised, non-blinded, phase 3, non-inferiority trial. Lancet Oncol 2017;18(3): p. 336–346.
20. Pettersson D, Lorinc E, Holm T, Iversen H, Cedermark B, Glimelius B, et al. Tumour regression in the randomized Stockholm III Trial of radiotherapy regimens for rectal cancer. Br J Surg. 2015;102(8):972–8. Discussion 8.
21. Pettersson D, Cedermark B, Holm T, Radu C, Pahlman L, Glimelius B, et al. Interim analysis of the Stockholm III trial of preoperative radiotherapy regimens for rectal cancer. Br J Surg. 2010;97(4):580–7.
22. Latkauskas T, Pauzas H, Gineikiene I, Janciauskiene R, Juozaityte E, Saladzinskas Z, et al. Initial results of a randomized controlled trial comparing clinical and pathological downstaging of rectal cancer after preoperative short-course radiotherapy or long-term chemoradiotherapy, both with delayed surgery. Color Dis. 2012;14(3):294–8.
23. Myerson RJ, Tan B, Hunt S, Olsen J, Birnbaum E, Fleshman J, et al. Five fractions of radiation therapy followed by 4 cycles of FOLFOX chemotherapy as preoperative treatment for rectal cancer. Int J Radiat Oncol Biol Phys. 2014;88(4):829–36.
24. Bujko K, Wyrwicz L, Rutkowski A, Malinowska M, Pietrzak L, Krynski J, et al. Long-course oxaliplatin-based preoperative chemoradiation versus 5 × 5 Gy and consolidation chemotherapy for cT4 or fixed cT3 rectal cancer: results of a randomized phase III study. Ann Oncol. 2016;27(5):834–42.
25. Nilsson PJ, van Etten B, Hospers GA, Pahlman L, van de Velde CJ, Beets-Tan RG, et al. Short-course radiotherapy followed by neo-adjuvant chemotherapy in locally advanced rectal cancer—the RAPIDO trial. BMC Cancer. 2013;13:279.
26. Folkesson J, Birgisson H, Pahlman L, Cedermark B, Glimelius B, Gunnarsson U. Swedish Rectal Cancer Trial: long lasting benefits from radiotherapy on survival and local recurrence rate. J Clin Oncol. 2005;23(24):5644–50.
27. Randomized study on preoperative radiotherapy in rectal carcinoma. Stockholm Colorectal Cancer Study Group. Ann Surg Oncol. 1996;3(5):423–30.
28. Marsh PJ, James RD, Schofield PF. Adjuvant preoperative radiotherapy for locally advanced rectal carcinoma. Results of a prospective, randomized trial. Dis Colon Rectum. 1994;37(12): 1205–14.

29. van Gijn W, Marijnen CA, Nagtegaal ID, Kranenbarg EM, Putter H, Wiggers T, et al. Preoperative radiotherapy combined with total mesorectal excision for resectable rectal cancer: 12-year follow-up of the multicentre, randomised controlled TME trial. Lancet Oncol. 2011; 12(6):575–82.
30. Sebag-Montefiore D, Stephens RJ, Steele R, Monson J, Grieve R, Khanna S, et al. Preoperative radiotherapy versus selective postoperative chemoradiotherapy in patients with rectal cancer (MRC CR07 and NCIC-CTG C016): a multicentre, randomised trial. Lancet. 2009;373(9666): 811–20.

Intersphincteric Resection: Perineal or Abdominal Dissection First?

30

Paula Loughlin, Quentin Denost, and Eric Rullier

Introduction

The management of rectal cancer continues to evolve. The increasing use of neoadjuvant chemoradiotherapy and improved understanding of what impacts oncological outcomes have led to sphincter-preserving surgery for low rectal cancer being possible for the majority. Not only is it technically feasible, it is associated with better oncological outcomes than abdominoperineal resection (APR) [1, 2], has less of a negative impact on sexual function [3], and avoids the need for a permanent stoma, in all but a minority. In this chapter we will discuss the rationale for its use, the technical details, and finally why we advocate for a perineal first approach.

Indications for Intersphincteric Resection

Oncological Rules for Rectal Cancer

Historically and conventionally, the decision to perform a sphincter-saving procedure is based on the distal resection margin, i.e., the distance between the lower edge of the tumor and the anal sphincter. In the 1980s, the acceptable distal margin decreased from 5 cm to 2 cm when it was established that the majority have no distal spread beyond 2 cm and that there was no association between a shorter distal resection margin and local recurrence or survival [4, 5]. More recently it has become

P. Loughlin
Department of Surgery, Altnagelvin Hospital, Derry, UK
e-mail: paula.loughlin@westerntrust.hscni.net; drpaulaloughlin@gmail.com

Q. Denost · E. Rullier (✉)
Department of Colorectal Surgery, Magellan Centre, Bordeaux University Hospital, Pessac 33600, France
e-mail: quentin.denost@chu-bordeaux.fr; eric.rullier@chu-bordeaux.fr

C.M. Schlachta, P. Sylla (eds.), *Current Common Dilemmas in Colorectal Surgery*,
https://doi.org/10.1007/978-3-319-70117-2_30

apparent that a 1 cm margin is adequate [6] largely as a result of the impact of neoadjuvant therapy. A review of 17 studies even suggests that in selected patients a margin of <1 cm does not compromise oncological outcomes [7]. Thus, decreasing the acceptable distal resection margin permitted performance of sphincter-saving surgery for mid-rectal cancer and in some low rectal cancers. By using the distal resection margin as the main oncologic rule, the limit for sphincter-saving resection is a patient with a tumor at less than 1 cm from the top of the anal sphincter or anal canal. This is what is recommended in most surgical guidelines [8].

In the 1990s, the circumferential resection margin (CRM) became the most important surrogate marker of surgical quality, showing a strong association between a CRM ≤ 1 mm and pelvic recurrence [9]. However, despite this new oncologic concept, and the evidence that shorter margins are acceptable, surgical practice has been slower to change, with high rates of APR still common [10]. We believe that modern practice should take into account both the distal resection margin and the CRM when planning the optimal management of low rectal cancer in order to adopt sphincter preservation as the gold standard for appropriately selected patients.

Surgical Options for Low Rectal Cancer

The surgical management of mid- and upper rectal cancers is well standardized with the adoption of partial mesorectal excision (PME) for upper third cancers and total mesorectal excision (TME) for those in the mid-rectum. Sphincter-sparing procedures are the norm for the majority. However, the management of low rectal cancer is a more complex issue, and despite the potential for sphincter preservation, APR is still considered by many to be the gold standard. There are, however, several other surgical options for low rectal cancer (Fig. 30.1).

Low anterior resection (LAR) with stapled low colorectal anastomosis is the most common procedure because it can be performed using the transabdominal route. In case of a narrow male pelvis or bulky tumor, a hand-sewn coloanal anastomosis is an alternative to stapling (Fig. 30.1b). According to Park's procedure, the anal canal is exposed with a Lone Star self-retaining retractor (CooperSurgical, Trumbull, Connecticut), and the distal rectal mucosa is excised. Then, the colon is pulled through the anal canal and sutured at the dentate line [11]. For tumors close to or partially invading the internal sphincter, partial or total ISR (intersphincteric resection) (Fig. 30.1c) is the only sphincter-preserving option that can achieve a negative resection margin. When reconstructing the rectum, a colonic J pouch or side-to-end anastomosis is used in preference to a straight anastomosis, especially following intersphincteric resection, where the risk of anal incontinence is higher than after a LAR [12].

The variation in rate of APR observed between hospitals in Europe and the United States reflects the heterogeneous surgical strategies employed in the management of low rectal cancer [10, 13]. This heterogeneity is related to the difference in training between surgeons, as well as the difference in experience, skill, and rectal cancer volume. However, we believe that these variations in the surgical treatment of low

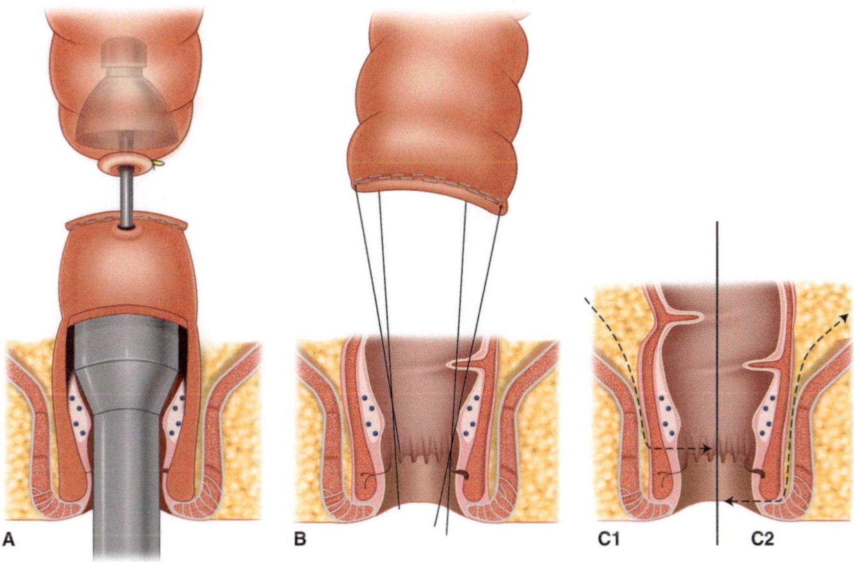

Fig. 30.1 Types of sphincter-saving procedures. (**a**) Stapled low colorectal anastomosis. (**b**) Hand-sewn coloanal anastomosis after rectal mucosectomy. (**c**) Partial (C1) and total (C2) intersphincteric resection. Modified from Seminars Colon & Rectum Surgery 2006 (Rullier et al.)

rectal cancer are mainly due to the lack of consensus regarding what constitutes a low rectal cancer and of standardization regarding its management.

Classification of Low Rectal Cancer and Standardization of Surgery

In Bordeaux, by standardizing the approach to low rectal cancer, we have challenged the concept that ultralow rectal cancers must be managed with APR [14]. We developed an anatomical classification to determine which surgical strategy should be used and demonstrated that most patients with low rectal cancers could be managed with a sphincter-preserving approach, without compromising oncological outcomes [15]. Low rectal cancers were classified into four distinct types, each type managed using one surgical technique (Fig. 30.2). Type I includes supra-anal tumors (>1 cm from the anal sphincter) and are treated by conventional coloanal anastomosis, type II are juxta-anal tumors (<1 cm from the anal sphincter) and treated by partial intersphincteric resection, type III are intra-anal tumors (internal sphincter invasion) treated by total intersphincteric resection, and type IV are transanal tumors (external sphincter or levator ani muscles invasion) treated by APR.

High-resolution magnetic resonance imaging is critical in determining the position of the tumor in relation to the anal sphincter and the levator ani muscles and therefore determines the type of low rectal cancer. Those who have a margin of

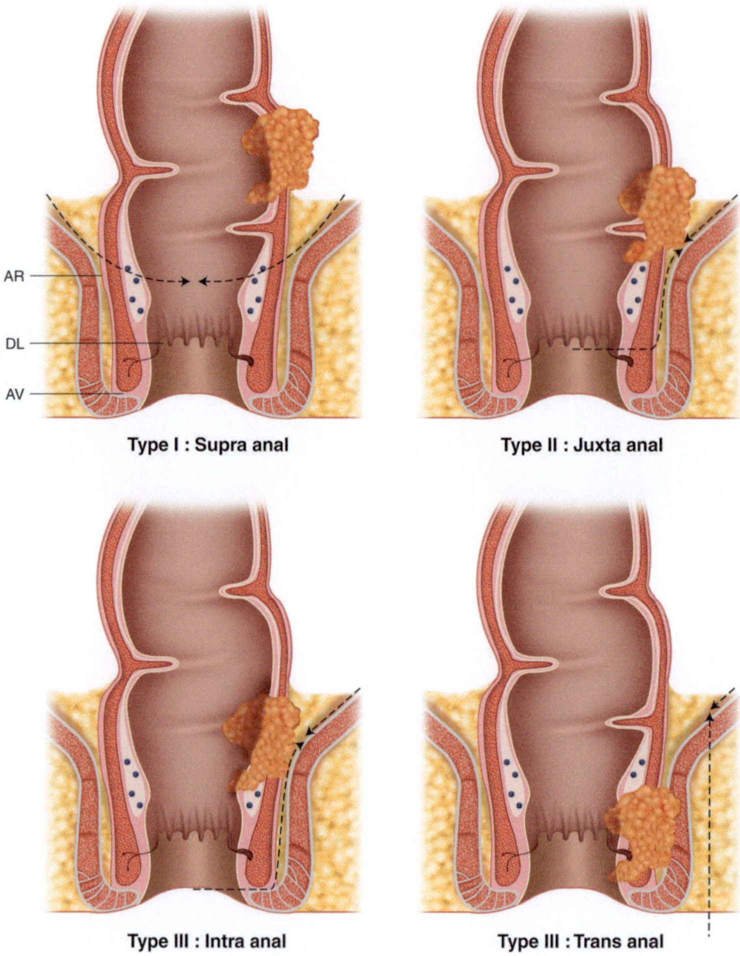

Fig. 30.2 Surgical classification of low rectal cancer. *AR* anal ring, *DL* dentate line, *AV* anal verge. Modified from Dis Colon Rectum 2013 (Rullier et al.)

>1 mm from the levator ani muscles with a clear intersphincteric plane are suitable for sphincter-preserving surgery, in the absence of any other contraindications. This classification therefore respects oncological principles with respect to both distal and circumferential resection margins.

The Role of Chemoradiotherapy in Sphincter-Preserving Surgery

Neoadjuvant chemoradiotherapy therapy for rectal cancer is the recommended standard for some T3 and most T4 tumors of the mid- and lower rectum. Neoadjuvant treatment can induce tumor downstaging, facilitating excision with clear margins [16, 17], and also significantly improving local control [18]. Our classification can therefore be used to reassess the tumor after neoadjuvant treatment. A repeat MRI should be performed 6–8 weeks after completion of treatment and in advance of surgery. Using MRI in low rectal cancer before and after neoadjuvant therapy, together with classification of low rectal cancer, can increase the chance of sphincter-saving surgery because the decision regarding the type of surgery is based on tumor response to treatment and not based on the original stage of the tumor.

Surgical Technique

The surgical technique of intersphincteric resection (ISR) consists of two phases, the abdominal dissection and the perineal dissection. Historically, the abdominal dissection is performed first. However, in recent years, initiation of the dissection via the transanal route has gained popularity, and we will discuss the potential benefits of this.

Abdominal Dissection First

In our hands, the abdominal dissection for TME surgery is done laparoscopically in most cases. The principles are the same as for open or robotic surgery. The standardized approach includes high ligation of the inferior mesenteric artery and full mobilization of the left colon and splenic flexure to ensure a tension-free coloanal anastomosis and the fact that the specimen will be removed transanally. The rectum is then mobilized in the TME plane, posteriorly and laterally, and dissection continues along the levator ani muscles to the top of the anal canal. This plane of dissection is anterior to the sheath of the pelvic floor, which covers the levator ani. If possible, the intersphincteric plane is initiated posteriorly (Fig. 30.3). Anteriorly, it is carried out close to the prostate, removing Denonvilliers' fascia (if the tumor is anterior), and continued to the top of the anal canal or the distal vagina. The technique includes preservation of the hypogastric and pelvic plexuses and the presacral nerves. The last 2–3 cm of the rectal dissection, i.e., the distal third of the TME procedure, is the most difficult part, due to limited exposure of the distal pelvis, the limited length of the laparoscopic instruments, and the proximity of the tumor where the mesorectum is lacking. By dissecting as low as possible with the objective of facilitating the perineal dissection, the risk of dissecting too close to the tumor and achieving an incomplete resection (R1 resection) increases. Other intraoperative risks include bleeding and potential pelvic nerve injury due to difficult transabdominal low rectal dissection.

The perineal dissection is performed after digital rectal examination to confirms that the abdominal dissection has reached the top of the anal ring. The perineal transanal dissection is carried out with conventional instruments, under direct vision. Laparoscopic TaTME [19] is not necessary. Indeed, the objective is to perform a short dissection to connect the previous abdominal dissection. The anal canal is exposed with a self-retaining retractor (Lone Star Retractor, Lone Star Medical Products Inc., Houston, TX). A gauze swab is placed into the rectal lumen to prevent

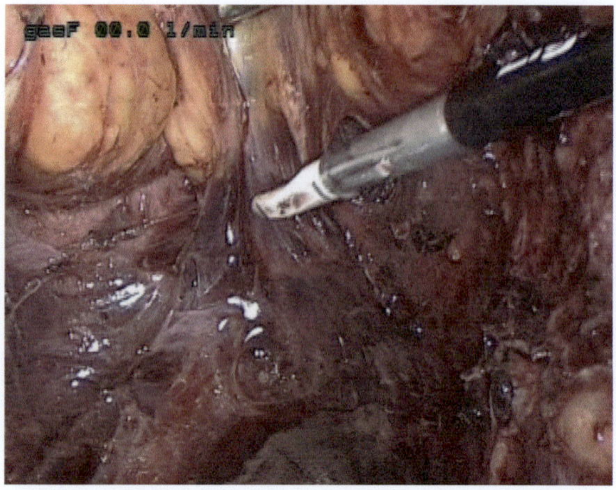

Fig. 30.3 Abdominal laparoscopic posterior dissection. Abdominal opening of the posterior intersphincteric plane by cutting the right coccygeorectal muscle

spillage of tumor cells or luminal contents. A full-thickness circumferential incision is then made with diathermy, at least 1 cm below the lower edge of the tumor. The level of transection is the dentate line for partial intersphincteric resection and 1–2 cm below the dentate line for total intersphincteric resection. In case of good response to neoadjuvant therapy, the decision between partial versus total intersphincteric resection is made according to reclassification of the tumor type based on post-neoadjuvant treatment imaging. After dissection of the distal 2 cm, the rectum is closed with a purse-string suture. Dissection is carried out posteriorly along the puborectalis muscle which facilitates identification of the correct plane of dissection and continued laterally along the fibers of the levator ani muscles. Dissection is extended behind the pelvic floor sheath (Waldeyer's fascia), for a few centimeters, which must be transected to join the abdominal dissection. The anterior dissection is carried out along the prostate or vagina to join the same plane from above. Care is taken to intermittently release retraction on the sphincter to prevent excessive stretching or injury. The rectum is then usually extracted transanally. The proximal sigmoid is divided and the rectum is reconstructed with a hand-sewn side-to-end or J pouch coloanal anastomosis. A loop ileostomy is fashioned as standard and closed after 2–3 months.

Recently, an alternative to conventional retractors and direct vision is to use single port and laparoscopic instruments [19–21]. However, we do not feel it is necessary in this case as only a few centimeters of distal rectum needs to be mobilized after the abdominal dissection is complete. This could be useful only in the case of a long anal canal and when the abdominal dissection cannot be completely achieved for technical reasons.

Perineal Dissection First

Gerard Marks et al. described the TATA (transanal transabdominal transanal) surgery for sphincter-saving surgery in low rectal cancer after high-dose irradiation [22]. They transected the rectum transanally, extending the low rectal dissection as high as possible with fingers before beginning the abdominal dissection. In Asia,

Teramoto et al. [23] proposed the same strategy in order to optimize the distal resection margin by using direct vision to guide the rectal transection. In Europe, we used intersphincteric resection for ultralow rectal cancer [24] and decided to begin LAR procedures by using the transanal step starting in the 2000s, after showing that the quality of the TME can be compromised during the conventional laparoscopic approach for low rectal dissection [25].

Technically, the principles of transanal low rectal dissection have been described above. We usually stop the transanal procedure when the dissection reaches the upper part of the tumor, i.e., usually at least 5 cm above the anal ring for low rectal cancer. In practice, part of the levator ani muscles has been dissected posteriorly and laterally, as well as most of the prostate or vagina. Interestingly, even by using conventional anal retractors and direct vision, it is possible to achieve dissection of the rectum up to 8–10 cm from the anal verge. In female and non-obese male patients, the cervix and the seminal vesicles can be reached with this approach. Recently some surgeons have used TaTME with a single port and laparoscopic instrument to perform the transanal dissection. Thus, by using TaTME one option is to perform a partial TME (only dissecting the distal rectum), and the other option is performing a total mesorectal excision transanally. However, it is unclear as to whether performing a full TME, via the transanal approach, is of any additional benefit.

After completing the distal rectal dissection transanally, the abdominal component is completed as described above except that the pelvic dissection stops when it joins the dissection from below. Connection between the perineal and the abdominal dissection sometimes needs to break the sheath of the pelvic floor (Waldeyer's fascia). Indeed, the plane of dissection is usually above the sheath during the abdominal step, whereas it is below it during the transanal step (Fig. 30.4). In all cases, completion of the perineal dissection of the distal rectum first facilitates the abdominal step.

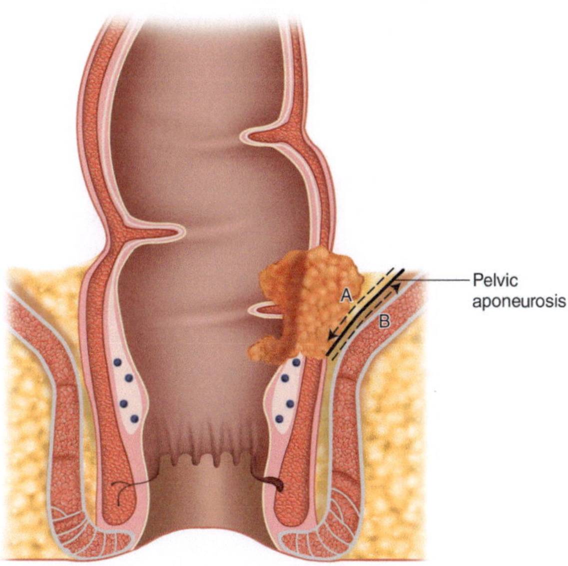

Fig. 30.4 Intersphincteric resection: A is the plane of abdominal low rectal dissection and B is the plane of transanal low rectal dissection. Modified from Annals of Surgery 2014 (Rullier et al.)

Advantages of a Perineal First Approach

The abdominal dissection of the lower third of the rectum is difficult due to the limitations in exposure of the pelvis. Moreover the plane of dissection is angulated due to the presence of the sacrum posteriorly and the genital organs anteriorly. The length of laparoscopic instruments can also be limited to dissect deep in the pelvis. These limitations are particularly problematic in male and obese patients and in case of bulky or low rectal tumors. Thus, several difficulties can occur during abdominal TME resulting in coning effect on the mesorectum, inadequate surgical margins, pelvic bleeding, nerve injuries, and difficulties with stapling of the low rectum. All these technical challenges may also increase the rate of conversion.

By using a transanal approach first to dissect the rectum and mesorectum, a longer distal resection margin (2.8 cm vs 1.7 cm; $p < 0.01$) [19] and a better quality of the mesorectum can be achieved [21]. Transecting the rectum transanally under direct vision as the first step probably facilitates achieving a negative distal resection margin. In a randomized trial comparing 100 patients treated with transanal versus laparoscopic distal rectal dissection for low rectal cancer, we observed a lower rate of positive circumferential margins (4% vs 18%; $p = 0.02$) in the transanal group. We hypothesized that the fact that the plane of the intersphincteric resection was behind the sheath of the levator ani muscles during the transanal dissection as opposed to above during the abdominal dissection, increasing the chances of achieving a negative margin after transanal approach [26]. This concept may only apply to cases of ultralow sphincter-saving resection for low rectal cancer, where transection of the rectum involves the anal canal and thus the transanal dissection is carried out along the fibers of the levator ani muscles.

When performing a conventional laparoscopic sphincter-saving procedure, the surgeon attempts low rectal stapling. However, this may be associated with technical difficulties inducing a higher number of firings, which can increase the rate of anastomotic leakage [27]. Using a transanal approach first avoids the intraoperative technical difficulty of distal rectal stapling. A new alternative combines transanal dissection with transanal stapling [28]. Finally all methods of sphincter-saving resection are technically possible in association with transanal TME, avoiding the difficulties of transabdominal distal rectal stapling.

Conversion is probably one of the main technical advantages of the transanal low rectal dissection first. In our randomized single institution trial, we observed a lower rate of conversion, although not significant (4% vs 10%), in the transanal group compared to the laparoscopic group [26]. This is in accordance with 1.4% vs 5.4% of conversion reported in a review comparing transanal with laparoscopic TME surgery [29]. Finally, other advantages of beginning by the transanal approach are shorter operative time [30], less fatigue for the surgeon [31], and theoretically safer surgery for the patient because the oncologic step is carried out at the beginning of the procedure.

Results of Intersphincteric Resection

Feasibility and Morbidity

Intersphincteric resection was first described by Schiessel in 1994 in Europe [32] and has subsequently been popularized by Rullier [14, 15, 17, 24, 26, 33]. In the United States, Gerard and John Marks have developed the same procedure [22]. Two reviews of intersphincteric resection reported an acceptable rate of morbidity, including 9.1% anastomotic leak and 0.8% mortality [34, 35]. In our personal experience of 303 patients treated by intersphincteric resection for low rectal cancer, the leak rate was 12% and mortality 0.3% (1/303) (unpublished data). We did not observe a significant difference between transanal and laparoscopic abdominal approach in our trial including 100 patients: overall morbidity 32% vs 44%, surgical morbidity Dindo 3–5 12% vs 14%, anastomotic leak 2% vs 10%, and urologic medical morbidity 6% vs 10%, respectively [26].

Oncological Results

In specialist hands the quality of surgery following intersphincteric resection is adequate, including a 1.7 cm mean distal resection margin with 97% R0 resection in a pooled analysis of 1289 patients from 14 studies [35]. The rate of local recurrence was 7% and the disease-free survival 79% after a median follow-up of 56 months. While some authors argue that intersphincteric resection should be reserved for T1and T2 tumors only [36], our experience has shown that with the use of neoadjuvant chemoradiotherapy, the procedure is oncologically safe for locally advanced tumors [17]. In Bordeaux from 1990 to 2014, we have performed 303 intersphincteric resections for low rectal cancer. There were 8 T1, 33 T2, 232 T3, and 30 T4, and 89% (n = 270) received preoperative radiochemotherapy. The average distal resection margin was 15 mm and the R0 resection rate was 86%. In the past, patients with R1 resection after neoadjuvant therapy had completion APR, whereas since 1995 they were observed. After a median follow-up of 62 months, the rate of local recurrence was 4.8% (14/303), and the disease-free survival was 73% (unpublished data). Our results are concordant with the long-term results of Schiessel et al. [37], reporting 5.3% local recurrence after a median follow-up of 72 months in 121 patients who had intersphincteric resection over a 16-year period.

Finally, in patients having intersphincteric resection, with perineal dissection completed first, there may be an oncological advantage. As previously described, during this approach, the plane of dissection is usually behind the aponeurosis of the pelvic floor (Waldeyer's fascia), in contrast to the abdominal dissection where it takes place anterior to it. In our hands, we observed a median difference of 2 mm in the circumferential resection margin between the two approaches, which translated to a significantly lower rate of CRM positivity in the perineal group [26]. However, this theoretical oncologic advantage has not yet impacted the oncologic outcomes with similar local recurrence rate at 3 years between groups (unpublished data).

Functional Results

Having established the oncological safety of intersphincteric resection, functional outcomes and quality of life are the next priority. While intersphincteric resection does avoid a permanent stoma, it is associated with the low anterior resection syndrome, dysfunctional defecation, and incontinence [35]. Symptoms are significantly worse in those who have had radiochemotherapy [38], a lower anastomosis [39], and anastomotic leak [40]. Quality of life globally is similar between intersphincteric resection and APR [3], although it can be impaired by defecatory problems during the first 6 months [41].

The main side effect of intersphincteric resection is fecal incontinence. A significant incontinence score (Wexner score >10) is observed in 47% of the cases after intersphincteric resection compared to 19% after a conventional LAR [42]. However, efficient treatment of refractory fecal incontinence after ultralow sphincter-saving surgery is available by using anterograde enema, which avoids a definitive colostomy in most cases [43].

The impact of the surgical approach (perineal versus abdominal) on functional outcomes after intersphincteric resection is unclear. Among the 100 patients included in our randomized trial comparing laparoscopic and transanal TME, 72 responded to questionnaires [44]. The bowel function was similar between the transanal and laparoscopic groups: LARS 36 versus 37 ($p = 0.94$) and anal continence Wexner score 9 versus 10 ($p = 0.79$). Similarly the urologic function did not differ: IPSS 5.5 versus 3.5, respectively ($p = 0.82$). However, at 1 year after surgery, sexual activity was present in 71% of the patients in the transanal group versus 39% in the laparoscopic group ($p = 0.02$), and erectile function was also better in men in the transanal group: IIEF 17 versus 7 ($p = 0.12$). The potential improvement of pelvic nerve preservation and genital function by using the perineal transanal dissection of the distal or the total mesorectum, however, needs to be confirmed by future studies.

Conclusion

Intersphincteric resection is a safe oncologic option in low rectal cancer. Indications are most low rectal cancers without invasion of the intersphincteric plane and levator ani muscles based on repeat MRI after completion of neoadjuvant chemoradiotherapy. The limitation of this approach is the risk of fecal incontinence, for which new treatments are available. However, the conventional abdominal laparoscopic intersphincteric resection is very challenging. Using the perineal transanal approach first facilitates the low rectal dissection in patients with difficult anatomy, limiting the rate of conversion and increasing chance of R0 resection. In addition, completing the perineal approach first may have functional advantages, but long-term follow-up studies are needed.

References

1. Rullier E, Sebag-Montefiore D. Sphincter saving is the primary objective for local treatment of cancer of the lower rectum. Lancet Oncol. 2006;7:769–71.
2. Kim C, Lee SY, Kim H, Kim YJ. Factors associated with oncologic outcomes following abdominoperineal or intersphincteric resection in patients treated with preoperative chemoradiotherapy. A propensity score analysis. Medicine (Baltimore). 2015;94(45):e2060.
3. Konanz J, Herrle F, Weiss C, Post S, Kienle P. Quality of life of patients after low anterior, intersphincteric, and abdominoperineal resection for low rectal cancer: a matched-pair analysis. Int J Color Dis. 2013;28:679–88.
4. Williams NS, Dixon MF, Johnston D. Reappraisal of the 5 centimetre rule of distal excision for carcinoma of the rectum: a study of distal intramural spread and of patients' survival. Br J Surg. 1983;70:150–4.
5. Pollett WG, Nicholls RJ. The relationship between the extent of distal clearance and survival and local recurrence rates after curative anterior resection for carcinoma of the rectum. Ann Surg. 1983;198(2):159–63.
6. Ueno H, Mochizuki H, Hashiguchi Y, Ishikawa K, Fujimoto H, Shinto E, et al. Preoperative parameters expanding the indication of sphincter preserving surgery in patients with advanced low rectal cancer. Ann Surg. 2004;239:34–42.
7. Bujko K, Rutkowski A, Chang GJ, Michalski W, Chmielik E, Kusnierz J. Is the 1-cm rule of distal bowel resection margin in rectal cancer based on clinical evidence? A systematic review. Ann Surg Oncol. 2012;19:801–8.
8. Lakkis Z, Manceau G, Bridoux V, Brouquet A, Kirzin S, Maggiore L, French Research Group of Rectal Cancer Surgery (GRECCAR) and the French National Society of Coloproctology (SNFCP). Management of rectal cancer: the 2016 French guidelines. Color Dis. 2017;19(2):115–22.
9. Quirke P, Durdey P, Dixon MF, Williams NS. Local recurrence of rectal adenocarcinoma due to inadequate surgical resection: histopathological study of lateral tumour spread and surgical excision. Lancet. 1986;1(38):996–9.
10. Morris E, Quirke P, Thomas JD, Fairley L, Cottier B, Forman D. Unacceptable variation in abdominoperineal excision rates for rectal cancer: time to intervene? Gut. 2008;57:1690–7.
11. Parks AG, Percy JP. Resection and sutured colo-anal anastomosis for rectal carcinoma. Br J Surg. 1982;69:301–4.
12. Hüttner FJ, Tenckhoff S, Jensen K, Uhlmann L, Kulu Y, Büchler MW, et al. Meta-analysis of reconstruction techniques after low anterior resection for rectal cancer. Br J Surg. 2015;102:735–45.
13. Ricciardi R, Roberts PL, Read TE, Marcello PW, Schoetz DJ, Baxter NN. Variability in reconstructive procedures following rectal cancer surgery in the United States. Dis Colon Rectum. 2010;53:874–80.
14. Rullier E, Denost Q, Laurent C. A concept of sphincter salvage in low rectal cancer. In: Schiessel R, Metzger P, editors. Intersphincteric resection for low rectal tumors. Wien: Springer; 2012. p. 111–9.
15. Rullier E, Denost Q, Vendrely V, Rullier A, Laurent C. Low rectal cancer: classification and standardization of surgery. Dis Colon Rectum. 2013;56:560–7.
16. Weiser MR, Quah HM, Shia J, et al. Sphincter preservation in low rectal cancer is facilitated by preoperative chemoradiation and intersphincteric dissection. Ann Surg. 2009;249:236–42.
17. Rullier E, Goffre B, Bonnel C, Zerbib F, Caudry M, Saric J. Preoperative radiochemotherapy and sphincter-saving resection for T3 carcinomas of the lower third of the rectum. Ann Surg. 2001;234:633–40.
18. McCarthy K, Pearson K, Fulton R, Hewitt J. Pre-operative chemoradiation for non-metastatic locally advanced rectal cancer. Cochrane Database Syst Rev. 2012;12:CD008368.
19. Sylla P, Rattner DW, Delgado S, Lacy AM. NOTES transanal rectal cancer resection using transanal endoscopic microsurgery and laparoscopic assistance. Surg Endosc. 2010;24:1205–10.

20. Fernández-Hevia M, Delgado S, Castells A, et al. Transanal total mesorectal excision in rectal cancer: short-term outcomes in comparison with laparoscopic surgery. Ann Surg. 2015;261:221–7.
21. Velthuis S, nieuwenhuis DH, Ruijter TE, Cuesta MA, Bonjer HJ, Sietses C. Transanal versus traditional laparoscopic total mesorectal excision for rectal carcinoma. Surg Endosc. 2014;28:3494–9.
22. Marks G, Mohiuddin M, Masoni L, Montori A. High-dose preoperative radiation therapy as the key to extending sphincter-preservation surgery for cancer of the distal rectum. Surg Oncol Clin North Am. 1992;1:71–86.
23. Teramoto T, Watanabe M, Kitajima M. Per anum intersphincteric rectal dissection with direct coloanal anastomosis for lower rectal cancer: the ultimate sphincter-preserving operation. Dis Colon Rectum. 1997;40(Suppl):S43–7.
24. Rullier E, Zerbib F, Laurent C, Bonnel C, Caudry M, Saric J, Parneix M. Intersphincteric resection with excision of internal anal sphincter for conservative treatment of very low rectal cancer. Dis Colon Rectum. 1999;42:1168–75.
25. Laurent C, Paumet T, Leblanc F, Denost Q, Rullier E. Intersphincteric resection for low rectal cancer: laparoscopic versus open surgery approach. Color Dis. 2011;14:35–43.
26. Denost Q, Adam J, Rullier A, Buscail E, Laurent C, Rullier E. Perineal transanal approach: a new standard for laparoscopic sphincter-saving resection in low rectal cancer, a randomized trial. Ann Surg. 2014;260:993–9.
27. Kim CW, Baek SJ, Hur H, Min BS, Baik SH, Kim NK. Anastomotic leakage after low anterior resection for rectal cancer is different between minimally invasive surgery and open surgery. Ann Surg. 2016;263:130–7.
28. Veltcamp Helbach M, Deijen CL, Velthuis S, Bonjer HJ, Tuynman JB, Sietses C. Transanal total mesorectal excision for rectal carcinoma: short-term outcomes and experience after 80 cases. Surg Endosc. 2016;30(2):464–70.
29. Deijen C, Tsai A, Koedam W, Hlebach V, Sietses C, Lacy A. Clinical outcomes and case volume effect of transanal total mesorectal excision for rectal cancer: a systematic review. Tech Coloproctol. 2016;20:811–24.
30. Kanso F, Maggiori L, Debove C, Chau A, Ferron M, Panis Y. Perineal or abdominal approach first during intersphincteric resection for low rectal cancer: which is the best strategy? Dis Colon Rectum. 2015;58:637–44.
31. Uhrich ML, Underwood RA, Standeven JW, Soper NJ, Engsberg JR. Assessment of fatigue, monitor placement, and surgical experience during simulated laparoscopic surgery. Surgical Endosc. 2002;16:635–9.
32. Schiessel R, Karner-Hanusch J, Herbst F, Teleky B, Wunderlich M. Intersphincteric resection for low rectal tumours. Br J Surg. 1994;81:1376–8.
33. Rullier E, Laurent C, Bretagnol F, Rullier A, Vendrely V, Zerbib F. Sphincter-saving resection for all rectal carcinomas. The end of the 2-cm distal rule. Ann Surg. 2005;241:465–9.
34. Tilney HS, Tekkis PP. Extending the horizons of restorative rectal surgery: intersphincteric resection for low rectal cancer. Color Dis. 2008;10:3–15.
35. Martin ST, Heneghan HM, Winter DC. Systematic review of outcomes after intersphincteric resection for low rectal cancer. Br J Surg. 2012;99:603–12.
36. Akasu T, Takawa M, Yamamoto S, Fujita S, Moriya Y. Incidence and patterns of recurrence after intersphincteric resection for very low rectal adenocarcinoma. J Am Coll Surg. 2007;205:642–7.
37. Schiessel R, Novi G, Holzer B, Rosen HR, Renner K, Hölbling N. Technique and long-term results of intersphincteric resection for low rectal cancer. Dis Colon Rectum. 2005;48:1858–65.
38. Saito N, Ito M, Kobayashi A, Nishizawa Y, Kojima M, Nishizawa Y, et al. Long-term outcomes after intersphincteric resection for low-lying rectal cancer. Ann Surg Oncol. 2014;21:3608–15.
39. Gamagami R, Istvan G, Cabarrot P, Liagre A, Chiotasso P, Lazorthes F. Fecal continence following partial resection of the anal canal in distal rectal cancer: long-term results after coloanal anastomoses. Surgery. 2000;127:291–5.

40. Yokata M, Ito M, Nishizawa Y, Kobayashi A, Saito N. The impact of anastomotic leakage on anal function following intersphincteric resection. World J Surg. 2017;41(8):2168–77. https://doi.org/10.1007/s00268-017-3960-4.
41. Kinoshita Y, Nokes K, Kawamoto R, Kanaoka M, Miyazono M, Nakao H, et al. Health-related quality of life in patients with lower rectal cancer after sphincter-saving surgery: a prospective 6-month follow-up study. Eur J Cancer Care. 2015;25. https://doi.org/10.1111/ecc.12417. [Epub ahead of print].
42. Bretagnol F, Rullier E, Laurent C, Zerbib F, Gontier R, Saric J. Comparison of functional results and quality of life between intersphincteric resection and conventional coloanal anastomosis for low rectal cancer. Dis Colon Rectum. 2004;47:832–8.
43. Didailler R, Denost Q, Loughlin P, et al. Anterograde enema after TME for rectal cancer: the last chance to avoid definitive colostomy for refractory LARS and fecal incontinence. Dis Colon Rectum. (in press).
44. Pontallier A, Denost Q, Van Geluwe B, Adam JP, Celerier B, Rullier E. Potential sexual function improvement by using transanal mesorectal approach for laparoscopic low rectal cancer excision. Surg Endosc. 2016;30:4924–33.

Assessing Anastomotic Integrity and Perfusion

31

Adam T. Stearns and John T. Jenkins

Introduction

Anastomotic complications remain a major cause of postoperative morbidity after colorectal surgery, with mortality rates after anastomotic leak ranging 6–22% [1, 2]. In addition to perioperative morbidity, anastomotic leak is associated with increased rates of local recurrence [3], permanent stoma [4], and reduced long-term survival [3] and quality of life [5]. Despite technological advances, anastomotic leak remains a common complication after colorectal surgery. In rectal cancer, large prospective randomized controlled trials and cohort studies describe anastomotic leak rates of 11–15% [6, 7]. Patient risk factors are multifactorial, including older age, male sex, smoking status, obesity, and nutritional status [8–11]. Technical factors, including local ischemia, tension, sepsis, and distal obstruction, increase the risk of leakage. Lastly, position of the anastomosis is relevant, with anastomoses less than 5 cm from anal verge being at higher risk [2], along with ileorectal anastomoses [1].

Anastomotic integrity depends on a patent and mechanically intact anastomosis, without bleeding or ischemia [12]. Compromise to integrity, ultimately presenting as an anastomotic leak, likely occurs very early in the postoperative course. Patients who subsequently develop an anastomotic leak have early elevations in peritoneal fluid biomarkers, detectable within 4 h of surgery [13, 14]. Clinically, however, anastomotic leak is not identified until much later, with mean time to recognition reported between 7.5 and 17.7 days postoperatively in recent large series [1, 15–18].

A.T. Stearns (✉)
Department of Surgery, Norfolk and Norwich University Hospitals NHS Foundation Trust, Norwich, Norfolk, UK
e-mail: adam.stearns@nnuh.nhs.uk

J.T. Jenkins
Department of Surgery, St. Marks Hospital, London, UK
e-mail: i.jenkins@nhs.net

C.M. Schlachta, P. Sylla (eds.), *Current Common Dilemmas in Colorectal Surgery*,
https://doi.org/10.1007/978-3-319-70117-2_31

Table 31.1 Summary of mechanisms for early detection of anastomotic dehiscence

Assessment of mechanical completeness
Completeness of "doughnuts"
Air-leak test
Air/gas insufflation
Patent blue dye
Endoscopic examination of anastomosis
Intraoperative assessment of perfusion
Fluorescence angiography
Indocyanine green-based microperfusion assessments
Measurements of tissue oxygen tension
Polarographic assessments of tissue oxygen tension
Assessments of vascular flow
Doppler ultrasound
Laser Doppler flowmetry
Biomarker evidence of anastomotic failure
Local evidence of ischemia (microdialysis catheters)
Local pH, lactate, lactate/pyruvate ratios
Inflammatory markers in peritoneal fluid
Matrix metalloproteinases MMP-8 and MMP-9
Lysozyme
Cytokines IL-6, IL-10, and tumor necrosis factor-α
Intraperitoneal evidence of loss of enteric barrier
Endotoxin (lipopolysaccharide)

Given the relatively late presentation of frank anastomotic leakage, and the morbidity associated with this, it is clear why early assessment of anastomotic integrity is extremely desirable. There is evidence that intraoperative clinical judgment is poor at predicting risk of anastomotic leak [19]. Objective and accurate tests that could predict this would permit early anastomotic revision or diversion, as appropriate. Conversely, early confirmation of anastomotic integrity may permit avoidance of diverting ostomies when these would otherwise traditionally be employed, for example, the "ghost ileostomy" in total mesorectal excision [20, 21].

It is likely that anastomotic leaks occur through at least three separate pathways. The first is a physically incomplete anastomosis at the time of surgery, caused by a technical failure (either surgical or stapler misfire). Secondly, there may be focal or segmental ischemia of the bowel wall. This may be caused by local vascular insufficiency or splanchnic vasoconstriction due to postoperative hypotension or inotropic support [22]. The consequence will be delayed necrosis and dehiscence of a part or all of the anastomosis. Finally, there may be a delayed mechanical disruption of the anastomosis in the context of tension or distal obstruction. There may be additional pathways also contributing to leakage.

Early determination of anastomotic integrity therefore requires assessment of each of these pathways. Thus, assessment can be categorized broadly into:

1. Assessment of mechanical completeness of the anastomosis at the time of surgery
2. Intraoperative assessment of perfusion of the juxta-anastomotic bowel
3. Postoperative biomarker evidence of intestinal ischemia or anastomotic disruption

These assessments are summarized in Table 31.1. It is important to note that as there are multiple pathways culminating in anastomotic leakage, any individual test for anastomotic integrity will not identify all patients at risk. For example, intraoperative tests of mechanical completeness (e.g., air-leak tests) will not identify patients with insufficient perfusion of the anastomosis who are at risk of delayed dehiscence. Conversely, tests assessing anastomotic perfusion will not identify leaks resulting from mechanically incomplete anastomoses.

This chapter will largely concentrate on intraoperative assessment of anastomotic integrity and evolving technologies for monitoring anastomotic integrity over the initial postoperative period, rather than discussing conventional techniques for demonstrating an established postoperative leak with conventional radiological imaging. Largely the evidence presented relates to rectal anastomoses, but some of the evidence is based on right-sided colonic or other gastrointestinal anastomoses.

Assessment of Mechanical Completeness

Intraoperative assessments of mechanical completeness are the most frequently used tests of anastomotic integrity. Most surgeons will assess integrity of the "doughnuts" produced when using a circular stapler and will perform an air-leak test or other form of mechanical assessment for anastomotic integrity.

Completeness of Doughnuts

Incomplete doughnuts resulting from the use of a circular stapler are a potential indicator of an incomplete anastomosis. In an early series of 82 patients, 68 patients had complete doughnuts [23]. None had an air-leak on testing; four of these patients (6%) subsequently developed anastomotic leakage. Of the 14 patients with disrupted doughnuts, 10 were intact on air-leak testing, none of whom subsequently developed an anastomotic leak. Of the four patients who did have an air leak, two subsequently developed an anastomotic leak. A similar small series showed incomplete doughnuts were strongly associated with intraoperative air leaks, although importantly 36% of patients with intraoperative air leaks did have complete doughnuts [24]; thus, complete doughnuts are not a reliable indicator of a mechanically sound anastomosis.

Air-Leak Test

Air-leak tests are widely performed, and most rectal surgeons will be familiar with the technique whereby air or gas is instilled into the rectum, with the anastomosis kept submerged under saline or water. A defect in the anastomosis is visualized by bubbles. The procedure is practiced in a highly variable manner, employing syringes with or without catheters, rigid sigmoidoscopy, or flexible endoscopes. The amount of air instilled is equally variable, with studies reporting insufflation between 60 mL and 400 mL gas [24, 25]. Variations of the technique use saline or an intraluminal dye such as patent blue dye diluted in 180–240 mL saline or water [26]. A recent meta-analysis of 17 cohort studies and trials, comprising 3994 patients, reported positive air-leak tests in 7.1% of anastomoses [27]. A positive air-leak test is strongly associated with postoperative anastomotic leak (Fig. 31.1). Postoperative anastomotic leak occurred in 10.6% of patients with a positive air-leak test, versus 4.6% with a negative air-leak test (odds ratio (OR) 2.65 [1.74, 4.05], $p < 0.0001$). Furthermore, in each case where there was a positive air-leak test, measures were taken to address the air leak. These varied from oversewing the defect to excising the anastomosis and refashioning, drain insertion, or diverting ileostomy. It is reasonable to assume that without such measures, the leak rate would be much higher.

However, there is less evidence that performing air-leak tests actually reduces overall postoperative anastomotic leak rates. Two randomized controlled trials (RCTs) have been performed, allocating patients to either intraoperative air-leak test or no intraoperative assessment of anastomotic integrity [28, 29]. A meta-analysis of these two trials (combined total of 203 patients) found the risk of postoperative anastomotic leak to be decreased from 16% in the untested group to 5.8% in the air-test group ($p = 0.024$) [12]. In contrast, a more recent meta-analysis including 7 cohort studies (total 9 studies, 2887 patients) suggested performing an air-leak test did not significantly influence overall postoperative anastomotic leak rate (OR 0.61 [0.32, 1.18], $p = 0.15$) [27]. These findings are skewed by one large

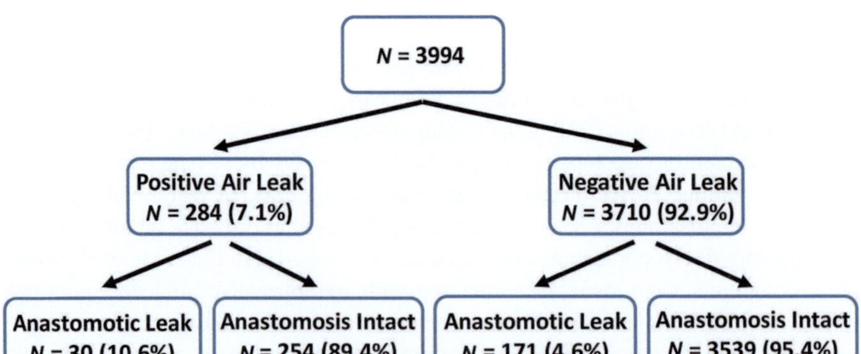

Fig. 31.1 Summary of meta-analysis of outcomes after positive and negative air-leak tests, showing increased rate of postoperative anastomotic leak after a positive intraoperative air-leak test. Modified from Wu et al. [27]

nonrandomized cohort study with 788 patients [30], which describes historical cohorts in a single institution before and after introduction of air-leak testing in 1995. The cohort study authors demonstrated a small increase in anastomotic leak rates in the cohort from 1995 to 2000 compared to that in the years 1987–1995, concluding that air-leak testing did not influence anastomotic leak rates. However, it is likely that there are numerous biases, not least a substantial increase in the rate of ultra-low resections performed between the two periods. Excluding this cohort study from the meta-analysis demonstrates a significant benefit from routine air-leak testing of anastomoses, halving postoperative anastomotic leak rates (OR 0.46 [0.29, 0.74], $p = 0.001$) [27].

The lack of definitive evidence for a benefit of air-leak testing in reducing post-operative anastomotic leak rate might be read as evidence to stop routine assessment of colorectal integrity. However, the authors (probably in common with most colorectal surgeons) would reject this, having identified and corrected significant anastomotic disruption that would otherwise have certainly resulted in gross post-operative anastomotic leakage. Probably of more importance is the recognition that anastomoses, which have had a positive air-leak test, remain at a significantly increased risk of postoperative leakage despite revision.

Intraoperative Endoscopic Assessment of Anastomosis

Direct luminal visualization of the anastomosis using intraoperative flexible endoscopy may identify and control hemorrhage from the anastomosis. Although anastomotic bleeding can usually be managed nonoperatively, it contributes to morbidity and delayed discharge and may be associated with increased anastomotic leak rates [31]. Routine colonoscopic evaluation identifies staple-line bleeding in 0.6 to 9.6% of cases [32]. In addition, insufflation allows an air-leak test to be performed under controlled conditions, with direct insufflation adjacent to the anastomosis. Other pathologies such as missed distal pathology and mucosal ischemia may also be identified [33].

Li et al. compared the use of routine intraoperative endoscopy versus selective intraoperative endoscopy in a small cohort study [33]. In patients routinely undergoing intraoperative endoscopy, luminal assessment identified significant pathology in 10.3% of patients (including anastomotic bleeding in 5.6%, air leaks in 2.8%, and missed polyps). In the comparison cohort, intraoperative endoscopy was performed selectively if felt indicated by the experienced staff surgeons. Selective endoscopy was performed in 22% of all patients, and identified significant pathology in 10% of patients examined (2.2% of all the patients undergoing surgery). Postoperatively, there was a 5.7-fold higher rate of anastomotic complications in patients examined selectively compared to those examined routinely (5.1% versus 0.9% respectively), although this did not quite meet significance given the small sample size. Of note, the identical rate of positive findings in the "routine" and "selective" endoscopy group (10.3% versus 10%) highlights the difficulty even very experienced surgeons face in subjectively identifying at-risk anastomoses. A similar result was observed in a second small-scale cohort study, with a small nonsignificant reduction in postoperative anastomotic bleeding after intraoperative endoscopy assessment [25]. However, a more recent report of routine intraoperative endoscopic evaluation in a much larger cohort of 415 consecutive patients only identified 1 patient with an anastomotic bleed (0.2%) and 15 patients with positive air leak on endoscopy (3.6%) [34]. It may be therefore that the benefits for intraoperative endoscopy have been overstated in the earlier small-scale cohort studies.

Intraoperative Assessment of Perfusion

Air-leak tests (or similar evaluations of mechanical integrity) assess anastomotic completeness at the time of surgery. However, a subgroup of patients who have a mechanically intact anastomosis at the time of surgery will nonetheless later develop a leak. It is likely that ischemia is a contributing factor to this phenomenon. Consequently, an assessment of the vascular perfusion of the bowel adjacent to the anastomosis is often performed, whether it be by assessing marginal artery bleeding, palpable pulsation, or color of the colonic wall or mucosa. Unfortunately, surgeons are not very accurate at predicting the risk of anastomotic leak [19], and therefore, efforts have been made to assess perfusion in an objective manner. This is all the more important in laparoscopic rectal surgery where, in contrast to open surgery, colonic division may occur shortly before formation of the anastomosis. This allows little time for demarcation to occur.

Indocyanine Green-Based Microperfusion Assessments

At present, the most widely reported objective assessment of intestinal perfusion uses indocyanine green fluorescence angiography (ICG-FA). ICG is a fluorescent marker, which when administered intravenously remains strictly in the intravascular compartment. It fluoresces when exposed to light in the near-infrared wavelength, and that fluorescence intensity correlates to tissue perfusion. A number of commercial endoscopes are now available which emit near-infrared light and can detect the resulting ICG fluorescence, including PINPOINT endoscopic fluorescence imaging system (NOVADAQ), SPIES (Karl Storz), Firefly (Intuitive Surgical, Inc.) and 1588 AIM ENV (Stryker). Prior to bowel division, ICG is administered intravenously, allowing assessment of the microperfusion of the bowel that will form the anastomosis, before transection of the bowel.

A recent systematic review of ICG in colorectal surgery examined 13 studies with a total of 992 patients [35]. These were all cohort studies and include the large PILLAR II trial [36]. This large trial reported outcomes of 139 patients undergoing left-sided resection, with intraoperative ICG perfusion assessment performed both laparoscopically and endoluminally. Meta-analysis demonstrated use of ICG-FA was associated with a highly significant reduction in leak rate from 7.6% to 3.8%. ICG-FA changed the transection point in up to 19% of resections [37] and influenced decision making (including avoidance of covering ileostomy) in up to 28% of patients [38]. However, the studies showed great heterogeneity, not least with how to manage a poorly perfused segment, and formal randomized controlled trials are clearly required to assess this further. This should be addressed somewhat by the PILLAR III randomized controlled trial (prematurely closed in 2017), which compared anastomotic leak rate after low anterior resection in patients who had intraoperative ICG perfusion assessment versus conventional surgery.

Unfortunately, the above techniques assessing microperfusion are currently largely focused on the colonic segment despite the likelihood that rectal microperfusion is at least as important if not more so than colonic. The rectal blood supply after anterior resection is restricted to inferior and medial rectal arteries but is not equally distributed throughout the rectum. The low rectum has a sparse network of intramural collaterals compared to the more densely vascularized middle and upper rectum [39]. This is particularly the case in the dorsocaudal part of the low rectum, and there is evidence of reduced perfusion in the posterior quadrant of the low rectum after TME (total mesorectal excision) surgery [40]. This may provide a biological explanation for why most leaks after low anterior resection occur posteriorly [41, 42]. With current technology, ICG-based assessment of low rectal microperfusion is likely to remain extremely challenging (particularly in the higher-risk male obese patient with a low anastomosis), and the options for revision if there are microperfusion deficiencies are limited in the context of TME surgery.

Other Methods of Assessing Anastomotic Perfusion

Aside from ICG-based technologies to assess anastomotic microperfusion, there is a wide variety of other technologies to objectively measure blood supply. However, these are largely limited to small case series or cohort studies and are best regarded as experimental at present. Tissue oxygenation has been assessed in a variety of manners. Use of a pulse oximeter has been proposed as an assessment of intestinal blood flow [43], but ultimately this reflects hemoglobin saturation (and thus central oxygenation) not tissue oxygen tension, and it is unlikely to differ to pulse oximetry measured at the limbs [44]. Direct measurements of tissue oxygen tension, using polarographic assessments with metal cathodes, give conflicting results. One study demonstrated decreased oxygen tension in patients who subsequently developed an anastomotic leak [45] and the other increased oxygen tension [46], leading to doubts about the role this may play in the etiology of anastomotic leakage. Spectrophotometry can measure the saturation of hemoglobin in the tissues (StO_2), either using visible light or near-infrared. The former penetrates approximately 2 mm into tissues, assessing StO_2 in the capillaries, while near-infrared penetrates deeper and thus assesses oxygenation in all vascular compartments. One study demonstrated that in anastomoses that healed without complication, an initially high StO_2 was observed, and this then climbed after fashioning the anastomosis [47]. In contrast, in anastomoses that ultimately leaked, the initial StO_2 was lower and did not rise after fashioning the anastomosis. However, there are a number of disadvantages with this technique, not least that there is no clear discriminator value of StO_2 below which an anastomosis can be predicted to leak, and the high cost of the equipment. Doppler ultrasound has been employed to assess adequacy of blood supply at the resection margins, and in a large series of 200 patients undergoing left-sided colonic or colorectal anastomoses, leak rates of 1% were achieved by assessing vascularity of the colon [48]. However, other authors have questioned if it contributes anything to clinical judgment [49]. Lastly, Laser Doppler flowmetry (LDF) is a technique that uses a monochromatic laser to assess number and velocity of erythrocytes moving in any given tissue, expressed as a quantifiable flow rate. Vignali et al. used LDF to measure transmural blood flow in the rectal stump before mobilization and after division [50]. In patients with an uncomplicated recovery, a 6.2% decrease in blood flow to the rectal stump was observed after resection. In patients who ultimately developed an anastomotic leak, a 16% fall in blood flow was observed after resection. Similar changes were observed in the proximal colonic end. Seike et al. used similar methods to assess changes in rectal microperfusion on clamping the inferior mesenteric artery [51]. They suggested that patients with a greater than 50% decline in perfusion on clamping the inferior mesenteric artery at origin should be considered for a low ligation below the origin of the left colic artery.

Biomarker Evidence of Anastomotic Failure

For those anastomoses that are mechanically intact at the time of surgery but subsequently dehisce due to local ischemia, a pathway may be proposed whereby initial local ischemia progresses to localized inflammation [52]. As cell death and necrosis occur and the anastomosis dehisces, bacterial contamination of the peritoneum will also occur. This is summarized in Fig. 31.2. Biomarkers may be present systemically, in peritoneal fluid, or in the local tissue.

Biomarker Evidence of Intestinal Ischemia

Systemic biomarkers of ischemia detectable in the blood (such as neutrophilia and metabolic acidosis), lactate and liver function tests are regularly assayed postoperatively. However, they have generally been shown to be of limited accuracy in predicting anastomotic leak [53]. Local changes may, however, be more accurate at identifying ischemia. Measurements using an intraluminal microdialysis catheter demonstrate a fall in pH as early as 24 h postoperatively in patients who subsequently developed an anastomotic leak [54], while increases in lactate and lactate/pyruvate levels have also been observed in such patients, often preceding clinical leaks by several days [55].

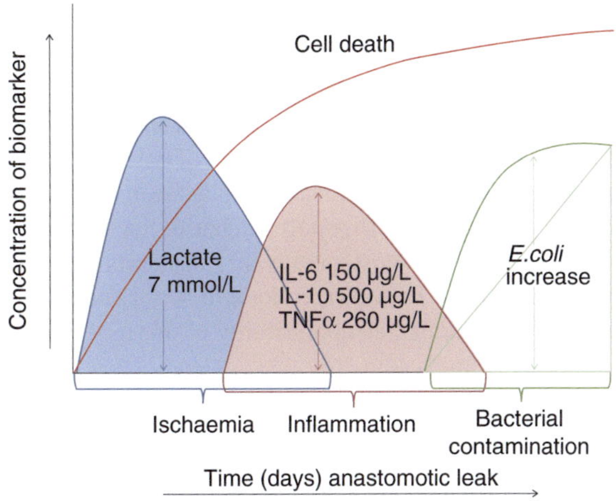

Fig. 31.2 Potential biomarker concentrations postoperatively in the development of an anastomotic leak. Modified from Hirst et al. [52]

Biomarker Evidence of Intestinal Inflammation

Inflammatory markers may be released into the systemic bloodstream or locally into peritoneal fluid. C-reactive protein has long been regarded as a useful indicator of postoperative complications and may be elevated in the days preceding presentation of an anastomotic leak [56, 57]. However, more recent studies have suggested that it is not reliable in detecting the presence of a minor leak and only reaches significance in predicting presentation of a major clinical leak [58].

Pelvic drains may be employed to assay peritoneal fluid for inflammatory markers, where they are found at much higher concentrations than in the bloodstream. Matrix metalloproteinases MMP-8 and MMP-9, involved in tissue repair and healing, are significantly raised in patients at 4 h post-surgery in patients who go on to develop an anastomotic leak [14]. Lysozyme, a marker of macrophage function, is elevated at day 1 postoperatively in patients who go on to develop an anastomotic leak [13]. Lastly, cytokines IL-6, IL-10, and tumor necrosis factor-α (TNF-α) have all been demonstrated to be elevated in peritoneal fluid of patients who develop an anastomotic leak, with significant elevations occurring as early as day 1 for IL-6 and day 2 for TNF-α [59]. Increases are dramatic, with 13.5-fold increases in TNF-α and 4.9-fold increases in IL-6 at 5 days postoperatively in patients who subsequently develop an anastomotic leak [59]. IL-10 also rises significantly by day 1 postoperatively [60].

Although measuring peritoneal fluid cytokines may seem a very specific and discriminatory method of detecting anastomotic leaks, they require expensive and specialized laboratory facilities. Furthermore, testing requires pelvic drains, which are less commonly used in the era of enhanced recovery.

Biomarker Evidence of Anastomotic Disruption and Leakage of Luminal Contents

Anastomotic failure would be expected to permit migration of luminal bacteria into the peritoneal cavity. Thus, detection of enteric, gram-negative bacteria in drain fluid may permit early identification of anastomotic dehiscence. Significantly elevated levels of endotoxin (lipopolysaccharide) within peritoneal drain fluid have been described at day 3 postoperatively in patients who subsequently develop an anastomotic leak [61]. However, endotoxin is not currently measured in clinical laboratories, and this limits the applicability of this as a biomarker at present [52].

Conclusion

Early detection of potential anastomotic failure, before the clinical presentation of an anastomotic leak, may allow timely intervention to prevent the short- and long-term consequences of this major complication. There is clear evidence that surgeons struggle identifying at-risk anastomoses [19, 33], and therefore, there is a strong argument that whichever method is employed for checking anastomotic integrity should be used routinely rather than selectively. Mechanical testing of anastomotic integrity, either with an air-leak test or with routine endoscopy, comes at little cost and probably reduces anastomotic leak rate. Routine assessments of microperfusion, such as ICG-FA, seem promising, at least in relation to the early data. They do however require more robust assessment of their efficacy in randomized controlled trials as an adjunct to mechanical testing. Lastly, biomarker assays pose a potential opportunity for early detection of anastomotic leak in the postoperative period. While the cost and logistic problems limit their widespread use at present, they may provide useful opportunities in the future.

While many of these technologies may appear expensive at present, they need to be viewed in the context of high frequencies of "unnecessary" diverting ileostomies (where the anastomosis heals completely intact) and the morbidity associated with ileostomies and their closure. It also needs to be viewed in the context of the short-term morbidity and long-term impact of anastomotic leakage on both oncological outcomes and overall quality of life.

References

1. Hyman N, Manchester TL, Osler T, Burns B, Cataldo PA. Anastomotic leaks after intestinal anastomosis: it's later than you think. Ann Surg. 2007;245(2):254–8.
2. Rullier E, Laurent C, Garrelon JL, Michel P, Saric J, Parneix M. Risk factors for anastomotic leakage after resection of rectal cancer. Br J Surg. 1998;85(3):355–8.
3. Mirnezami A, Mirnezami R, Chandrakumaran K, Sasapu K, Sagar P, Finan P. Increased local recurrence and reduced survival from colorectal cancer following anastomotic leak: systematic review and meta-analysis. Ann Surg. 2011;253(5):890–9.
4. Chiu A, Chan HT, Brown CJ, Raval MJ, Phang PT. Failing to reverse a diverting stoma after lower anterior resection of rectal cancer. Am J Surg. 2014;207(5):708–11. Discussion 711.

5. Marinatou A, Theodoropoulos GE, Karanika S, Karantanos T, Siakavellas S, Spyropoulos BG, Toutouzas K, Zografos G. Do anastomotic leaks impair postoperative health-related quality of life after rectal cancer surgery? A case-matched study. Dis Colon Rectum. 2014;57(2):158–66.
6. Pigazzi A, Luca F, Patriti A, Valvo M, Ceccarelli G, Casciola L, Biffi R, Garcia-Aguilar J, Baek JH. Multicentric study on robotic tumor-specific mesorectal excision for the treatment of rectal cancer. Ann Surg Oncol. 2010;17(6):1614–20.
7. Senagore A, Lane FR, Lee E, Wexner S, Dujovny N, Sklow B, Rider P, Bonello J. Bioabsorbable staple line reinforcement in restorative proctectomy and anterior resection: a randomized study. Dis Colon Rectum. 2014;57(3):324–30.
8. Lipska MA, Bissett IP, Parry BR, Merrie AE. Anastomotic leakage after lower gastrointestinal anastomosis: men are at a higher risk. ANZ J Surg. 2006;76(7):579–85.
9. Yamamoto S, Fujita S, Akasu T, Inada R, Moriya Y. Risk factors for anastomotic leakage after laparoscopic surgery for rectal cancer using a stapling technique. Surg Laparosc Endosc Percutan Tech. 2012;22(3):239–43.
10. Frasson M, Flor-Lorente B, Rodriguez JL, Granero-Castro P, Hervas D, Alvarez Rico MA, Brao MJ, Sanchez Gonzalez JM, Garcia-Granero E. Risk factors for anastomotic leak after colon resection for cancer: multivariate analysis and nomogram from a multicentric, prospective, national study with 3193 patients. Ann Surg. 2015;262(2):321–30.
11. Richards CH, Campbell V, Ho C, Hayes J, Elliott T, Thompson-Fawcett M. Smoking is a major risk factor for anastomotic leak in patients undergoing low anterior resection. Color Dis. 2012;14(5):628–33.
12. Nachiappan S, Askari A, Currie A, Kennedy RH, Faiz O. Intraoperative assessment of colorectal anastomotic integrity: a systematic review. Surg Endosc. 2014;28(9):2513–30.
13. Miller K, Arrer E, Leitner C. Early detection of anastomotic leaks after low anterior resection of the rectum. Dis Colon Rectum. 1996;39(10):1081–5.
14. Pasternak B, Matthiessen P, Jansson K, Andersson M, Aspenberg P. Elevated intraperitoneal matrix metalloproteinases-8 and -9 in patients who develop anastomotic leakage after rectal cancer surgery: a pilot study. Color Dis. 2010;12(7 Online):e93–82.
15. Alves A, Panis Y, Pocard M, Regimbeau JM, Valleur P. Management of anastomotic leakage after nondiverted large bowel resection. J Am Coll Surg. 1999;189(6):554–9.
16. Bellows CF, Webber LS, Albo D, Awad S, Berger DH. Early predictors of anastomotic leaks after colectomy. Tech Coloproctol. 2009;13(1):41–7.
17. Telem DA, Chin EH, Nguyen SQ, Divino CM. Risk factors for anastomotic leak following colorectal surgery: a case-control study. Arch Surg. 2010;145(4):371–6. Discussion 376.
18. Feo LJ, Jrebi N, Asgeirsson T, Dujovny N, Figg R, Hoedema R, Slay H, Kim D, Luchtefeld M. Anastomotic leaks: technique and timing of detection. Am J Surg. 2014;207(3):371–4. Discussion 374.
19. Karliczek A, Harlaar NJ, Zeebregts CJ, Wiggers T, Baas PC, van Dam GM. Surgeons lack predictive accuracy for anastomotic leakage in gastrointestinal surgery. Int J Color Dis. 2009;24(5):569–76.
20. Gulla N, Trastulli S, Boselli C, Cirocchi R, Cavaliere D, Verdecchia GM, Morelli U, Gentile D, Eugeni E, Caracappa D, Listorti C, Sciannameo F, Noya G. Ghost ileostomy after anterior resection for rectal cancer: a preliminary experience. Langenbeck's Arch Surg. 2011;396(7):997–1007.
21. Mori L, Vita M, Razzetta F, Meinero P, D'Ambrosio G. Ghost ileostomy in anterior resection for rectal carcinoma: is it worthwhile? Dis Colon Rectum. 2013;56(1):29–34.
22. Zakrison T, Nascimento BA Jr, Tremblay LN, Kiss A, Rizoli SB. Perioperative vasopressors are associated with an increased risk of gastrointestinal anastomotic leakage. World J Surg. 2007;31(8):1627–34.
23. Lazorthes F, Chiotassol P. Stapled colorectal anastomoses: peroperative integrity of the anastomosis and risk of postoperative leakage. Int J Color Dis. 1986;1(2):96–8.
24. Griffith CD, Hardcastle JD. Intraoperative testing of anastomotic integrity after stapled anterior resection for cancer. J R Coll Surg Edinb. 1990;35(2):106–8.
25. Shamiyeh A, Szabo K, Ulf Wayand W, Zehetner J. Intraoperative endoscopy for the assessment of circular-stapled anastomosis in laparoscopic colon surgery. Surg Laparosc Endosc Percutan Tech. 2012;22(1):65–7.

26. Chen CW, Chen MJ, Yeh YS, Tsai HL, Chang YT, Wang JY. Intraoperative anastomotic dye test significantly decreases incidence of anastomotic leaks in patients undergoing resection for rectal cancer. Tech Coloproctol. 2013;17(5):579–83.
27. Wu Z, van de Haar RC, Sparreboom CL, Boersema GS, Li Z, Ji J, Jeekel J, Lange JF. Is the intraoperative air leak test effective in the prevention of colorectal anastomotic leakage? A systematic review and meta-analysis. Int J Color Dis. 2016;31(8):1409–17.
28. Ivanov D, Cvijanovic R, Gvozdenovic L. Intraoperative air testing of colorectal anastomoses. Srp Arh Celok Lek. 2011;139(5–6):333–8.
29. Beard JD, Nicholson ML, Sayers RD, Lloyd D, Everson NW. Intraoperative air testing of colorectal anastomoses: a prospective, randomized trial. Br J Surg. 1990;77(10):1095–7.
30. Schmidt O, Merkel S, Hohenberger W. Anastomotic leakage after low rectal stapler anastomosis: significance of intraoperative anastomotic testing. Eur J Surg Oncol. 2003;29(3):239–43.
31. Choi DH, Hwang JK, Ko YT, Jang HJ, Shin HK, Lee YC, Lim CH, Jeong SK, Yang HK. Risk factors for anastomotic leakage after laparoscopic rectal resection. J Korean Soc Coloproctol. 2010;26(4):265–73.
32. Ishihara S, Watanabe T, Nagawa H. Intraoperative colonoscopy for stapled anastomosis in colorectal surgery. Surg Today. 2008;38(11):1063–5.
33. Li VK, Wexner SD, Pulido N, Wang H, Jin HY, Weiss EG, Nogeuras JJ, Sands DR. Use of routine intraoperative endoscopy in elective laparoscopic colorectal surgery: can it further avoid anastomotic failure? Surg Endosc. 2009;23(11):2459–65.
34. Kamal T, Pai A, Velchuru VR, Zawadzki M, Park JJ, Marecik SJ, Abcarian H, Prasad LM. Should anastomotic assessment with flexible sigmoidoscopy be routine following laparoscopic restorative left colorectal resection? Color Dis. 2015;17(2):160–4.
35. Degett TH, Andersen HS, Gogenur I. Indocyanine green fluorescence angiography for intraoperative assessment of gastrointestinal anastomotic perfusion: a systematic review of clinical trials. Langenbeck's Arch Surg. 2016;401(6):767–75.
36. Jafari MD, Wexner SD, Martz JE, McLemore EC, Margolin DA, Sherwinter DA, Lee SW, Senagore AJ, Phelan MJ, Stamos MJ. Perfusion assessment in laparoscopic left-sided/anterior resection (PILLAR II): a multi-institutional study. J Am Coll Surg. 2015;220(1):82–92. e81
37. Jafari MD, Lee KH, Halabi WJ, Mills SD, Carmichael JC, Stamos MJ, Pigazzi A. The use of indocyanine green fluorescence to assess anastomotic perfusion during robotic assisted laparoscopic rectal surgery. Surg Endosc. 2013;27(8):3003–8.
38. Grone J, Koch D, Kreis ME. Impact of intraoperative microperfusion assessment with Pinpoint Perfusion Imaging on surgical management of laparoscopic low rectal and anorectal anastomoses. Color Dis. 2015;17(Suppl 3):22–8.
39. Allison AS, Bloor C, Faux W, Arumugam P, Widdison A, Lloyd-Davies E, Maskell G. The angiographic anatomy of the small arteries and their collaterals in colorectal resections: some insights into anastomotic perfusion. Ann Surg. 2010;251(6):1092–7.
40. Rutegard M, Hassmen N, Hemmingsson O, Haapamaki MM, Matthiessen P, Rutegard J. Anterior resection for rectal cancer and visceral blood flow: an explorative study. Scand J Surg. 2016;105(2):78–83.
41. Rutegard M, Rutegard J. Anastomotic leakage in rectal cancer surgery: the role of blood perfusion. World J Gastrointest Surg. 2015;7(11):289–92.
42. Vogel P, Klosterhalfen B. The surgical anatomy of the rectal and anal blood vessels. Langenbecks Arch Chir. 1988;373(5):264–9.
43. MacDonald PH, Dinda PK, Beck IT, Mercer CD. The use of oximetry in determining intestinal blood flow. Surg Gynecol Obstet. 1993;176(5):451–8.
44. Hadley GP, Mars M. Limitations of oximeters. Pediatr Surg Int. 2003;19(1–2):130.
45. Sheridan WG, Lowndes RH, Young HL. Tissue oxygen tension as a predictor of colonic anastomotic healing. Dis Colon Rectum. 1987;30(11):867–71.
46. Jacobi CA, Zieren HU, Zieren J, Muller JM. Is tissue oxygen tension during esophagectomy a predictor of esophagogastric anastomotic healing? J Surg Res. 1998;74(2):161–4.
47. Karliczek A, Benaron DA, Baas PC, Zeebregts CJ, Wiggers T, van Dam GM. Intraoperative assessment of microperfusion with visible light spectroscopy for prediction of anastomotic leakage in colorectal anastomoses. Color Dis. 2010;12(10):1018–25.

48. Ambrosetti P, Robert J, Mathey P, Rohner A. Left-sided colon and colorectal anastomoses: Doppler ultrasound as an aid to assess bowel vascularization. A prospective evaluation of 200 consecutive elective cases. Int J Color Dis. 1994;9(4):211–4.
49. Bulkley GB, Zuidema GD, Hamilton SR, O'Mara CS, Klacsmann PG, Horn SD. Intraoperative determination of small intestinal viability following ischemic injury: a prospective, controlled trial of two adjuvant methods (Doppler and fluorescein) compared with standard clinical judgment. Ann Surg. 1981;193(5):628–37.
50. Vignali A, Gianotti L, Braga M, Radaelli G, Malvezzi L, Di Carlo V. Altered microperfusion at the rectal stump is predictive for rectal anastomotic leak. Dis Colon Rectum. 2000;43(1):76–82.
51. Seike K, Koda K, Saito N, Oda K, Kosugi C, Shimizu K, Miyazaki M. Laser Doppler assessment of the influence of division at the root of the inferior mesenteric artery on anastomotic blood flow in rectosigmoid cancer surgery. Int J Color Dis. 2007;22(6):689–97.
52. Hirst NA, Tiernan JP, Millner PA, Jayne DG. Systematic review of methods to predict and detect anastomotic leakage in colorectal surgery. Color Dis. 2014;16(2):95–109.
53. Corke C, Glenister K. Monitoring intestinal ischaemia. Crit Care Resusc. 2001;3(3):176–80.
54. Millan M, Garcia-Granero E, Flor B, Garcia-Botello S, Lledo S. Early prediction of anastomotic leak in colorectal cancer surgery by intramucosal pH. Dis Colon Rectum. 2006;49(5):595–601.
55. Ellebaek Pedersen M, Qvist N, Bisgaard C, Kelly U, Bernhard A, Moller Pedersen S. Peritoneal microdialysis. Early diagnosis of anastomotic leakage after low anterior resection for rectosigmoid cancer. Scand J Surg. 2009;98(3):148–54.
56. Almeida AB, Faria G, Moreira H, Pinto-de-Sousa J, Correia-da-Silva P, Maia JC. Elevated serum C-reactive protein as a predictive factor for anastomotic leakage in colorectal surgery. Int J Surg. 2012;10(2):87–91.
57. Woeste G, Muller C, Bechstein WO, Wullstein C. Increased serum levels of C-reactive protein precede anastomotic leakage in colorectal surgery. World J Surg. 2010;34(1):140–6.
58. Garcia-Granero A, Frasson M, Flor-Lorente B, Blanco F, Puga R, Carratala A, Garcia-Granero E. Procalcitonin and C-reactive protein as early predictors of anastomotic leak in colorectal surgery: a prospective observational study. Dis Colon Rectum. 2013;56(4):475–83.
59. Cini C, Wolthuis A, D'Hoore A. Peritoneal fluid cytokines and matrix metalloproteinases as early markers of anastomotic leakage in colorectal anastomosis: a literature review and meta-analysis. Color Dis. 2013;15(9):1070–7.
60. Matthiessen P, Strand I, Jansson K, Tornquist C, Andersson M, Rutegard J, Norgren L. Is early detection of anastomotic leakage possible by intraperitoneal microdialysis and intraperitoneal cytokines after anterior resection of the rectum for cancer? Dis Colon Rectum. 2007;50(11):1918–27.
61. Junger W, Junger WG, Miller K, Bahrami S, Redl H, Schlag G, Moritz E. Early detection of anastomotic leaks after colorectal surgery by measuring endotoxin in the drainage fluid. Hepato-Gastroenterology. 1996;43(12):1523–9.

Laparoscopic TME: Is There a Verdict?

32

James Fleshman and Katerina Wells

Introduction

Total mesorectal excision (TME), as initially fostered through Europe by Heald, is directly responsible for low rates of local recurrence and improved postoperative outcomes [1]. Level 1 data is emerging supporting the feasibility of laparoscopy for TME; however, the oncologic efficacy of laparoscopy is unclear [2, 3]. Emerging technology including robotics and transanal TME offers alternative methods of resection. Current experience supports the use of these modalities provided operative principles of good surgical resection are adhered to. The key to maintaining the highest standards in this shifting surgical environment is accreditation of centers specializing in rectal cancer care.

Operative Principles

Laparoscopic TME begins at the sacral promontory, by sharply incising the areolar tissue behind the mesorectal envelope. This is the guiding plane investing the mesorectum allowing for safe circumferential dissection from the pelvic brim to the pelvic floor (Fig. 32.1).

The pelvic splanchnic nerves and ureters are positioned laterally and are protected from dissection with the help of the magnified laparoscope view. The anterolateral ligaments containing the middle hemorrhoidal vessels and splanchnic nerve branches are identified with medial traction of the rectum using laparoscopic graspers (Fig. 32.2).

The ligaments should be divided away from the lateral pelvic sidewall to prevent damage to the nerve trunks. Sharp or cautery devices allow for precise dissection.

J. Fleshman • K. Wells (✉)
Department of Surgery, Baylor University Medical Center, Dallas, TX, USA
e-mail: James.Fleshman@bswhealth.org; Katerina.wells@bswhealth.org

C.M. Schlachta, P. Sylla (eds.), *Current Common Dilemmas in Colorectal Surgery*,
https://doi.org/10.1007/978-3-319-70117-2_32

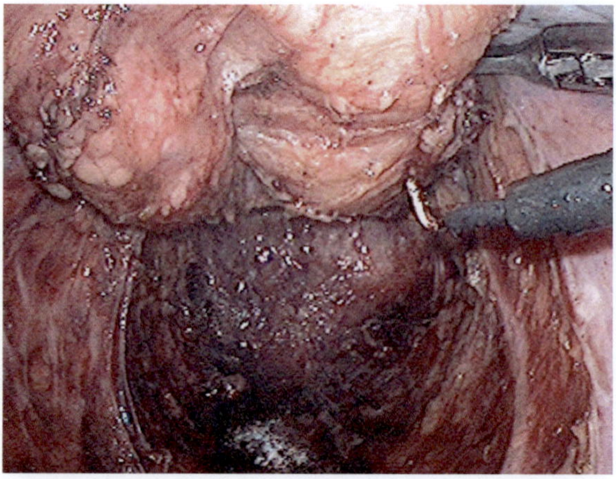

Fig. 32.1 Posterior dissection of the mesorectum

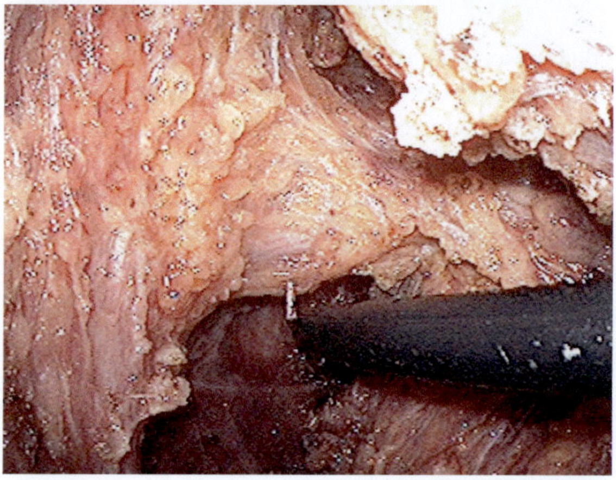

Fig. 32.2 Lateral dissection of the mesorectum

For posterior tumors, anterior dissection begins immediately behind Denonvilliers' fascia, preserving nerves of sexual function traveling to the bladder, prostate, and sexual organs (Fig. 32.3).

For anterior tumors, dissection includes Denonvilliers' fascia, exposing the seminal vesicles or posterior vaginal wall to ensure a clear anterior margin at the expense of potential damage to the nerves of urogenital function. Dissection proceeds until the pelvic floor is reached, aided by magnified visualization of the coccyx and fascia of the levator musculature with the laparoscope. Dissection extends into the upper anal canal if ultralow resection is needed. The completed TME is a circumferentially encased fascial envelope with a bilobed configuration of the posterior mesorectum. In tumor specific TME (TSTME), the mesorectum is transected at the appropriate distal margin at a right angle to the axis of the mesorectum without coning of the mesorectum in the vicinity of the tumor. The integrity of the mesorectum is graded with complete and near complete considered acceptable (Fig. 32.4).

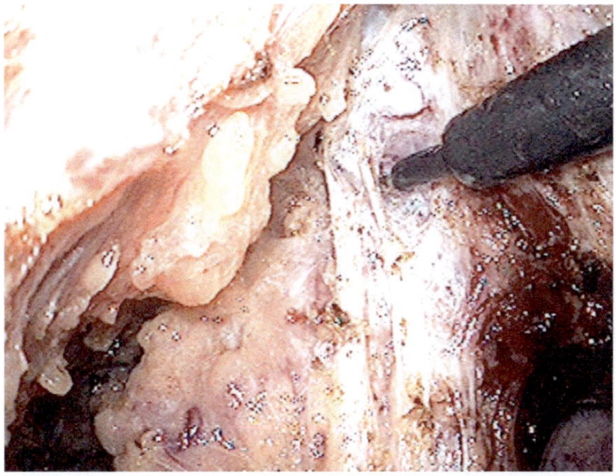

Fig. 32.3 Anterior dissection of Denonvilliers' fascia

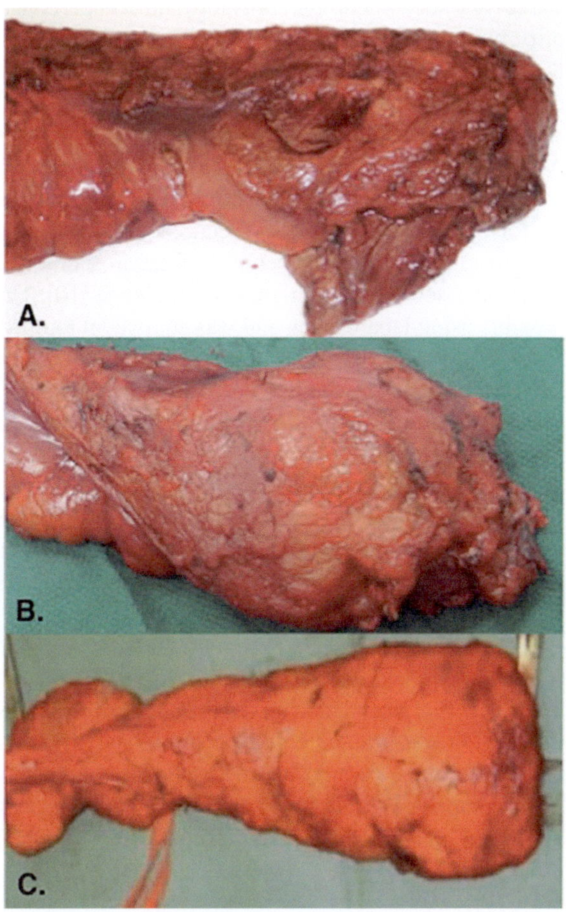

Fig. 32.4 TME grading. (**a**) Incomplete TME. (**b**) Near-complete TME. (**c**) Complete TME

Trials

Oncologic Outcomes

Multiple nonrandomized studies support the use of laparoscopy for rectal cancer [4–6]. There is also now a body of Level 1 data evaluating the surgical and oncologic efficacy of this technique. The earliest randomized controlled, multicenter trial is the UK MRC CLASICC trial reported in the early 2000s. In subset analysis of rectal cancer patients (50% of the study population), CRM positivity was greater in the laparoscopic group (12%) than in the open group (6%), however not statistically significant. Conversion was high and associated with greater postoperative complications [7]. A trend toward improved early survival was observed in the laparoscopic group; however, 3-year OS, DFS, and local recurrence (9.7% laparoscopic vs. 10.1% open) were similar [8].

The COLOR II trial was conducted in 30 centers across Europe and included 1044 patients randomized in a 2:1 fashion to laparoscopic versus open resection. Three-year local recurrence was low and comparable at 5.0%, within the noninferiority margin of 5%. Three-year OS and 3-year DFS were similar with improved DFS among stage II patients treated with laparoscopic resection. Approximately 30% of included patients had stage I disease, and only half received neoadjuvant chemoradiotherapy. Less than 30% of patients had lesions within <5 cm from the AV [9]. Acceptable TME was 92% (laparoscopic) and 94% (open) with 100% negative distal margins and 10% positive CRM for both groups. However, CRM positivity for open resection of low rectal cancers was high at 22%, attributed to better visualization of the lower pelvis with laparoscopy [9]. The rate of conversion was 16% and associated with higher BMI and age [10]. The trial concluded that TME is possible using laparoscopy and was equivalent to open resection.

In 2014, the COREAN trial was a smaller noninferiority study including stage II and III mid- to low rectal cancers (0–9 cm from the AV) randomized to laparoscopic versus open resection using a noninferiority margin of 15%. Conversion was exceedingly low at 1.2% with acceptable TME in 92% (laparoscopic) and 88% (open), $p = 0.41$. There was no difference in CRM positivity between laparoscopic (2.9%) or open (4.1%) techniques, $p = 0.77$ [11]. Of note, the mean BMI of patients was 24, which is not generalizable to Western populations. Stage-specific analysis showed similar DFS, OS, and local recurrence rates between groups [12].

In 2015, the Australian Laparoscopic Compared with open Low Anterior Resection Trial (ALaCaRT) reported on their experience of 26 accredited surgeons from 24 centers in Australia and New Zealand. ALaCaRT was a randomized, noninferiority trial intended to model the protocol of ACOSOG Z6051 (outlined below). Conversion was low at 9% with no significant difference in the short-term outcomes between groups. Composite successful resection was 82% (CRM negative 93%, TME complete 87%, DM negative 99%) in the laparoscopic group and 89% (CRM negative 97%, TME complete 92%, DM negative 99%) in the open group with a difference in risk of −7.0% (95% CI, −12.4 to infinity; $p = 0.38$) which failed to exclude the margin of noninferiority of $\Delta = -8\%$. Based on these findings, laparoscopic rectal resection cannot be considered noninferior to open surgery, and caution is needed before uniformly applying this technique for the management of rectal cancer [3]. Long-term oncologic outcomes are currently being acquired.

The concept of composite pathologic outcomes for successful resection was established in the design of ACOSOG Z6051 wherein 35 centers in the USA and Canada compared open ($n = 222$) and laparoscopic ($n = 242$) TME. Conversion was low at 11.3%. Composite successful resection was 81.7% (CRM negative 87.9%, TME complete 92.1%, DM negative 98.3%) in the laparoscopic group and 86.9% (CRM negative 92.3%, TME complete 95.1%, DM negative 98.2%) in the open group; this did not support noninferiority (difference, −5.3%; one-sided 95% CI, −10.8% to infinity; $p = 0.41$). Similarly, this trial could not support the use of laparoscopic resection for patients with stage II/III rectal cancer based on inferior rates of successful resection [2].

Meta-analysis of the outcomes of COLOR II, COREAN, ALaCaRT, and ACOSOG Z6051 is anticipated following completion of reporting. It is the expectation that the deficiencies identified on composite pathologic outcomes will not translate into a clinically significant oncologic disadvantage, supporting laparoscopy as valuable tool for rectal cancer surgery.

Short-Term Outcomes

The short-term benefits of laparoscopy are clearly demonstrated. In a 2014 Cochrane review of 14 studies and 3528 rectal cancer patients, there is moderate-quality evidence that laparoscopy affords shorter hospital stay by 2 days (95% CI -3.22 to −1.10) and shorter time to defecation by almost 1 day (95% CI −1.17 to −0.54), with fewer wound infections (OR 0.68; 95% CI 0.50 to 0.93), bleeding complications (OR 0.30; 95% CI 0.10 to 0.93), and similar 30-day morbidity (OR 0.94; 95% CI 0.8 to 1.1) compared to open resection. Laparoscopic resection also afforded lower analgesic use and pain scores, and length of incision was significantly shorter by 12 cm (MD −12.83; 95% CI −14.87 to −10.80) [6]. In a more recent meta-analysis by Zheng et al. including 38 studies and 13,408 patients, similar benefits of decreased complications and early recovery with laparoscopic technique were realized at the expense of significantly increased operative times (MD = 37.23 min, 95% CI 28.88–45.57, $p < 0.0001$) [13].

In addition to the immediate surgical advantages, Strouch et al. demonstrated that laparoscopy was an independent predictor of time to postoperative chemotherapy by 25 days (50.1 days (laparoscopic) versus 75.2 days (open), $p < 0.0001$) due to the early recovery afforded by this approach. This outcome measure may be a more valuable measure of short-term benefit by its potential to translate into long-term oncologic advantage [14].

Functional Outcomes

Multiple trials report comparable rates of male and female sexual dysfunction between open versus laparoscopic resection [15]. In the MRC CLASICC trial, however, overall sexual function was worse with laparoscopy owing to higher rates of TME in the laparoscopic group (80% versus 62% open), which was an independent predictor of male sexual dysfunction on multivariate analysis [16]. Comparison of genitourinary function from the COLOR II trial found no difference in erectile dysfunction or micturition symptoms; however, an overall twofold increase in erectile dysfunction postoperatively was reported. The functional assessment group represented only 62.7% of the original cohort with lower rates of leak and radiotherapy compared to nonrespondents, suggesting that these rates are underestimates [17]. The COREAN trial reported better physical functioning, less fatigue, fewer micturition and GI and defecatory problems compared to open resection. Short- and long-term sexual function were similar between groups [11]. ACOSOG Z6051 awaits secondary outcomes of quality-of-life assessments [2].

Robotic Proctectomy

The benefits of robotic proctectomy are realized in the articulating instruments that improve retraction and maneuverability in the pelvis which are an advantage over rigid in-line laparoscopic instruments. Relative comfort of the robotic console also results in less surgeon fatigue compared to laparoscopy [18]. The technical advantage offered by the robotic platform is supported by a low rate of conversion and acceptable pathologic outcomes compared to laparoscopy. In review of the National Cancer Database (NCDB) comparing laparoscopic resection ($n = 5447$) versus robotic resection ($n = 956$), conversion was 9.5% (robotic) versus 16.4% (laparoscopic), $p < 0.001$ with similar margin status, and 30-day outcomes [19]. Baik et al. supports these findings along with shorter length of hospital stay (5.7 ± 1.1 (robotic) versus 7.6 ± 3 days (laparoscopic), $p = 0.001$) [20]. In a randomized controlled trial of 163 patients by Kim et al., the rate of acceptable TME was high across groups (98.5% robotic versus 100% laparoscopic, $p = 0.599$). Postoperative quality-of-life scoring was also similar with sexual function at 12 months favoring robotic resection [21]. The oncologic efficacy of robotic proctectomy is also supported; Saklani et al. report 3-year local recurrence of 2.7% robotic versus 6.3% laparoscopic, $p = 0.420$ with comparable rates of 3-year disease-free and overall survival [22]. Among patients undergoing ultralow TME (avg distance from AV 4.39 ± 2.25 robotic and 5.52 ± 3.74 laparoscopic), Baek et al. report equivalent postoperative outcomes, 3-year local recurrence, and overall and disease-free survival between robotic and laparoscopic resection [23].

The Robotic or Laparoscopic Anterior Rectal Resection trial (ROLARR) is a randomized controlled trial comparing robotic to laparoscopic resection with the primary endpoint of conversion and additional oncologic, safety, and quality-of-life secondary endpoints. Early data reports conversion of 12.2% (laparoscopy) versus

8.1% (robotic). Though robotic resection failed to meet superiority by this primary endpoint, obesity was a factor for conversion in the laparoscopic group only, suggesting that robotic surgery may offer an advantage in the obese pelvis. Robotic procedures had average OR times that were 40 minutes longer compared to laparoscopy. Secondary endpoints including rate of TME, CRM positivity, and intraoperative complications were comparable [24]. We currently await long-term outcomes and anticipate further Level 1 data following completion of COLRAR (Trial to Assess Robot-assisted Surgery and Laparoscopy-assisted Surgery in Patients With Mid- or Low Rectal Cancer) which is a similar Korean multicenter randomized controlled trial currently in accrual [25].

Transanal TME

In response to the technical challenge of the low pelvis, a combined transanal and transabdominal approach to produce a transanal total mesorectal excision (taTME) is an emerging technique. The transanal-transabdominal (TATA) approach was introduced by Marks in the 1980s, offering TEMS-based resection of ultralow tumors with hand-sewn coloanal anastomosis for sphincter preservation [26, 27]. Further adaptations evolved from attempts at a NOTES technique for colon resection described by Whiteford [28]. The TAMIS platform with routine laparoscopic equipment allowed for greater flexibility in surgical technique [29]. Mutch et al. demonstrated successful transanal anterior resection, mobilization of the splenic flexure, and devascularization and extraction of the resection specimen using a GelPort platform in the anus and laparoscopic equipment in a cadaver model [30]. Following extensive experience in a porcine model [31], Sylla and Lacy reported successful completion of the taTME procedure in a living patient with good margins and postoperative outcomes.

Guiding principles of the taTME include transanal placement of a gas-tight purse-string suture in the anal canal above the intended distal margin of resection. Rectal division begins distal to the purse string until the mesorectal plane "holy plane" is entered. Point of entry begins at 5 or 7 o'clock and is then propagated posteriorly, anteriorly, and finally laterally where dissection is most challenging. Transabdominal resection is performed with a laparoscopic approach, though robotic-assisted transabdominal resection is also described [32]. Transanal dissection can precede, follow, or occur in concert with transabdominal dissection depending on institutional resources. TaTME promises an advantage for low or ultralow rectal cancers, distorted anatomy secondary to neoadjuvant therapy, the narrow male pelvis, significant visceral obesity (BMI > 30), and in cases of prostatic hypertrophy [33]. The ETAP-GRECCAR 11 Trial is a multicenter randomized controlled trial currently underway that is designed to evaluate the efficacy of taTME against laparoscopic TME [34]. Similarly, the COLOR III trial is an international multicenter randomized controlled trial currently in accrual, comparing taTME against laparoscopic TME with the primary endpoint of positive CRM. It is the expectation that taTME will afford lower rates of CRM positivity and enable sphincter preservation particularly for low- and mid-rectal lesions [35]. Outcomes are also collected in the taTME registry hosted by the OSTRiCh (Optimizing Surgical Treatment of Rectal Cancer) national clinical collaborative [36].

National Accreditation Program for Rectal Cancer (NAPRC)

Whatever the advances in operative techniques for rectal cancer surgery, complete TME remains the goal. Defining operative benchmarks and establishing accreditation of complex/high-risk operations to specialized centers is the way to standardize a high level of quality via real-time auditing. Through OSTRiCh recommendations to the ACS Commission on Cancer (CoC), the National Accreditation Program for Rectal Cancer (NAPRC) was developed to employ a multidisciplinary, evidence-based approach to guide the processes of rectal cancer care [37].

Part of this process includes designation of high-risk procedures, including TME, to specialized centers with high-volume surgeons to ensure that surgical standards are consistently achieved. This is controversial as the absolute number of cases needed to overcome the learning curve for proficiency remains unclear. Historically, high-volume surgeons (>20 cases) had fewer complications and need for post-procedural interventions compared to lower-volume surgeons [38]. A more recent database analysis supports that surgeons with a cumulative 5-year experience of >25 rectal resections had significantly lower rates of major events (OR = 0.82) and surgical complications (OR 0.71) [39]. There are very few reports on the learning curve for laparoscopic resection of the rectum. In the randomized controlled trials outlined above, high volume was a requirement for participation. Z6051 required that surgeons be credentialed for laparoscopic and open TME rectal resection and submit 20 operative and path reports as well as an unedited recording of a laparoscopic pelvic dissection for review. ROLARR required 30 rectal cancer resections per surgeon prior to credentialing. Certainly the excellent results reported in recent literature have become the expectation for clinical practice, and colorectal surgeons who intend to manage rectal cancer should, therefore, undergo the same degree of scrutiny.

Conclusions

Total mesorectal excision through a minimally invasive approach is feasible in the hands of the experienced surgeon. Currently short-term outcomes through minimally invasive techniques approach those of open resection; however, we await oncologic outcomes and meta-analysis of the most recent randomized controlled trials. Until then, laparoscopic TME should be used judiciously. Emerging technologies including robotic surgery and taTME offer alternative strategies for achieving the goal of a high-quality oncologic resection. As the landscape of rectal cancer surgery evolves, the necessary constant needs to be multidisciplinary oversight with rectal cancer surgery limited to a body of surgeons and surgical centers experienced in this high-risk procedure.

References

1. Heald RJ, Husband EM, Ryall RD. The mesorectum in rectal cancer surgery—the clue to pelvic recurrence? Br J Surg. 1982;69(10):613–6.
2. Fleshman J, Branda M, Sargent DJ, Boller AM, George V, Abbas M, et al. Effect of laparoscopic-assisted resection vs open resection of stage II or III rectal cancer on pathologic outcomes. JAMA. 2015;314(13):1346.
3. Stevenson ARL, Solomon MJ, Lumley JW, Hewett P, Clouston AD, Gebski VJ, et al. Effect of laparoscopic-assisted resection vs open resection on pathological outcomes in rectal cancer. JAMA. 2015;314(13):1356.
4. Fleshman JW, Wexner SD, Anvari M, LaTulippe JF, Birnbaum EH, Kodner IJ, et al. Laparoscopic vs. open abdominoperineal resection for cancer. Dis Colon Rectum. 1999;42(7):930–9.
5. Feliciotti F, Guerrieri M, Paganini AM, De Sanctis A, Campagnacci R, Perretta S, et al. Long-term results of laparoscopic versus open resections for rectal cancer for 124 unselected patients. Surg Endosc. 2003;17(10):1530–5.
6. Vennix S, Pelzers L, Bouvy N, Beets GL, Pierie J-P, Wiggers T, et al. Laparoscopic versus open total mesorectal excision for rectal cancer. Cochrane Database Syst Rev. 2014;58(4):CD005200.
7. Guillou PJ, Quirke P, Thorpe H, Walker J, Jayne DG. Short-term endpoints of conventional versus laparoscopic-assisted surgery in patients with colorectal cancer (MRC CLASICC trial): multicentre, randomised controlled trial. Lancet. 2005;365(9472):1718–26.
8. Green BL, Marshall HC, Collinson F, Quirke P, Guillou P, Jayne DG, et al. Long-term follow-up of the Medical Research Council CLASICC trial of conventional versuslaparoscopically assisted resection in colorectal cancer. Br J Surg. 2012;100(1):75–82.
9. Bonjer HJ, Deijen CL, Abis GA, Cuesta MA, van der Pas MHGM, de Lange-de Klerk ESM, et al. A randomized trial of laparoscopic versus open surgery for rectal cancer. N Engl J Med. 2015;372(14):1324–32.
10. Pas MHGM, Deijen CL, Abis GSA, Klerk ESML-D, Haglind E, Fürst A, et al. Conversions in laparoscopic surgery for rectal cancer. Surg Endosc. 2016;31(5):2263–70.
11. Kang S-B, Park JW, Jeong S-Y, Nam BH, Choi HS, Kim D-W, et al. Open versus laparoscopic surgery for mid or low rectal cancer after neoadjuvant chemoradiotherapy (COREAN trial): short-term outcomes of an open-label randomised controlled trial. Lancet Oncol. 2010;11(7):637–45.
12. Jeong S-Y, Park JW, Nam BH, Kim S, Kang S-B, Lim S-B, et al. Open versus laparoscopic surgery for mid-rectal or low-rectal cancer after neoadjuvant chemoradiotherapy(COREAN trial): survival outcomes of an open-label, non-inferiority, randomised controlled trial. Lancet Oncol. 2014;15(7):767–74.
13. Zheng J, Feng X, Yang Z, Hu W, Luo Y, Li Y. The comprehensive therapeutic effects of rectal surgery are better in laparoscopy: a systematic review and meta-analysis. Oncotarget. 2017;8(8):12717–29.
14. Strouch MJ, Zhou G, Fleshman JW, Birnbaum EH, Hunt SR, Mutch MG. Time to initiation of postoperative chemotherapy. Dis Colon Rectum. 2013;56(8):945–51.
15. Celentano V, Cohen R, Warusavitarne J, Faiz O, Chand M. Sexual dysfunction following rectal cancer surgery. Int J Color Dis. 2017;32(11):1523–30.
16. Jayne DG, Brown JM, Thorpe H, Walker J, Quirke P, Guillou PJ. Bladder and sexual function following resection for rectal cancer in a randomized clinical trial of laparoscopicversus open technique. Br J Surg. 2005;92(9):1124–32.
17. Andersson J, Abis G, Gellerstedt M, Angenete E, Angerås U, Cuesta MA, et al. Patient-reported genitourinary dysfunction after laparoscopic and open rectal cancer surgery in a randomized trial (COLOR II). Br J Surg. 2014;101(10):1272–9.
18. Pigazzi A, Ellenhorn JDI, Ballantyne GH, Paz IB. Robotic-assisted laparoscopic low anterior resection with total mesorectal excision for rectal cancer. Surg Endosc. 2006;20(10):1521–5.
19. Speicher PJ, Englum BR, Ganapathi AM, Nussbaum DP, Mantyh CR, Migaly J. Robotic low anterior resection for rectal cancer. Ann Surg. 2015;262(6):1040–5.

20. Baik SH, Kwon HY, Kim JS, Hur H, Sohn SK, Cho CH, et al. Robotic versus laparoscopic low anterior resection of rectal cancer: short-term outcome of a prospective comparative study. Ann Surg Oncol. 2009;16(6):1480–7.
21. Kim MJ, Park SC, Park JW, Chang HJ, Kim DY, Nam BH, et al. Robot-assisted versus laparoscopic surgery for rectal cancer: a phase II open label prospective randomized controlled trial. Ann Surg. 2017. https://doi.org/10.1097/SLA.0000000000002321. [Epub ahead of print].
22. Saklani AP, Lim DR, Hur H, Min BS, Baik SH, Lee KY, et al. Robotic versus laparoscopic surgery for mid–low rectal cancer after neoadjuvant chemoradiation therapy: comparison of oncologic outcomes. Int J Color Dis. 2013;28(12):1689–98.
23. Baek SJ, AL-Asari S, Jeong DH, Hur H, Min BS, Baik SH, et al. Robotic versus laparoscopic coloanal anastomosis with or without intersphincteric resection for rectal cancer. Surg Endosc. 2013;27(11):4157–63.
24. Collinson FJ, Jayne DG, Pigazzi A, Tsang C, Barrie JM, Edlin R, et al. An international, multicentre, prospective, randomised, controlled, unblinded, parallel-group trial of robotic-assisted versus standard laparoscopic surgery for the curative treatment of rectal cancer. Int J Color Dis. 2011;27(2):233–41.
25. COLRAR. https://clinicaltrials.gov/ct2/show/NCT01423214.
26. Marks G, Mohiuddin M, Goldstein SD. Sphincter preservation for cancer of the distal rectum using high dose preoperative radiation. Int J Radiat Oncol Biol Phys. 1988;15(5):1065–8.
27. Marks JH, Frenkel JL, D'Andrea AP, Greenleaf CE. Maximizing rectal cancer results: TEM and TATA techniques to expand sphincter preservation. Surg Oncol Clin N Am. 2011;20(3):501–20. viii–ix.
28. Whiteford MH, Denk PM, Swanström LL. Feasibility of radical sigmoid colectomy performed as natural orifice translumenal endoscopic surgery (NOTES) using transanal endoscopic microsurgery. Surg Endosc. 2007;21(10):1870–4.
29. Atallah S, Albert M, Larach S. Transanal minimally invasive surgery: a giant leap forward. Surg Endosc. 2010;24(9):2200–5.
30. Fajardo AD, Hunt SR, Fleshman JW, Mutch MG. Transanal single-port low anterior resection in a cadaver model. Surg Endosc. 2010;24(7):1765.
31. Sylla P, Sohn DK, Cizginer S, Konuk Y, Turner BG, Gee DW, et al. Survival study of natural orifice translumenal endoscopic surgery for rectosigmoid resection using transanal endoscopic microsurgery with or without transgastric endoscopic assistance in a swine model. Int J Color Dis. 2010;25(8):2022–30.
32. Bravo R, Trépanier JS, Arroyave MC, Fernández-Hevia M, Pigazzi A, Lacy AM. Combined transanal total mesorectal excision (taTME)with laparoscopic instruments and abdominal robotic surgery in rectal cancer. Tech Coloproctol. 2017;21(3):233–5.
33. Motson RW, Whiteford MH, Hompes R, Albert M, Miles WFA, Expert Group. Current status of trans-anal total mesorectal excision (TaTME) following the second international consensus conference. Color Dis. 2016;18(1):13–8.
34. Lelong B, de Chaisemartin C, Meillat H, Cournier S, Boher JM, Genre D, et al. A multicentre randomised controlled trial to evaluate the efficacy, morbidity and functional outcome of endoscopic transanal proctectomy versus laparoscopic proctectomy for low-lying rectal cancer (ETAP-GRECCAR 11 TRIAL): rationale and design. BMC Cancer. 2017;30:1–8.
35. COLOR III. https://clinicaltrials.gov/ct2/show/NCT02736942.
36. OSTRiCh. https://tatme.ostrichconsortium.org.
37. NAPRC. https://www.facs.org/quality-programs/cancer/naprc.
38. Billingsley KG, Morris AM, Green P, Dominitz JA, Matthews B, Dobie SA, et al. Does surgeon case volume influence nonfatal adverse outcomes after rectal cancer resection? J Am Coll Surg. 2008;206(6):1167–77.
39. Yeo HL, Abelson JS, Mao J, O'Mahoney PRA, Milsom JW, Sedrakyan A. Surgeon annual and cumulative volumes predict early postoperative outcomes after rectal cancer resection. Ann Surg. 2017;265(1):151–7.

Index

C.M. Schlachta, P. Sylla (eds.), *Current Common Dilemmas in Colorectal Surgery*,
https://doi.org/10.1007/978-3-319-70117-2

MIX
Papier aus verantwortungsvollen Quellen
Paper from responsible sources
FSC® C105338

If you have any concerns about our products,
you can contact us on
ProductSafety@springernature.com

In case Publisher is established outside the EU,
the EU authorized representative is:
Springer Nature Customer Service Center GmbH
Europaplatz 3, 69115 Heidelberg, Germany

Printed by Libri Plureos GmbH
in Hamburg, Germany